Register Now for
to Your

MW01056055

SPRINGER PUBLISHING COMPANY
CONNECT™

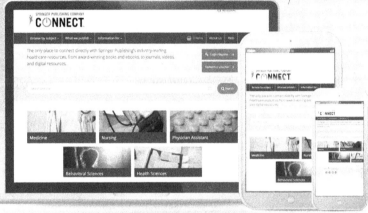

Your print purchase of *Leadership and Systems Improvement for the DNP*
includes online access to the contents of your book—increasing accessibility,
portability, and searchability!

Access today at:

**http://connect.springerpub.com/content/book/978-0-8261-8863-2
or scan the QR code at the right with your smartphone
and enter the access code below.**

E3CS05E6

*Scan here for
quick access.*

SPC

SPRINGER PUBLISHING COMPANY
View all our products at springerpub.com

LEADERSHIP AND SYSTEMS IMPROVEMENT FOR THE DNP

Gail E. Armstrong, PhD, DNP, ACNS-BC, CNE, is a professor at Oregon Health & Science University School of Nursing, where she is the assistant dean of the DNP program. Dr. Armstrong holds both a bachelor's and a master's degree in literature, a master's degree in nursing (with an adult clinical nurse specialist focus), a doctor of nursing practice degree, and a PhD in nursing science.

Dr. Armstrong was an early graduate of the Nursing Doctorate Program at the University of Colorado, which later transitioned into the Doctor of Nursing Practice Program. Dr. Armstrong's long-term nursing practice was in medical/surgical nursing before she became an advanced practice nurse. Dr. Armstrong's recent practice was with the Institute of Healthcare Quality, Safety and Efficiency (IHQSE) in Denver. This regional institute offers a 12-month training program for interprofessional teams of clinicians. This program trains teams in the areas of systems leadership, process improvement, and patient safety. Dr. Armstrong's teaching in IHQSE focuses on content specific to systems leadership interprofessional teams, teamwork, culture, creating a just culture, and change fatigue. Dr. Armstrong also worked on a 4-year, $11 million grant by the Center for Medicare & Medicaid Services to help prepare primary care and specialty care practices in Colorado for value-based payment models. This grant focused on clinical transformation and Dr. Armstrong worked with practices and practice facilitators to improve teamwork within a practice.

Dr. Armstrong's scholarship focuses on the integration of updated quality and safety content in nursing curricula; effective, interprofessional collaboration on healthcare teams; and preparing DNP graduates for systems leadership.

Sharon Sables-Baus, PhD, MPA, RN, PCNS-BC, CPPS, FAAN, is an associate professor with the University of Colorado and has appointments at both the College of Nursing and the School of Medicine's Department of Pediatrics. At the College of Nursing, Dr. Sables-Baus teaches in the DNP program. She has experience in healthcare systems leadership positions supported by an earned MPA. A fellowship in the American Academy of Nursing acknowledges her cumulative impact on the nursing profession. Dr. Sables-Baus is a certified pediatric clinical nurse specialist with a clinical background in acute care. Dr. Sables-Baus has earned an endorsement as a certified professional in patient safety (CPPS) by the Certification Board for Professionals in Patient Safety (CBPPS), recognizing professional competency in patient safety science and application. Her leadership on patient safety was recognized with an invitational book chapter on high-reliability organizations (HROs).

Dr. Sables-Baus has vast experience leading research, program evaluations, as well as quality-improvement projects. Her research has been translated into practice across disciplines, and has received international, national, and local recognition, including funding, recognition from the National Heart Institute, and the Colorado 2012 Nightingale Luminary Award. Dr. Sables-Baus's quality-improvement projects have been timely; the most recent improved outcomes for infants exposed to substances while in utero. She was also funded with a grant to lead a quality-improvement project examining outcomes of a safety coaching program. Dr. Sables-Baus's aptitude to form effective interdisciplinary partnerships is the hallmark of her work as both a clinical and academic leader. She has worked to break down silos and shift paradigms using a participatory leadership process to redesign health systems to focus on safe care and patient-centered outcomes.

LEADERSHIP AND SYSTEMS IMPROVEMENT FOR THE DNP

Gail E. Armstrong, PhD, DNP, ACNS-BC, CNE

Sharon Sables-Baus, PhD, MPA, RN, PCNS-BC, CPPS, FAAN

Editors

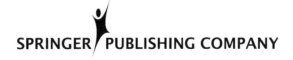

SPRINGER PUBLISHING COMPANY

Springer Publishing Company, LLC
11 West 42nd Street
New York, NY 10036
www.springerpub.com
http://connect.springerpub.com

Acquisitions Editor: Joseph Morita
Compositor: Exeter Premedia Services Private Ltd.

ISBN: 978-0-8261-8846-5
ebook ISBN: 978-0-8261-8863-2
Instructor's Manual ISBN: 978-0-8261-6426-1
Instructor's PowerPoints ISBN: 978-0-8261-6425-4
DOI: 10.1891/9780826188632

Instructor's Materials: Qualified instructors may request supplements by emailing textbook@springerpub.com.

19 20 21 22 23 / 5 4 3 2 1

The author and the publisher of this Work have made every effort to use sources believed to be reliable to provide information that is accurate and compatible with the standards generally accepted at the time of publication. The author and publisher shall not be liable for any special, consequential, or exemplary damages resulting, in whole or in part, from the readers' use of, or reliance on, the information contained in this book. The publisher has no responsibility for the persistence or accuracy of URLs for external or third-party Internet websites referred to in this publication and does not guarantee that any content on such websites is, or will remain, accurate or appropriate.

Library of Congress Cataloging-in-Publication Data

Names: Armstrong, Gail E., editor. | Sables-Baus, Sharon, editor.
Title: Leadership and systems improvement for the DNP / Gail E. Armstrong,
   Sharon Sables-Baus, editors.
Description: New York, NY: Springer Publishing Company, LLC, [2020] |
   Includes bibliographical references and index.
Identifiers: LCCN 2019017498| ISBN 9780826188465 | ISBN 9780826188632 (ebook)
   | ISBN 9780826164261 (Instructor's manual)
Subjects: | MESH: Advanced Practice Nursing—education | Education, Nursing,
   Graduate | Leadership | Program Evaluation—methods | Evidence-Based
   Nursing—education
Classification: LCC RT71 | NLM WY 128 | DDC 610.73071/1—dc23
LC record available at https://lccn.loc.gov/2019017498

Contact us to receive discount rates on bulk purchases.
We can also customize our books to meet your needs.
For more information please contact: sales@springerpub.com

Gail E. Armstrong: https://orcid.org/0000-0002-1274-5267
Sharon Sables-Baus: https://orcid.org/0000-0002-7979-5226

Publisher's Note: **New and used products purchased from third-party sellers are not guaranteed for quality, authenticity, or access to any included digital components.**

Printed in the United States of America.

This book is dedicated to the memory of Dr. Vicki Erickson, PhD, PNP, FAANP, who generously led many nursing doctorate (ND) students at the University of Colorado through the transition of becoming DNPs. Dr. Erickson was an effective advocate at the regional and national level for practice doctorate students, advanced-practice nurses, and practice faculty.
—Gail E. Armstrong

To my husband, Terry—it's a privilege to share my life with you—and to all new nursing graduates for fueling the flame of caring, compassion, and competence that sustain the nursing profession.
— Sharon Sables-Baus

CONTENTS

Contributors   ix
Foreword   Gwen Sherwood, PhD, RN, FAAN, ANEF   xi
Preface   xv

I. IMPROVEMENT AND LEADERSHIP IN NURSING

1. The History and Future of the DNP in Nursing   3
    Gail E. Armstrong and Deborah Lindell

2. Effective Leadership   23
    Peggy Jenkins

3. Leadership and Systems Thinking   43
    Mary A. Dolansky

4. Quality Improvement: The Essentials   61
    Sharon Sables-Baus and Gail E. Armstrong

5. Leading Process Improvement   77
    Sarah J. Caffrey

6. Improvement, Evidence-Based Practice, and Research   95
    Mary Beth Flynn Makic

7. Leading With Quality Metrics   109
    Gail E. Armstrong, Jennifer Disabato, Scott Harpin, Kim Paxton, and Laura Rosenthal

8. Leadership and Team Science   133
    Rebecca S. Miltner, Cori Johnson, and Kathleen E. Miltner

9. Leading Program Evaluation   147
    Sharon Sables-Baus

10. Improvement and Big Data   171
    John M. Welton, Sharon Sables-Baus, and Catherine Kleiner

11. Value-Based Payment Models in Healthcare   189
    Barbara J. Martin

II. THE DNP PROJECT

12. The DNP Project—The Essentials   **221**
    Tammy Spencer

13. Using an Evidence-Based Approach to Develop a DNP Project   **251**
    Jennifer Disabato

14. Finding Evidence to Improve Processes   **277**
    Rebecca S. Graves

15. Cost Analysis in DNP Projects   **295**
    Amy J. Barton and Pamela Jones

16. The DNP Project Deliverables: Sustainability and Spread   **309**
    Noreen Heer Nicol and Sharon Sables-Baus

17. Answers to Case Study Questions   **323**

Index   *341*

CONTRIBUTORS

Gail E. Armstrong, PhD, DNP, ACNS-BC, CNE, Professor, Oregon Health & Science University School of Nursing, Portland, Oregon

Amy J. Barton, PhD, RN, FAAN, ANEF, Professor, University of Colorado, College of Nursing, Centennial, Colorado

Sarah J. Caffrey, Deming Scholars MBA, American College of Healthcare member; Director, Supply Chain Department, University of Colorado Hospital, Denver, Colorado

Jennifer Disabato, DNP, RN, CPNP-BC, AC, Assistant Professor, University of Colorado, College of Nursing, Denver, Colorado

Mary A. Dolansky, PhD, RN, FAAN, Associate Professor, Frances Payne Bolton School of Nursing, Case Western Reserve University, Cleveland, Ohio

Rebecca S. Graves, MLS, AHIP, Educational Services Librarian, Health Sciences Library, University of Missouri, Columbia, Missouri

Scott Harpin, PhD, MPH, RN, APHN-BC, FSAHM, Associate Professor, University of Colorado, College of Nursing, Denver, Colorado

Peggy Jenkins, PhD, RN, Assistant Professor, University of Colorado, College of Nursing, Denver, Colorado

Cori Johnson, DNP, CRNP, AGNP-C, Instructor, University of Alabama at Birmingham, School of Nursing, Pelham, Alabama

Pamela Jones, PhD, Assistant Professor, University of Colorado, College of Nursing, Elizabeth, Colorado

Catherine Kleiner, PhD, RN, Director, Research, Innovation, and Professional Practice, Children's Hospital of Colorado, Aurora, Colorado

Deborah Lindell, DNP, MSN, RN, CNE, ANEF, FAAN, Associate Professor, Frances Payne Bolton School of Nursing, Case Western Reserve University, Solon, Ohio

Mary Beth Flynn Makic, PhD, RN, CCNS, CCRN-K, FAAN, FNAP, Professor, University of Colorado, College of Nursing, Arvada, Colorado

Barbara J. Martin, MSN, MPH, ACNP-BC, RN, PhD student, University of Colorado, College of Nursing, Denver, Colorado

Kathleen E. Miltner, MS, CRNP, AGNP-C, CNS-C, Acute Care Nurse Practitioner with Medstar Health, Severn, Maryland

Rebecca S. Miltner, PhD, RN, CNL, NEA-BC, Associate Professor, University of Alabama at Birmingham, School of Nursing, Hoover, Alabama

Noreen Heer Nicol, PhD, RN, FNP, NEA-BC, Associate Professor, University of Colorado, College of Nursing, Morrison, Colorado

Kim Paxton, DNP, APRN, ANP-BC, LHIT-C, Assistant Professor, University of Colorado, College of Nursing, Castle Pines, Colorado

Laura Rosenthal, DNP, ACNP, FAANP, Associate Professor, University of Colorado, College of Nursing, Denver, Colorado

Sharon Sables-Baus, PhD, MPA, RN, PCNS-BC, CPPS, FAAN, Associate Professor, University of Colorado, College of Nursing, Greenwood Village, Colorado

Tammy Spencer, DNP, RN, ACNS-BC, CCNS, CNE, Assistant Professor, University of Colorado, College of Nursing, Denver, Colorado

John M. Welton, PhD, RN, FAAN, Professor, University of Colorado, College of Nursing, Parker, Colorado

FOREWORD

Nursing education and nursing practice are like mirrors; what happens in one influences and drives developments in the other. Increasing complexities of nursing practice, healthcare delivery, payment systems, technology, and knowledge development are drivers of current shifts in the healthcare market; these in turn have led to advancing roles and responsibilities for nurses that require higher education. This text effectively addresses many of these shifts. The rapid expansion of the DNP degree reflects the need for nurses in advanced clinical roles who demonstrate skills to design and lead new approaches from a systems perspective; however, the rapid expansion of the DNP did not always allow for thoughtful role delineation and evidence-based curricular approaches. This thoughtful book from DNP leaders pulls together information from across systems leadership to define the parameters of DNP education, improvement projects both for academic credit but also for system redesign, and competencies expected of DNP graduates.

The need for expanding advanced practice nursing education is rooted in several reports. Since the 2000 Institute of Medicine (IOM) report *To Err Is Human* (IOM, 2000), the public has become increasingly aware of quality concerns in healthcare. The 2001 follow-up report by the IOM, *Crossing the Quality Chasm*, described the STEEEP model, a quality-improvement framework to measure **s**afety, **t**imeliness, **e**fficiency, **e**ffectiveness, **e**quity, and **p**erson-centeredness as key factors in healthcare quality. The depth of the quality problem, however, has confounded solutions. Amid calls to transform health professions education (IOM, 2003), the QSEN project (Quality and Safety Education for Nursing) went a step further to elucidate the six competencies essential for all health professionals for both prelicensure and graduate levels: person-centered care, teamwork and collaboration, quality improvement, evidence-based practice, safety, and informatics (Cronenwett et al., 2007, 2009). The objective statements describing the knowledge, skills, and attitudes for the graduate competencies have often lagged behind implementation of the prelicensure competencies. This book integrates these improvement frameworks, offering a substantial contribution in producing practitioners with the skills to address the continuing concerns of preventable patient harm, using a systems approach.

Still we need to rethink how we design and deliver healthcare as well as how we prepare healthcare professionals. The Institute for Healthcare Improvement (IHI) Quadruple Aim follows a systems approach that focuses on enhancing the patient experience, improving population health, reducing costs of care, and improving the work life of providers, an update of the Triple Aim that adds care and concern for providers (IHI, 2014). Professionals appreciate the value of working in organizations focused on quality; we all like the satisfaction that comes from good work. Reflective practitioners engaged in their work focus on the how and the why of the care they deliver adding to the meaning realized from their work. Too often nurses follow first-order problem-solving whereby workarounds become the norm: they see a problem and seek a single-incident solution versus righting the system. Using a systems approach, those who are prepared with second-order problem-solving apply systems thinking to identify flaws in process designs, trace the action pathway, and develop reliable systems with predictable results and see the end result of processes that work. This text prepares DNP students and graduates through broad explication of complex systems, systems thinking, and complexity leadership.

Predictable results are another identifying characteristic of high-reliability organizations (HROs), which are based on a systems approach and human factors design. Nurses with advanced education in systems thinking and processes can apply second-order problem-solving to rectify ill-designed processes, lack of standardization, and poorly functioning teams. To achieve these aims and alleviate preventable harm, nurses must accept and embrace new models of leadership that move beyond the managerial horizontal approaches; vertical leadership development reinforces reflective practices for thinking deeply about care provided and the systems that surround daily work. This text addresses these new, necessary competencies, culling expertise from a wide variety of chapter authors.

This ground-breaking book helps fill these gaps in defining leadership development for DNP graduates and their role in leading system redesign improvement. The change in expanding nurses' role of delivering patient care to leading changes in systems of care represents a shifting paradigm. To fill these emerging roles requires leadership development in complex adaptive systems to examine the numerous places where care lacks standardization such as handoffs, hierarchical relationships, medication administration, and organizational structures. The lens of complexity shifts the role of leadership to embrace both second-order problem-solving and vertical development; the leader is not focused on providing answers but creates an environment in which all providers are engaged in improvements (Cohen & Smetzer, 2016). This text leads DNP students, faculty, and graduates through germane content to create these vitally needed practice environments.

This book also provides clear explication of the differences between the research-focused PhD and the clinically focused DNP, and ways they can integrate. The DNP focus is translation of evidence-based practice guide-lines and research into practice, process-improvement projects, and evaluation/assessment of outcomes, whereas the PhD prepares nurse scientists who develop the evidence through research. Both degrees have critical roles in the expanse of healthcare if we are to achieve the quality and safety goals set out in the 2001 IOM report, *Crossing the Quality Chasm*. By delivering up-to-date information about improvement work in healthcare systems for DNP students and graduates, this must-read book for faculty, students, and clinicians offers hope for achieving the quality goals that will provide the right care for the right patient at the right time, every time.

Gwen Sherwood, PhD, RN, FAAN, ANEF
Professor Emeritus, University of North Carolina at Chapel Hill
Co-Investigator of Quality and Safety Education for Nurses

REFERENCES

Cohen, M. R., & Smetzer, J. L. (2016). Reporting and second-order problem solving can turn short-term fixes into long-term remedies. *Nurse Advise ERR, 14*(7), 1–3.

Cronenwett, L., Sherwood, G., Barnsteiner, J., Disch, J., Johnson, J., Mitchell, P., . . . Warren, J. (2007). Quality and safety education for nurses. *Nursing Outlook, 55*(3), 122–131. doi:10.1016/j.outlook.2007.02.006

Cronenwett, L., Sherwood, G., Pohl, J., Barnsteiner, J., Moore, S., Sullivan, D. T., . . . Warren, J. (2009). Quality and safety education for advanced practice nursing practice. *Nursing Outlook, 57*(6), 338–348. doi:10.1016/j.outlook.2009.07.009

Institute for Healthcare Improvement. (2014). The Triple Aim or the Quadruple Aim. Retrieved from http://www.ihi.org/communities/blogs/the-triple-aim-or-the-quadruple-aim-four-points-to-help-set-your-strategy

Institute of Medicine. (2000). *To err is human*. Washington, DC: National Academies Press.

Institute of Medicine. (2001). *Crossing the quality chasm*. Washington, DC: National Academies Press.

Institute of Medicine. (2003). *Health professions education: A bridge to quality*. Washington, DC: National Academies Press.

PREFACE

DNP programs are rapidly expanding in number and scope. October 2018 statistics from the American Association of Colleges of Nursing (AACN) indicate that 336 DNP programs exist in all 50 states, with 121 programs in the planning stage. In the proximate future, there will be more than 450 DNP programs in the United States, with a high degree of variation among them. Although all DNP programs use the AACN DNP Essentials to guide their curricula, interpretation and implementation of the Essentials vary tremendously. Due to this variability, several challenges are endemic to DNP programs: DNP faculty have a wide variety of preparation for teaching DNP students and overseeing DNP projects, DNP students matriculate from diverse educational and clinical backgrounds, and the roles into which a DNP graduate is promoted are poorly defined.

One consistent element of most DNP programs is the curricular structure of an integrative curriculum, where a DNP student systematically builds skills to envision, research, plan, execute, and evaluate a final DNP project. This integrative curricular model has a variety of names in DNP programs, often with consecutively linked classes (e.g., *DNP project, leading transformation, integrative DNP course, translating evidence into practice, DNP leadership*). *Leadership and Systems Improvement for the DNP* is a textbook specifically designed to provide a substantive and rigorous faculty guide for key elements to include in a DNP integrative curriculum.

A high priority for DNP faculty is to be able to proficiently lead DNP students through a well-constructed, clinically relevant curriculum, which culminates in a relevant, rigorous, well-executed DNP project. Limited up-to-date and practical resources exist that support DNP faculty and students throughout the duration of a DNP curriculum, provide an evidence-based scaffold upon which DNP projects with differing foci can be developed, and provide strategic resources for a DNP nurse's ongoing career. *Leadership and Systems Improvement for the DNP* is a resource for DNP faculty that spans the duration of a DNP program, from early in a DNP student's coursework, beyond graduating with the DNP degree.

Leadership and Systems Improvement for the DNP is a text that DNP students will find extremely useful throughout and beyond their DNP program to guide them in understanding the work of a nurse leader, to orient them as to how to execute a successful DNP project, as well as being a valuable resource for the long-term work in systems leadership. The content of this text is updated, timely, and includes some of the most important topics for DNP students to read, think about, and integrate into their professional framework.

The first 11 chapters of the text cover topics that provide important context for the DNP as a systems leader. Often the DNP student transitions from a clinical role into a leader role. These chapters ground DNP students in the scope of necessary skills for their future work, and provides high-quality resources they will use long into their DNP leadership practice. The first chapter covers the rarely examined history of the DNP degree and grounds the DNP student in a firm understanding of the degree's recent evolution. Many DNP texts contain chapters on quality improvement (QI); however, this text builds on that foundational knowledge (Chapter 4) and further expands one's QI understanding through chapters on the difference between improvement, evidence-based practice, and quality improvement (Chapter 6), quality metrics (Chapter 7), and the difference between quality improvement and process improvement (Chapter 5). This text focuses on contemporary approaches and topics relevant to a DNP graduate's work as a systems leader, including effective leadership (Chapter 2), leadership and systems thinking (Chapter 3), and leadership and team science (Chapter 8). Many DNPs will work in clinical arenas where program evaluation is part of their leadership (Chapter 9). Some DNPs will be using big data in their leadership work (Chapter 10), and all DNP students and graduates need to be aware of the current shifts in the U.S. healthcare system specific to value-based payment models (Chapter 11).

The second section of the book shares DNP project models from the current literature and offers content to support DNP students as they envision, research, plan, execute, and evaluate a final DNP project. These chapters provide guidance and standards for students, advisors, and DNP faculty as DNP students engage with all phases of the DNP project. Topics in this section include the essentials of an evidence-based DNP project (Chapter 12), finding evidence for a DNP project (Chapter 14), using an evidence-based practice approach throughout a DNP project (Chapter 13), cost analyses to support a DNP project (Chapter 15), and sustainability and spread of a DNP project (Chapter 16).

Unique features of this text include clear identification of the American Association of College of Nursing DNP Essentials addressed in each chapter. These clear links between content in *Leadership and Systems Improvement for the DNP* and AACN DNP Essentials enables a DNP program to clearly plan and design curricular outcome for accreditation requirements. This text includes case studies at the end of each chapter, with answers to study questions found in the final chapter. These case studies facilitate learning through application for the DNP student throughout the DNP curriculum.

This text includes an online instructor's manual with ancillary materials for faculty. Instructor support materials include PowerPoint slides for each chapter; these slides can be used in a variety of learning modalities (e.g., online, face to face, or in a hybrid course) and can be adjusted for individual faculty preferences. Other instructor support materials include online resources for each chapter. These online resources will expand the scope of each chapter, offering current, relevant resources for further exploration of a chapter's topics. Faculty will also have access to learning activities for each chapter. These learning activities can be used in online or face-to-face classes and facilitate application of the chapter's content in assignments that are specific to a DNP student's DNP project, or work as a systems leader. The case studies from the text are also available online, so faculty can reproduce them in a variety of formats that are convenient for their own teaching. *Qualified instructors may obtain access to a supplementary Instructor's Manual and PowerPoints by emailing textbook@springerpub.com.*

The DNP is an emerging degree in nursing. *Leadership and Systems Improvement for the DNP* is a textbook that invites DNP faculty and students into an expansive vista of how DNP students can be taught during the DNP program, providing the necessary tools, evidence, and strategies for this view. This text also offers a clear picture of the potentially critical impact of the future work of DNP graduates as healthcare systems leaders.

Gail E. Armstrong
Sharon Sables-Baus

ACKNOWLEDGEMENTS

Thanks to Jason Weiss, M.Ed., Program Manager for the Colorado Collaborative for Nursing Research, for your valuable and timely assistance with editing.

IMPROVEMENT AND LEADERSHIP
IN NURSING

THE HISTORY AND FUTURE OF THE DNP IN NURSING

GAIL E. ARMSTRONG | DEBORAH LINDELL

INTRODUCTION

The clinical doctorate model of education, also called the *practice doctorate*, is a model shared by most practice professions. The clinical doctorate is designed to be the terminal degree to prepare one for the highest level of clinical practice within one's profession. Table 1.1 outlines the clinical doctorate degree in a variety of clinical professions.

Nursing has had a turbulent history regarding a lack of agreement on one model for the clinical doctorate. This chapter outlines that history, clarifying the influences that led to this tumultuous history. The standardized model for the DNP degree was formally introduced in 2004 in a position statement by the American Association of Colleges of Nursing (AACN; 2004). Since the appearance of this cornerstone document, the rapid growth of DNP programs and graduates speak to an alignment of timing, ideas, and needs in the healthcare system. Current leadership trends in healthcare indicate that the needs for the clinical leadership offered by DNP graduates will only increase in the future.

Confusion About Nursing's Non-PhD Doctorate

Leadership within the nursing profession is shared by several professional organizations (e.g., the American Nurses Association [ANA], the AACN, the National League for Nursing [NLN], the National Organization of Nurse Practitioner Faculty [NONPF], the National Association of Clinical Nurse Specialists [NACNS]). Without one unifying professional

TABLE 1.1 CLINICAL PROFESSIONS AND CORRESPONDING CLINICAL DOCTORATE DEGREES

Profession	Clinical Doctorate Degree	Degree Abbreviation
Medicine	Doctor of Medicine	MD
Dentistry	Doctor of Dental Medicine	DDM
Veterinary medicine	Doctor of Veterinary Medicine	DVM
Optometry	Doctor of Optometry	OD
Osteopathy	Doctor of Osteopathy	DO
Public health	Doctor of Public Health	DrPH
Pharmacy	Doctor of Pharmacy	PharmD
Psychology	Doctor of Psychology	PsyD
Physical therapy	Doctor of Physical Therapy	DPT

voice, nursing has lacked a single clinical doctorate model to address the needed clinical leadership within the profession, outside of the PhD in nursing, a doctorate clearly focused on generating and advancing nursing research. Several models emerged over many years, offering differing elements of what educational leaders believed was needed. As early as 1979, a variety of non-PhD doctoral degrees emerged in nursing, including the doctor of nursing science (DNS, DNSc), doctor of science in nursing (DSN), and the nursing doctorate (ND). Sandra Edwardson offered a concise classification of doctoral degrees in nursing (Figure 1.1). Edwardson's proposed model (2004) is similar to models suggested by the AACN at the same time.

The ND Degree

The ND degree is the clearest predecessor to the DNP, aiming to provide clinical nurse leaders. Although there were never more than a handful of

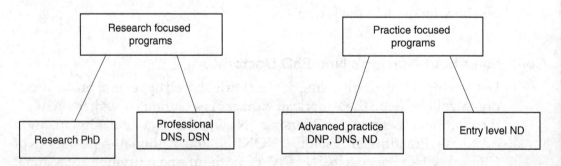

FIGURE 1.1 Classification of NDs.

Source: From Edwardson, S. R. (2004). Matching standards and needs in doctoral education in nursing. *Journal of Professional Nursing, 20*(1), 40–46. doi:10.1016/j.profnurs.2003.12.006

ND degrees at U.S. nursing schools, there was notable variation among the existing programs. In the 2004 AACN position statement outlining the DNP, the lack of uniformity among existing ND programs was cited as a guiding factor in the development of the DNP model (AACN, 2004). To highlight the variations in the ND degree, two early ND models will be examined in depth: (a) Case Western Reserve University and (b) University of Colorado.

The Evolution of the Professional Doctorate (ND) at Case Western Reserve University

Laying the Foundation (1935–1960)

During the 1960s and 1970s, visionary nurse scholars began to articulate their views of nursing as both a profession and a discipline. Their views of nursing differed according to their experiences in practice, education, and perspectives of health, persons, and the environment. Dr. Rozella Schlotfeldt, RN, PhD, FAAN, was noted to be "an original thinker, outstanding scholar, and an educator having innovative, progressive, and sometimes startling concepts for nursing" (Safier, 1977, p. 334). Schlotfeldt's vision for advancing the discipline of nursing focused on nursing education and had several elements, of which the "cornerstone" was the ND, a postbaccalaureate professional doctorate, as preparation for entry into nursing practice (Center for the Study of Nursing, n. d.).

Schlotfeldt was born in Iowa in 1914 and earned a BS degree in nursing, after which she worked as a direct-care RN, head nurse, combined instructor–supervisor, and Army nurse in Germany. Following World War II, Schlotfeldt served in faculty roles at two universities prior to pursuing her PhD at the University of Chicago. In 1960, following completion of her PhD and 3 years as associate dean for research and development at Wayne State University, Schlotfeldt was appointed dean and professor of nursing at the Frances Payne Bolton (FPB) School of Nursing, Case Western Reserve University (CWRU) in Cleveland, OH.

A "Plan for Progress" of Nursing Education (1960–1978)

From the time Schlotfeldt first worked as a nurse educator in 1939, she began "thinking about better ways to combine teaching and practice while experimenting with creative approaches that held promise for improving nursing care" (Center for the Study of Nursing, n. d.). She pursued these interests during her doctoral study and, as dean at CWRU, articulated her "Plan for Progress" of nursing education: (a) collaboration between academic and healthcare organizations, (b) faculty roles, (c) her view of nursing, and (d) educational preparation for nursing practice. Schlotfeldt believed that academic and healthcare organizations should collaborate to implement faculty roles that integrated education, research, and practice. In regard to the focus of nursing, Schlotfeldt frequently described her views as aligned with those of Nightingale that nursing is "the helping profession whose primary practice concern is to promote the gamut of health-seeking behaviors of human beings in the several environments" (Schlotfeldt, 1976, p. 105). The fourth part of Schlotfeldt's vision was that "if nursing is to become a full-fledged professional discipline," then its practitioners need a full-fledged, professional program of study, with entry at the postbaccalaureate level (Schlotfeldt, 1978, p. 302). In the *American Journal of Nursing*, she noted: "My view is that all programs of professional study in nursing should be intellectually demanding and that they should warrant the award of the professional doctorate in nursing—the ND degree" (Schlotfeldt, 1976, p. 107).

During 1960 through 1972, and following her deanship at CWRU, Schlotfeldt was a prolific writer and speaker on her vision of nursing education and educational preparation for nursing practice. Moreover, she was a strong advocate for the changes needed within nursing to achieve her vision. At CWRU, under Schlotfeldt and her successor, Dean Janetta MacPhail (1972–1982), the leadership and faculty of the Frances Payne Bolton School of Nursing, initiated changes that reflected elements of the plan for progress. In 1972, the PhD program was established (third in the country) and, in collaboration with University Hospitals of Cleveland, faculty received dual appointments integrating the three roles described earlier.

Launching of the First Professional Doctorate (ND) Program (1978–1989)
In 1978, the CWRU nursing faculty prepared and distributed a "formal document describing the new Doctor of Nursing (ND) program" (Fitzpatrick, 1986, p. 4). In 1979, the BSN program was closed and the first nursing professional doctorate program was launched.

The initial ND program lasted six semesters over three academic years and, by 1981, was accredited by the NLN. The concept of the professional doctorate was disseminated widely in popular and professional literature. In the *CWRU General Bulletin of 1983 to 1985* (CWRU, 1983, p. 287), the ND program was described as "the basic program for entry into professional nursing practice. This program leads to the ND degree and prepares individuals as generalists with the knowledge, skills, and values necessary to enter first-level positions in a variety of healthcare settings and to be licensed as registered nurses. . . . The sequencing of educational offerings is comparable to the educational preparation offered in other practice professions such as medicine, dentistry, law and pharmacy. The professional doctorate (ND, MD, DDS, JD, PharmD) is the degree necessary for entry into professional practice. ND graduates could transition into the MSN or PhD programs."

In 1986, Dean Joyce Fitzpatrick reported that the program had reached the halfway point projected as necessary for acceptance of the new program and there were 134 ND graduates. She acknowledged the ND program had encountered "unpredicted resistances and changes in patterns

TABLE 1.2 ND CURRICULUM, 1986

Year	Overview of ND Curriculum, 1986
1	Foundations of the Discipline I & II, Foundations of Nursing Practice, Health Promotion and Maintenance I & II, Health Restoration & Support I
2	Health Restoration & Support I: a multidisciplinary course in ethics, nursing theory, and research with MSN students during which students will develop a proposal; includes clinical practice with concentrated opportunities to integrate knowledge and skills (20–24 hr per week)
3	Systematic study and/or practice in nursing in one of the four focal areas of choice: Organizational Theories, Information Systems. Two clinical research seminars in which students (a) implement and write an individual report of a pilot study or (b) develop an individual in-depth paper on an aspect within the proposal such as concept, method, or tool
	91–97 total credits

Source: Case Western Reserve University. (n.d.). *General Bulletin, 1991–93: Undergraduate Programs, Graduate Programs*, Professional Schools. Cleveland, OH: Author.

of healthcare delivery and education that directly or indirectly influenced program development" (Fitzpatrick, 1986, p. 8). Based on formative feedback from faculty and students and findings of a formal external evaluation, the curriculum was modified frequently "to develop more fully the program focus as a professional doctorate" (Fitzpatrick, 1986, p. 8).

Schlotfeldt's views of nursing practice, refined in the "Health Seeking Nursing Model," were integral to the ND curriculum. *Nursing* was defined as the "art and science of assisting people to enhance their health-seeking behaviors as they strive to attain, maintain, or regain optimal health" and as "a fully autonomous practice profession, a scholarly discipline, and an integral part of the healthcare system" (Glazer & Pressler, 1989, p. 242). Table 1.2 provides an overview of the ND curriculum in 1986.

The Case Western ND Program Is Restructured (1990)
In 1990, in response to the evaluation findings, the faculty completely restructured the ND program and reinstituted the BSN program with an emphasis on acute and critical care. The revised ND was "a clinical doctorate designed for baccalaureate prepared college graduates from a variety of disciplines . . . and for BSN and MSN prepared nurses who desired advanced clinical knowledge" (CWRU, n.d., p. 388). The program was "characterized by educational depth and emphasis on advanced practice nursing, inquiry and management" (CWRU, n.d., p. 388). As noted in Table 1.3, the revised ND program differed from the 3-year ND in several key respects.

The ND Program Evolves (1990–2005)
From 1990 to 2005, the ND program continued in two phases: prelicensure and postlicensure. Administratively, a director of the ND program

TABLE 1.3 COMPARISON OF 3-YEAR AND 4-YEAR DNP PROGRAMS

	"Original" ND (1979–1990)	Restructured ND (1990–2009)
Length of curriculum	3 years	4 years (first 2 years prelicensure)
Outcome of prelicensure phase	"Knowledge, skills, and values for clinical practice, clinical scholarship, and for a professional career" (Fitzpatrick, 1986, p. 9)	Levels I and II: An entry-level RN ready to move directly into levels III and IV (CWRU, 1993–1995)
Outcome of full program	3-year ND degree; same as prelicensure phase	4-year ND degree: Students can apply for the MSN; in levels III and IV, students prepare as an APN in a primary care specialty; the APN courses are integrated with 24 credits of professional doctorate courses and a clinical research thesis (CWRU, 1993–1995)
Pathway options	Single pathway to ND isfull-time participation	Multiple pathways: (A) nonnursing baccalaureate graduates can enter at level I (prelicensure) and complete levels I–IV, (B) RNs with the BSN can enter at level III (APN and doctorate), and (C) RNs with the MSN can enter at level IV (doctoral); in addition, levels III and IV can be completed part time or full time (CWRU, 1993–1995); the post-MSN ND curriculum had a clinical focus or "practice doctorate"

APN, advanced practice nurse.

was responsible for the prelicensure and post-MSN components. A separate director was responsible for the MSN program, including students enrolled in postlicensure advanced practice nursing (APN) courses.

Prelicensure component. Upon completion of the prelicensure curriculum, students received a certificate of professional nursing (CPN), participated in the School of Nursing's pinning ceremony, could apply for RN licensure in most states, and were expected to continue on to the MSN/ND. The curriculum was updated as indicated by evaluation findings (e.g., adding courses in genetics and health and aging). The most significant change (2003) revised the curriculum to four semesters, for 16 continuous months of study. Enrollment remained steady with a dramatic increase for the classes starting in 2003 to 2005. Approximately 65% of CPN recipients proceeded into the MSN program within 2 years of receiving the CPN; however, few proceeded onto the ND (C. Quinn, personal communication, May 15, 2007).

Postlicensure component. Over time, some MSN and all post-MSN courses were revised from meeting regularly over a semester to an executive or "intensive" format that allowed flexibility for nurses in full-time positions. Enrollment in the post-MSN ND was limited until 2005, when it significantly increased following several key changes: (a) the post-MSN ND graduate was seen as prepared to teach in pre-RN, MSN, and ND programs and the ND curriculum was revised to have two "tracks"—clinical leadership and educational leadership; (b) the program built on the "intensive" format by implementing a highly successful model of off-site cohorts; (c) funding to support post-MSN students; and (d) in line with national trends, the ND was officially revised to the post-MSN DNP. Previous ND graduates who held the MSN could apply to convert their ND degree to the DNP. Administratively, the pre- and post-MSN components of the ND program were divided to have separate directors and were designated as graduate entry ND and post-MSN ND programs.

The DNP Program: 2005–2018

Graduate Entry DNP Program. As nursing evolved, recipients of the CPN experienced limitations of opportunities in education and practice. In 2009, the curriculum was heavily revised, returned to 4 semesters, 2 academic years; clinical hours were increased by 25% to over 1000, and the CPN was replaced with the Master of Nursing (MN) degree. Several years later, in response to ongoing evaluation, admission to the graduate entry nursing program was changed to the MN and MSN only with students strongly encouraged to consider the DNP, PhD, or DNP/PhD and a concentration in "Leadership for Quality Improvement" was added. CCNE accreditation was achieved in 2015 and enrollment remains steady.

Post-MSN DNP Program. The DNP program was accredited by the Commission on Collegiate Nursing Education (CCNE) in 2011, the intensive and cohort formats continue, funding support is available for nurse educators, the "research study or thesis" has transitioned to a "scholarly project," and enrollment remains robust.

Today, CWRU's Frances Payne Bolton School of Nursing continues to be a leader in nursing education with both the DNP and MSN programs highly ranked (#5 and #6, respectively) by US News and World Report Education (2018). Faculty use a continuous-improvement approach to consider internal and external evaluation findings and to revise all of its programs, including the Graduate-Entry Nursing and Post-MSN DNP, accordingly.

The Evolution of the ND at the University of Colorado

Dr. Jean Watson served as dean of the University of Colorado School of Nursing (CU SON) from 1983 to 1990 and was the visionary leader driving CU's ND program. Much of Jean Watson's thinking about the ND at Colorado was built on the foundation of the ND at Case Western by Rozella Schlotfeldt (Watson & Bevis, 1990). Jean Watson's theoretical work, which centers on nursing as the art and science of human caring, had a strong impact on the philosophical foundations of Colorado's ND program. Colorado accepted its first ND students in 1990 and continued until 2005, whereupon it transitioned into a DNP program. Colorado's ND program was designed to prepare a broadly educated and technically competent,caring, professional nurse to practice with extended responsibilities, among diverse populations and clinical settings in order to address increasingly complex healthcare needs.

Dr. Watson's guiding ideas for Colorado's ND were based on future trends in healthcare: increased acuity in hospitalized patients, increase in scope of care provided in the home by home-care nurses, an increased emphasis on wellness care, an increased focus on models that provide patient-centered care, and emerging roles for nurses to coordinate care for patients across time and across settings (Watson, 1989). Watson (1988) proposed that the elements found in Table 1.4 provide the educational base for Colorado's ND.

TABLE 1.4 WATSON'S CORE COMPONENTS OF THE UNIVERSITY OF COLORADO'S ND PROGRAM

Element	Educational Component
Foundation	A more extensive liberal arts foundation focused on understanding of and appreciation for cultural diversity and on the human subjective dimensions of health–illness, caring, healing experiences, and needs Core knowledge underpinning biomedical science, social behavioral sciences, and organizations/systems management theory and practice
Clinical preparation	Preparation in critical thinking and advanced problem solving, contributing to clinical judgments and independent decision-making
Decision-making model	Extensive preparation in philosophical and ethical decision-making skills based on the ethics of human caring, which addresses both health policy and contextual, compassionate, relational, ethical dilemmas as well as knowledge of the traditional rationalistic approach to principled biomedical ethics and traditional health policy positions
Caring core	Exploration of the contextual value-laden relationship theory that is associated with human caring and healing transactions, emphasizing self-care and more autonomous decision-making processes
Curriculum	A curriculum based on human science and nursing theory that incorporates the latest research and practice knowledge of human caring, healing, and health and emphasizes the relationship between human and system caring approaches and health/healing outcomes

Source: From Watson, J. (1988). Human caring as moral context for nursing education. *Nursing and Health Care*, 9(8), 423–425.

A vital aspect of Watson's image of the career professional nurse was that the ND graduate would help address the fragmentation of care and isolation of the patient and family. With augmenting complexity in the healthcare system, Watson knew that this fragmentation and unintended segregation of the patient and family from the care team would increase. Watson imagined a new level of professional nurse whot would follow patients and families across time and across settings. "The ND regulates and monitors the highest level of professional care between and among multiple health personnel; coordinates, educates, counsels and advises the patient and family regarding different treatment protocols" (Watson, 1989, p. 370). The increasing complexity of the future U.S. healthcare system was becoming evident, and Watson wanted to educate highly functioning nurse clinicians whose education included explicit focus on the complexity of emerging healthcare systems, had the broad view of healthcare policy, but was patient/family centered in their core values and practice center. "The ND personalizes complex, acute and chronic healthcare needs, including symptom management, demystifying the medical world, and instructing patients on how to optimize self-care and inner healing resources, including better use of the traditional (medical) system (Watson, 1989, p. 374). Watson hoped to graduate clinicians whose education promoted both human care and the management of human caring systems.

Colorado developed its ND program, planning to be a model for other schools considering the practice doctorate model. The ND program at Colorado was selected by the Helene Fuld Health Trust in New York as a national demonstration program for postbaccalaureate caring and healing health curriculum, awarding CU over $500,000 for the implementation of the ND program. From its earliest planning, Watson included regional clinical agencies in the exploration and planning of the curriculum. The goal was not only to transform the model for clinical doctorate education, but also to design and test new care-delivery models with innovative roles for doctorally prepared nurses. Watson was also active in coordinating the ND model with other statewide projects, funded by The Colorado Trust, to develop a new articulation model to link all nursing education programs in the state, for more seamless progression from associate nursing degree programs to the ND (Watson & Phillips, 1992).

A unique characteristic of Colorado's model was its strong clinical preparation. Baccalaureate preparation provides students with approximately 750 hours of clinical practicum; Colorado's ND program included more than 3,800 hours of clinical practicum. Longer clinical rotations as well as two intensive clinical experiences contributed to the strong clinical proficiency of ND graduates. Colorado developed an ND professional residency, which was 1 calendar year of full-time practice, incorporating 1,960 hours of clinical practice into the ND degree. After graduation, many ND graduates begin their practice at the site that sponsored their residency.

The University of Colorado's ND curriculum was based on an academic, professional educational model that parallels the preparation of other clinical doctorates in health professions with respect to the nature and degree of educational preparation. Similar to the clinical doctorate in medicine, pharmacy, or dentistry, the University of Colorado's ND provided core clinical preparation during the program's first 2 years, developed the student's professional practice in the third year, and culminated in a clinically based residency in the fourth year.

The original ND curriculum was focused on four basic core areas: clinical sciences, clinical arts and humanities caring, health professional and ethical foundations, and discipline-specific human caring nursing. In the first 10 years of Colorado's ND program, courses were rearranged, renamed, and reconfigured to keep up with changing nursing education standards. These curricular changes are outlined in Table 1.5.

TABLE 1.5 COMPARISON OF THE UNIVERSITY OF COLORADO ND CURRICULUM 1990–1999

	Original ND Curriculum (1990)	ND Curriculum (1999)
Year 1	Philosophy, ethics, and science of human caring in nursing	Reflective practice
		Discipline and practice of nursing
	Clinical inquiry	Clinical inquiry
	Anatomy and physiology	Anatomy and physiology
	Health assessment and promotion	Health assessment and promotion
	Health assessment clinical practicum	Health assessment clinical practicum
	Microbiology	Microbiology and infectious diseases
	Primary care	Pathophysiology
	Primary care clinical practicum	Pharmacology
	Caring in art	Nursing interventions—arts and skills
	Caring in music	Nursing care of adults and older adults (Med/Surg I)
		Med/Surg I clinical practicum
		Caring in literature
		Nursing theory
Year 2	Nursing care of childbearing families	Nursing care of childbearing families
	Nursing care of children	Nursing care of children
	OB and pediatric clinical practicum	OB and pediatric clinical practicum
	Mental health nursing	Mental health nursing
	Mental health clinical practicum	Mental health clinical practicum
	Clinical externship	Clinical externship

(continued)

TABLE 1.5 COMPARISON OF THE UNIVERSITY OF COLORADO ND CURRICULUM 1990–1999 (*continued*)

	Original ND Curriculum (1990)	ND Curriculum (1999)
	Practice and disciplinary role socialization	ND clinical seminar
	Pathophysiology	Health systems and policy issue
	Pharmacology	Caring in art and music
	Caring in literature	Primary healthcare nursing
		Nursing care of adults (Med/Surg II)
		Med/Surg II clinical practicum
		Interdisciplinary ethics
	Eligible for NCLEX	**Eligible for NCLEX**
Year 3	Evaluation methodologies	
	Case management	Case management
		Care management
	Clinical practicum for case management	Clinical practicum for case/care management
	Public health nursing	Public health nursing
		Clinical practicum for public health nursing
	Health systems and policy issues	Inferential statistics
	Elective	Advanced assessment
		Human technology interface
	Professional residency	Introduction to ND residency
Year 4	Professional residency	Professional residency
		Capstone project

OB, obstetric.

Colorado also placed clear emphasis on the rigor of the ND's Capstone Project, requiring that ND students spend their 4-year residency completing a Capstone project that is focused on system improvement, care management across settings, care management across time, or strategies contributing to emerging patient-centered care models. These Capstone projects are showcased each May, as ND students are about to graduate. Table 1.6 provides examples of ND Capstone projects between 1998 and 2005.

AACN's Position Statement on the Practice Doctorate

Within the nursing literature of the 1990s and early 2000s, there was ongoing disagreement about the most beneficial model to use for a nursing practice doctorate degree. As early as 1993, there was a call for a clear model of a nursing clinical doctorate for the 21st century (Starck, Duffy, &

TABLE 1.6 EXAMPLES OF THE UNIVERSITY OF COLORADO ND CAPSTONE PROJECTS

Year	Title of Capstone Project
1998	Cost Analysis of a Medicaid Prenatal Care Coordinator Program
1998	Comparison of Community Care Management Programs
1998	Promoting Self-Efficacy Through Care Coordination and Community Links
1999	Needs Assessment for a Women's Health Clinic in Rural Colorado
1999	Case Complexity in Short-Term Disability Care
1999	Evaluation of a Pediatric Asthma Management Program
2003	Utilization Trends of a Rural COPD Population
2003	Establishment and Evaluation of a Case Management Program to Assist Clients in Obtaining a PCP or Health Insurance
2004	Family Presence During Resuscitation and/or Invasive Procedures: A Survey of Health Care Providers, Patients, and Families
2004	Health Literacy in a Diabetic Population in a VA System in Eastern Colorado
2005	Evaluation of an Emergency Department Nurse Case Manager Program
2005	Sedation Assessment Practices Among Experienced CICU Nurses
2005	Developing a Program to Promote Education and Implementation of Advanced Directives in a Chronic Dialysis Setting

CICU, cardiac intensive care unit; COPD, chronic obstructive pulmonary disease; PCP, primary care physician; VA, Veterans Affairs.

Vogler, 1993). The focus and intensity of this disagreement heated up as awareness grew that the existing ND programs lacked a consistent model. In 2003, the NONPF published an opinion, stemming from the work of a task force, aptly titled, "The Practice Doctorate in Nursing: Future or Fringe?" (Marion et al., 2003). The growing need for expert clinical teachers and clinicians was not being adequately met by existing graduate nursing education models, and NONPF, along with professional organization and educational institutional partners, began calling for a new, standardized model that would prepare graduates for future needs in healthcare (Marion et al., 2003).

In 2004, AACN shifted the conversation with y its position statement on the practice doctorate (AACN, 2004). This game-changing position statement emerged from a 2002 task force that was established to compare the various models of clinical or practice doctoral programs, to examine various models, and to make recommendations. The task force reviewed the literature, established a collaborative relationship with NONPF, interviewed key informants, and held open discussions at several nursing education conferences. Along with the task force's formal recommendations (Table 1.7), this statement recommended that the DNP replace the master's degree as preparation for advanced practice nurses (APNs). This recommendation later crystallized into a suggestion that schools of nursing move to eliminate their master's programs by 2015. Table 1.7 summarizes the 13 formal recommendations proposed within the AACN (2004) position statement.

TABLE 1.7 SUMMARY OF AACN RECOMMENDATIONS FOR THE DNP DEGREE

	Recommendation
1	The task force recommends that the terminology used in practice doctorate, be used in instead of clinical doctorate
2	The practice-focused doctoral program follow a distinct model of doctoral education that provides an additional option for attaining a terminal degree in the discipline
3	Practice-focused doctoral programs prepare graduates for the highest level of nursing practice beyond the initial preparation in the discipline
4	Practice-focused doctoral nursing programs include seven essential areas of content (which were developed to become the DNP Essentials)
5	Practice doctoral nursing programs should include development and/or validation of expertise in at least one area of specialized advanced nursing practice
6	Practice-focused doctoral nursing programs prepare leaders for nursing practice; the practice doctorate prepares individuals at the highest level of practice and is the terminal practice degree
7	One degree title should be chosen to represent practice-focused doctoral programs that prepare graduates for the highest level of nursing practice
8	The DNP is the degree associated with practice-focused doctoral nursing education
9	The ND degree should be phased out
10	The practice doctorate should be the graduate degree for advanced nursing practice preparation, including but not limited to the four current APN roles: clinical nurse specialist, nurse anesthetist, nurse midwife, and nurse practitioner
11	A transition period should be allowed to provide master's degrees to nurses who wish to obtain the practice doctorate degree using a mechanism to earn a practice doctorate in a relatively streamlined fashion, with credit given for previous graduate study and practice experience; the transition mechanism should provide multiple points of entry, standardized validation of competencies, and be time-limited
12	Research-focused doctoral programs are encouraged to offer additional coursework and practical experience that prepares graduates to fill the role of nurse educator
13	Practice-focused doctoral programs need to be accredited by a nursing accrediting agency recognized by the U.S. Secretary of Education

AACN, American Association of Colleges of Nursing.

Source: From American Association of Colleges of Nursing. (2004). AACN position statement on the practice doctorate in nursing. Retrieved from http://www.aacnnursing.org/DNP/Position-Statement

Support for AACN's Statement on the Practice Doctorate

With the publication of AACN's position statement, nursing literature experienced an eruption of responses, both in support of the DNP and challenging the emerging model. As it was a partner in the development of AACN's recommendations, NONPF continued its support for the DNP model. The NACNS identified the paucity of national dialogue that led to AACN's position statement as well as a lack of differentiation between master's-prepared APNs and DNP- prepared APNs. NACNS ultimately committed to contributing to the emerging model by developing a doctoral-level clinical nurse specialist curriculum (NACNS, 2005).

Not all nursing leaders were supportive of AACN's DNP model. Dracup, Cronenwett, Meleis, and Benner (2005) worried that the DNP would threaten the work of PhD graduates and the advancement of theory-based science in nursing. In addition, these prestigious nursing leaders worried about a decline in already negligible PhD program admissions, and whether the addition of a practice doctorate would increase the chasm between nursing practice and nursing research. Last, there was unease that the new degree would cause confusion among healthcare colleagues and the public (Dracup et al., 2005). These same authors offered additional concerns in 2011, focusing on the impact of the DNP on the nursing workforce. In 2011, reservations were expressed about the impact of the DNP elongating the preparation for APNs, thereby decreasing the APN workforce at a time in history when there was an increased need for APNs (Cronenwett et al., 2011).

A common criticism of AACN's 2004 position statement was the suggested deadline of 2015 for schools of nursing across the country to replace their master's programs with the DNP as preparation for APNs. Many identified complex logistics, significant cost, and the lack of available nursing faculty to teach in practice-doctorate programs (Chase & Pruitt, 2006; Cronenwett et al., 2011; Ketefian & Redman, 2015). AACN contracted with Rand Health, a leading organization in health policy research, to investigate schools' progress toward this 2015 goal. Rand's report (Auerbach et al., 2015) identified several facilitators toward schools transitioning to the DNP (mostly focused on increased demand by healthcare systems and students) and several barriers to this transition (internal and institutional barriers such as approval, cost, faculty, resources, and securing clinical sites). History has indicated that these concerns about the feasibility of all nursing schools transitioning to the DNP were indeed valid, as schools of nursing continue to offer master's degrees.

Rapid Growth of DNP Programs

Despite lack of agreement about many aspects of the DNP degree, DNP programs continue to flourish. Data from June 2017 indicate that there are

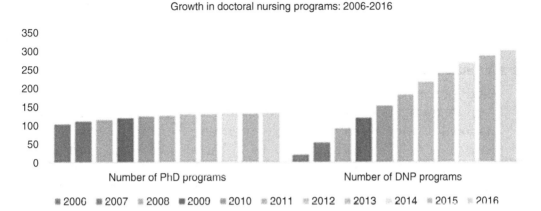

FIGURE 1.2 AACN growth in DNP programs 2006 to 2016.

Source: From American Association of Colleges of Nursing. (2017). Fact sheet: The doctor of nursing practice (DNP). Retrieved from http://www.aacnnursing.org/News-Information/Fact-Sheets/DNP-Fact-Sheet

303 DNP programs in all the states in the United States, and 124 new programs in the planning stages. From 2015 to 2016, DNP graduates increased from 4,100 to 4,855 (AACN, 2017). Figure 1.2 compares the growth in DNP programs compared to PhD in nursing pPrograms from 2006 to 2016.

FUTURE COLLABORATION BETWEEN DNP AND PhD NURSES

From its inception, concerns about the impact of the DNP degree on the PhD degree and the APN workforce have abounded. The loudest concerns identified a worry that the DNP degree would detract from the PhD preparation and slow the development of knowledge in the nursing discipline (Edwardson, 2010). Ongoing growth of DNP programs indicate that the DNP degree is in nursing education to stay; a commonly identified and exciting frontier explores models oft effective collaboration between DNP-prepared nurses and PhD-prepared nurses. What might effective collaborative models look like? One definition of *collaboration* is a model in which both sides value each other's power with acknowledgment and acceptance of the other's areas of responsibility, thereby forming a true partnership (Dougherty & Larson, 2005). Current thinking about effective collaboration between PhD-prepared and DNP-prepared nurses focuses on each understanding the other's preparation and expertise and developing models in which differing areas of specialty are maximally used. Emerging models emphasize the complementary nature of the two-degree preparations, with an understanding that because the DNP is in its infancy, effective strategies are only beginning to surface. How do

DNP- and PhD-prepared nurses effectively collaborate, and how might these models evolve in the future?

DNPs in Nursing Education

DNP-prepared nurses are rapidly entering nursing academia. Many nursing programs must limit their admissions due to the well-documented national nursing faculty shortage. According to AACN's report on 2016 to 2017 enrollment and graduations in baccalaureate and graduate programs in nursing, U.S. nursing schools turned away 64,067 qualified applicants from baccalaureate and graduate nursing programs in 2016 due to a variety of contributing factors, including the faculty shortage (AACN, 2014). The national faculty shortage was identified as the prevailing reason responding schools did not accept all qualified applicants into baccalaureate programs (AACN, 2014).

A recent 2016 study indicates that most nursing programs are adding DNPs to their faculty, both on tenure and nontenure tracks, with DNP-prepared faculty experiencing challenges around scholarship (Oermann, Lynn, & Agger, 2016). Another 2016 study interviewed nursing faculty, examining determinants for effective DNP/PhD nurse faculty collaboration. This study revealed five predominant themes: (a) ongoing confusion about the training and role of the DNP prepared nurse, even among DNPs; (b) inconsistent use of the word *research* with DNP nurses; (c) opportunities for collaboration (e.g., committee work); (d) research teams in which the DNP-prepared nurse brings clinical expertise and the PhD brings research expertise; and (e) lack of structural support for effective collaboration and identification of the contribution of personal characteristics to effective collaboration (e.g., respect, clinical interest, time, and mutual goals; Staffileno, Murphy, & Carlson, 2016). Buchholz, Yingling, Jones, and Tenfelde (2015) explore whether collaborative opportunities during foundational coursework in DNP and PhD programs would facilitate better understanding of the distinct preparations. Coenrollment of the PhD and DNP students in courses, such as nursing inquiry and analytic methods, create opportunities for academic socialization and the development of collaborative working relationships (Buchholz et al., 2015). DNP-prepared nurses are actively joining nursing faculty across the United States, and more work needs to be done to explore and disseminate effective, productive, and mutual models of DNP/PhD nurse faculty collaboration.

DNP/PhD Nurse Collaboration in Practice

A commonly emphasized synergy facilitating DNP/PhD nurse collaboration focuses on the necessary paradigm shift that addresses the growth of DNP programs concurrent with the need to improve practice expertise and move the translation of evidence into practice more efficiently (Brown & Crabtree, 2013). Courtney and colleagues developed a valuable model that explains the ways in which DNP and PhD scholars are similar in their pursuit of active scholarship, but have different areas of expertise. Their model (Figure 1.3) emphasizes that the DNP and PhD have different, but equally important, foci in the scholarly activities they undertake, which lead to the development of practice science (Buchholz et al., 2013).

Dr. Peggy Jenkins, from the University of Colorado College of Nursing in Aurora, Colorado, has also explored elements of effective collaboration between the DNP and PhD nurses in the practice setting. Table 1.8 examines Jenkins's model for effective doctoral nurse collaboration when focused on a similar clinical question.

CONCLUSIONS

Despite the ongoing dialogue about the benefit of the DNP model, and tremendous variation in DNP program structure, curricula, and outcomes, DNP programs remain on the rise. The continual rapid growth of DNP

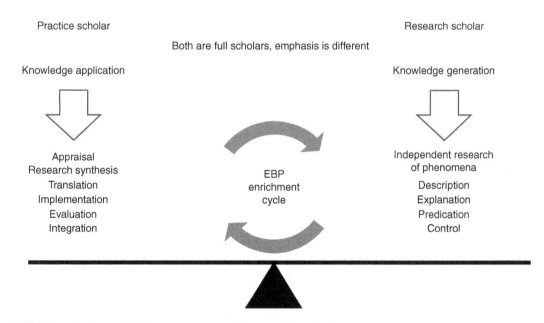

FIGURE 1.3 A model for practice and research scholarship.

EBP, evidence-based practice.

Source: From Buchholz, S. W., Budd, G. M., Courtney, M. R., Neiheisel, M. B., Hammersla, M., & Carlson, E. D. (2013). Preparing practice scholars: Teaching knowledge application in the Doctor of Nursing Practice curriculum. *Journal of the American Association of Nurse Practitioners, 25*(9), 473–480. doi:10.1002/2327-6924.12050

TABLE 1.8 JENKINS'S MODEL FOR EFFECTIVE DOCTORAL NURSE COLLABORATION

DNP Leader Role	PhD Leader Role	Collaboration
Formulate a PICO question asking whether richer skill mix has a positive effect on a certain patient population on her unit.	Formulate a research question asking what skill mix of RNs most positively correlates with desired patient outcomes.	Share questions so both aims contribute to a similar problem, one from the current system context and one from a larger, potentially generalizable context.
Search and evaluate the evidence for studies related to the question.	Conduct a literature search noting gaps in knowledge related to RN skill mix and patient outcomes.	Work together to identify gaps in knowledge. Collaborate in reviewing evidence using PhD expertise in analyzing research studies, finding high-quality evidence to implement in practice.
Use implementation framework to guide change of practice.	Use scientific research process to design a research study.	Communicate plans, timelines, and milestones. Adjust based on shifting practice context.
Organize a diverse team of key stakeholders.	Organize a research team to writea proposal and obtain funding.	Include common members on both teams for knowledge sharing and to link work.
Implement/evaluate change on unit.	Conduct a research study.	Transfer knowledge and expertise between teams.
Disseminate change process used and processes of implementation.	Disseminate results of a research study.	Present results internally/externally and publish together.

PICO, patient/problem,intervention,comparison, outcome.
Source: Developed by Peggy Jenkins, PhD, RN.

programs indicates that the DNP degree and DNP graduates are addressing current needs in the healthcare system. The DNP degree is a relatively new degree in nursing and is clearly an educational preparation in its infancy. The need for DNP graduates is impacted by healthcare system trends in quality, patient safety, patient-centered care, value-based payment models, process improvement, and sustainability of improvement within complex systems. The need to educae all DNP graduates in all spheres of systems leadership is becoming increasingly evident. The content of this text addresses these vital academic and clinical areas of opportunity.

REFERENCES

American Association of Colleges of Nursing. (2004). AACN position statement on the practice doctorate in nursing. Retrieved from http://www.aacnnursing.org/DNP/Position-Statement

American Association of Colleges of Nursing. (2014). Nurse faculty shortage. Retrieved from https://www.aacnnursing.org/News-Information/Fact-Sheets/Nursing-Faculty-Shortage

American Association of Colleges of Nursing. (2017). Fact sheet: The doctor of nursing practice (DNP). Retrieved from http://www.aacnnursing.org/News-Information/Fact-Sheets/DNP-Fact-Sheet

Auerbach, D. I., Martsolf, G. R., Pearson, M. L., Taylor, E. A., Zaydman, M., Muchow, A. N., . . . Lee, Y. (2015). The DNP by 2015: A study of the institutional, political, and professional issues that facilitate or impede establishing a post-baccalaureate doctor of nursing practice program. *Rand Health Quarterly, 5*(1), 3.

Brown, M., & Crabtree, K. (2013). The development of practice scholarship in DNP programs: A paradigm shift. *Journal of Professional Nursing, 29*, 330–337. doi:10.1016/j.profnurs.2013.08.003

Buchholz, S. W., Budd, G. M., Courtney, M. R., Neiheisel, M. B., Hammersla, M., & Carlson, E. D. (2013). Preparing practice scholars: Teaching knowledge application in the doctor of nursing practice curriculum. *Journal of the American Association of Nurse Practitioners, 25*(2013), 473–480. doi:10.1002/2327-6924.12050

Buchholz, S. W., Yingling, C., Jones, K., & Tenfelde, S. (2015). DNP and PhD collaboration: Bringing together practice and research expertise as predegree and postdegree scholars. *Nurse Educator, 40*(4), 203–206. doi:10.1097/NNE.0000000000000141

Case Western Reserve University. (1983). *Case Western Reserve University Bulletin: Undergraduate Programs, Professional Schools, Graduate Programs, 1983–85, 7*(4). Cleveland, OH: Author.

Case Western Reserve University. (1985). *Case Western Reserve University General Bulletin: Undergraduate Programs, Professional Schools, Graduate Programs, 1985–87, 9*(5). Cleveland, OH: Author.

Case Western Reserve University. (n.d.). *General Bulletin, 1991–93: Undergraduate Programs, Graduate Programs, Professional Schools.* Cleveland, OH: Author.

Center for the Study of the History of Nursing. (n.d.). *Biography/History, Rozella M. Schlotfeldt papers.* Philadelphia, PA: School of Nursing, University of Pennsylvania. Retrieved from http://dla.library.upenn.edu/dla/pacscl/ead.html?q=rozella%20schlotfeldt&id=PACSCL_UPENN_BATES_MC113&

Chase, S. K., & Pruitt, R. H. (2006). The practice doctorate: Innovation or disruption? *Journal of Nursing Education, 45*(5), 155–161.

Cronenwett, L., Dracup, K., Grey, M., McCauley, L., Meleis, A., & Salmon, M. (2011). The Doctor of Nursing practice: A national workforce perspective. *Nursing Outlook, 59*, 9–17. doi:10.1016/j.outlook.2010.11.003

Dougherty, M., & Larson, E. (2005). A review of instruments measuring nurse-physician collaboration. *Journal of Nursing Administration, 35*, 244–253. doi:10.1097/00005110-200505000-00008

Dracup, K., Cronenwett, L., Meleis, A. I., & Benner, P. E. (2005). Reflections on the doctorate of nursing practice. *Nursing Outlook, 53*(4), 177–182. doi:10.1016/j.outlook.2005.06.003

Edwardson, S. R. (2004). Matching standards and needs in doctoral education in nursing. *Journal of Professional Nursing, 20*(1), 40–46. doi:10.1016/j.profnurs.2003.12.006

Edwardson, S. R. (2010). Doctor of philosophy and doctor of nursing practice as complementary degrees. *Journal of Professional Nursing, 26*(3), 137–140. doi:10.1016/j.profnurs.2009.08.004

Fitzpatrick, J. (1986). *The ND Program: Integration of past and future.* Cleveland, OH: Case Western Resrve University.

Glazer, G., & Pressler, J. (1989). Schlotfeldt's health seeking model. In J. Fitzpatrick & A. Whall (Eds.), *Conceptual models of nursing: Analysis & application* (2nd ed., pp. 241–253). Norwalk, CT: Appleton & Lange.

Ketefian, S., & Redman, R. W. (2015). A critical examination of developments in nursing doctoral education in the United States. *Revista Latino-Americana de Enfermagem, 23*(3), 363–371. doi:10.1590/0104-1169.0797.2566

Marion, L., Viens, D., O'Sullivan, A. L., Crabtree, K., Fontana, S., & Price, M. M. (2003). The practice doctorate in nursing: Future or fringe? *Topics in Advanced Practice Nursing, 3*(2). Retrieved from https://www.medscape.com/viewarticle/453247

National Association of Clinical Nurse Specialists. (2005). White paper on the nursing practice doctorate. *Clinical Nurse Specialist, 19*(4), 215–218. doi:10.1097/00002800-200507000-00014

Oermann, M. H., Lynn, M. R., & Agger, C. A. (2016). Hiring intentions of directors of nursing programs related to DNP- and PhD-prepared faculty and roles of faculty. *Journal of Professional Nursing, 32*(3), 173–177. doi:10.1016/j.profnurs.2015.06.010

Safier, G. (1977). *Contemporary American leaders in nursing: An oral history*. New York, NY: McGraw-Hill.

Schlotfeldt, R. (1976). Rozella Schlotfeldt Says . . . *American Journal of Nursing, 76*(1), 105–107.

Schlotfeldt, R. (1978). The professional doctorate: Rationale and characteristics. *Nursing Outlook, 26*(5), 302–311.

Staffileno, B. A., Murphy, M. P., & Carlson, E. (2016). Determinants for effective collaboration among DNP- and PhD-prepared faculty. *Nursing Outlook, 65*(1), 94–102. doi:10.1016/j.outlook.2016.08.003

Starck, P. L., Duffy, M. E., & Vogler, R. (1993). Developing a nursing doctorate for the 21st century. *Journal of Professional Nursing, 9*(4), 212–219. doi:10.1016/8755-7223(93)90038-E

Watson, J. (1988). Human caring as moral context for nursing education. *Nursing and Health Care, 9*(8), 423–425.

Watson, J. (1989). The future-in-the making: Creating the new age. In E. O. Bevis (Ed.), *Toward a caring curriculum: A new pedagogy for nursing* (pp. 369–376). New York, NY: NLN Press.

Watson, J., & Bevis, E. O. (1990). Nursing education: Coming of age in a new age. In N. L., Chaska (Ed.), *The nursing profession: Turning points* (pp. 100–105). St. Louis, MO: Mosby

Watson, J., & Phillips, S. (1992). A call for educational reform: Colorado nursing doctorate model as exemplar. *Nursing Outlook, 40*(1), 20–26.

2

EFFECTIVE LEADERSHIP

PEGGY JENKINS

This chapter addresses the following DNP American Association of Colleges of Nursing (AACN) Essentials:

II. Organizational and Systems Leadership for Quality Improvement and Systems Thinking
V. Healthcare Policy for Advocacy in Healthcare
VI. Interprofessional Collaboration for Improving Patient and Population Health Outcomes

INTRODUCTION

What kind of clinical leadership is needed to effectively improve systems in healthcare? Advanced practice RNs (APRNs) are important contributors who provide guiding ideas for systems improvement; they also lead systems improvement work in a variety of clinical settings. Nursing is in a unique position across the continuum of care, and leaders have an opportunity to collaborate to envision and implement new care models focused on health promotion for diverse populations of patients.

LEADERSHIP THEORY

Leadership literature is vast and definitions are abundant. Contemporary concepts used to describe nurse leadership include *esthetic* (Mannix, Wilkes, & Daly, 2015), *authentic* (Dirik & Seren Intepeler, 2017; Perry, 2017), *servant* (Hanse, Harlin, Jarebrant, Ulin, & Winkel, 2016; Savel & Munro, 2017), *socially responsible* (Read, Pino Betancourt, & Morrison, 2016), and *resonant* (Cummings, 2004; Laschinger, Wong, Cummings, & Grau, 2014), to name a few. Transformational leadership has been predominant in nursing literature (Clavelle, 2012; Masood & Afsar, 2017; Spano-Szekely, Quinn Griffin, Clavelle, & Fitzpatrick, 2016), and the concept was recently further explained (Fischer, 2016). Fischer noted the limited operational definition and unclear underlying constructs. Her definition offered "an integrative style of leadership as well as a set of competencies" (p. 2650). Competencies of the transformational leader include emotional intelligence, enthusiasm to inspire/motivate, and collaborative communicator/coach/mentor.

Leadership is a specialty of some APRNs. Leadership is included in master's and doctor of nursing practice (DNP) programs that focus on health systems. APRNs with clinical focus learn leadership concepts, and the AACN views both master's and doctoral students' comprehension of leadership concepts as essential. Given the vast knowledge base available about leadership and the fact that it is considered an essential requirement by accreditating agencies, what are the knowledge, skills, and attitudes required for DNP-prepared nurse leaders? What role will the DNP-prepared nurse leader play in the future healthcare system, the profession, and the discipline of nursing?

INTEGRATIVE LEADERSHIP FRAMEWORK

A paradigm shift has occurred in the ontology and epistemology of nursing, healthcare, and other disciplines with regard to integrating and appreciating multiple ways of being and knowing (Drath et al., 2008). Globalization and the convergence of multiple cultures, beliefs, mind-sets, and values are driving forces contributing to this alteration in thinking about nursing. As the diversity of the healthcare workforce expands, it is hard to hold onto only one way of thinking Nursing is a multiparadigmatic discipline that is well positioned to lead healthcare using an integrative leadership framework.

Ken Wilber (2001) asserts that knowledge formation is a process of integration, and multiple ways of knowing are valid. Wilber uses a four-quadrant model consisting of individual (top) and collective (bottom) knowing on a vertical plane, with subjective (left) and objective (right) knowing on the horizontal plane (Figure 2.1). He places various scientific schools of thought within one of the four quadrants, for instance, behaviorism is the science of individual behavior measured objectively (the top right quadrant). Systems theory is an objective study of the collective (the bottom right quadrant). Interpretive paradigms fall into subjective individual (the top left quadrant, i.e., Jung) and subjective collective quadrants (the bottom left, i.e., Gadamer). Wilber's purpose is to model the complexity of the ways individuals and groups continuously interact and to value the understanding

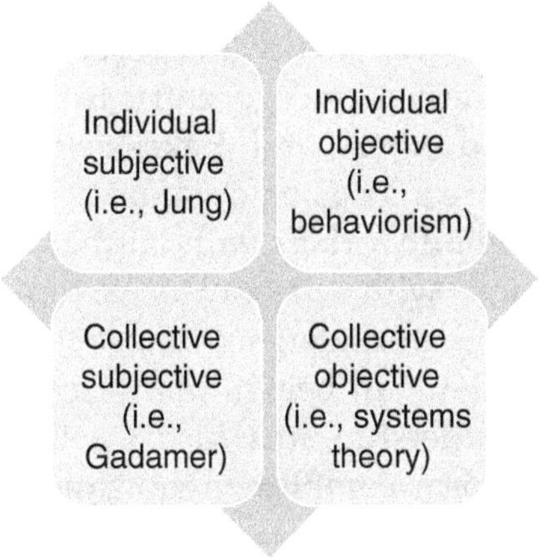

Individual subjective (i.e., Jung)	Individual objective (i.e., behaviorism)
Collective subjective (i.e., Gadamer)	Collective objective (i.e., systems theory)

FIGURE 2.1 Wilber's Integrative Model for Knowledge Development.

Source: From Wilber, K. (2001). The eye of spirit: An integral vision for a world gone llightly mad (3rd ed.). Boston, MA: Shambhala. © 2001, 2004 by Ken Wilber. Reprinted by arrangement with The Permissions Company, LLC, on behalf of Shambhala Publications Inc., Boulder, Colorado, www.shambhala.com.

gained from multiple perspectives. Wilber's model depicts the dynamic interplay between the individual and collective awareness, and the individual and collective realms that continuously influence systems and leaders.

In an integrated framework, use of one's preferred worldview only is not an option as multiple paradigms are included in the construct. Integrated frameworks merge numerous constructs and models to explain complex systems, organizations, teams, and individuals. Jarrin (2012) redefines nursing metaparadigm concepts (nursing, environment, person, nurse) through use of integral science. She gives examples of interior/exterior constructs of individuals/collective contributing to contextual knowing and being. Jarrin's purpose is to advance the science of nursing using a model grounded in contemporary integral science to guide understanding of the essence and experience of nursing for practice, research, and education. Her conceptualization of holistic nursing and need for optimal work environments for patient healing informs DNP leaders working with diverse patients and complex organizations.

Anderson and Adams (2016) synthesized studies and experiences of leadership spanning more than 30 years to create an integral model for mastering leadership, which can be useful to guide DNP leadership development. *Task* and *relationship* are two key constructs in their model. Leaders who effectively accomplish tasks while also establishing strong relationships are highly effective. The authors cite studies dating back to 1950 at Ohio State in which *task* and *relationship* account best for leadership effectiveness. When a leader focuses too much on tasks and not enough on relationships, he or she is not as successful. Nurse researchers substantiate the claim that a leader with a balanced focus on task and relationships has better job satisfaction and organizational commitment, is empowered, productive, and fosters teamwork(Cummings et al., 2010).

In addition to task and relationship concepts, the stages of leader development are key constructs in Anderson and Adams's mastering leadership model (2016). Developmental stages are universal in that they cross cultures and genders. As leaders develop, they move through personal transformation, which the authors describe as five levels of leadership: (a) egocentric, (b) reactive, (c) creative, (d) integral, and (e) unitive. The egocentric leader is self-centered, does not desire to understand others, and makes selfish decisions. Examples of egocentric leadership are a focus on organizational profit at the expense of environment, or laying off workers without regard to their welfare. Reactive leaders make decisions with a narrow focus, typically for self-preservation. Creative leaders seek to understand those they lead and work to develop the organization. Human beings rarely reach the highest level of consciousness, unitive leadership, in which mastery of complexity occurs. Integral leaders transform complex organizations because they combine creative behaviors with a universal systems view. They envision organizational effectiveness in the context of larger systems embedding the organization. The integral leader is concerned with global health and the connectedness of everything and understands the difference between reactive and creative behaviors (Table 2.1).

Fifty-thousand managers evaluated optimal leadership characteristics needed for organizations to thrive (Anderson & Adams, 2016). There was a negative correlation between reactive and creative styles of leadership, the more reactive one is, the less creative ($r = -0.76$). Creative styles correlated positively with effective leadership. To be specific, relating ($r = 0.85$), systems awareness ($r = 0.84$), authenticity ($r = 0.78$), self-awareness ($r = 0.76$), and achieving ($r = 0.61$) were skills most highly correlated with leadership efficacy. Reactive tendencies correlated negatively with effective leadership.

TABLE 2.1 REACTIVE VERSUS CREATIVE LEADERSHIP BEHAVIORS

Reactive Behaviors	Creative Behaviors
Complying	Relating
Protecting	Self-awareness
Controlling	Authentic
Conservative	Systems awareness
Pleasing	Achieving
Passive	Caring connection
Distant	Fosters team play
Critical	Collaborative
Arrogant	Mentoring/developing
Autocratic	Interpersonal intelligence
Ambitious	Selfless leader
Driven	Balance
Perfect	Composure

Source: From Anderson, R. J., & Adams, W. A. (2016). Mastering leadership: An integrated framework for breakthrough performance and extraordinary business results. Hoboken, NJ: Wiley.

Specifically, complying ($r = -0.63$), protecting ($r = -0.56$), and controlling ($r = -0.41$) were reactive behaviors most negatively correlated with success. Only about 20% of adults move from reactive to creative leadership, and very few leaders move to the integral and unitive level, yet creative, integral, and unitive leaders are necessary to transform organizations.

Learning to lead at higher levels takes a lot of work, yet continual personal growth is possible through discipline, focus, intention, experience, and exposure to leadership models. It is important for seasoned leaders to begin to develop novice, aspiring leaders early in their careers to help them achieve higher level skills. DNP nurse leaders work to develop themselves and to understand how to advance nurses in the organization.

MODEL TO DEVELOP FUTURE NURSE LEADERS

Although philosophies, theories, and definitions of leadership abound, there are universal concepts important for DNP-prepared leaders to grasp. The "great man" theory, or belief that leaders are born, has been replaced by the view that leadership is a set of skills that can be learned. Leadership, in all instances, begins with self-discovery. A model for developing DNP leadership contains personal power at its core (Figure 2.2). Leaders develop personal power to empower others, who innovate change and transform organizations. In the following sections, four key constructs of the model are explained: (a) personal power, (b) empowerment, (c) innovation, and (d) transformation. Effective DNP nurse leaders learn to integrate competencies consistent with all four constructs.

Personal Power

> *Experience is what you have when you didn't get what you want.*
> —R. Pausch and J. Zaslow

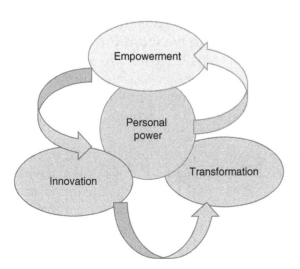

FIGURE 2.2 Model for DNP leadership.
Source: Developed by Peggy Jenkins, PhD, RN.

Power is a concept defined in multiple ways, that has traditionally been regarded negatively as a coercive or manipulative force. Some leaders choose to use a destructive, intimidating style of power, which is ineffective. Power has a facilitative capacity, and when used correctly illuminates and develops the strengths of oneself and others. Hagberg's definition of power (2003) focuses on leaders using both their inclination for action as well as their reflective ability in providing effective leadership. Personal power increases as one gains wisdom and the appreciation that leadership never involves self-interest. Having a title does not make one a leader. See Table 2.2 for definitions of Hagberg's six stages of personal power.

Stages of Personal Power

During the first stage of personal power, leaders are powerless. While in this phase, a nurse cannot lead. Here, egocentric actions are manipulative, and effort is invested in forcing others to conform. A minimal amount of self-awareness limits this leader's growth and there is no capacity to help others develop. Increasing personal power can be facilitated through a focus on self-awareness, leadership education, confronting one's fears, and by gaining support to increase one's personal power.

At the second stage of personal power, nurse leaders form relationships with mentors. They are gaining self-esteem and know reaching out to build skills is not a sign of weakness, but an indication of strength. The leader embraces constructive feedback for growth. The nurse with strong clinical skills often needs more expertise to be an effective leader and through learning develops leadership knowledge, skills, and attitudes.

The third stage of personal power is achieved by many nurses when they accept formal leadership positions. This leader may have completed a DNP, gained confidence to manage others, is often an expert clinician, and has the ambitious to advance in her or his career. Leaders at this stage will grow through experience, as it is often through the most difficult encounters that leaders gain wisdom. Leaders in stage three tend to look for others to blame if something goes wrong. To move forward, the nurse leader must reflect honestly and identify areas for personal growth. This journey of inward reflection and growth can take a long time, especially if the nurse leader is not encouraged to progress.

The fourth stage of personal power is the first in which leaders develop wisdom and focus more on one's team than on themselves. The leader has probably spent years in formal leadership positions and learned through successes and failures. These leaders understand their own leadership style and often become mentors to others. The fourth-stage leader generously uses empowerment as his or her focus is on

TABLE 2.2 HAGBERG'S SIX STAGES OF PERSONAL POWER

Description	Stage of Personal Power	Characteristics	Ways to Move Forward
Powerlessness	One	Manipulative, low self-esteem, uninformed, secure and dependent, need to learn leadership skills	Increase self-esteem, find support, confront fears, change jobs
Power by association	Two	Learning culture/organizational rules, dependent on supervisor/leader, more externally than internally powerful	Develop relationships with mentors, seek feedback, obtain education credentials, build networks, develop broader competency in leadership
Power by achievement	Three	Egocentric, competitive, expert, ambitious, charismatic	Self-reflection, seek wise mentors, build networks, focus on the present
Power by reflection	Four	Competent, reflective, strong, skilled at mentoring, showing true leadership, comfortable with personal style	Forgive others, seek silence, let go, experience loss, glimpse wisdom
Power by purpose	Five	Self-accepting, calm, visionary, humble, empowers others, spiritual, confident of life purpose	Moves forward in individual ways
Power by wisdom	Six	Comfortable with paradox, unafraid, quiet in service, ethical, on the universal plane	

Source: From Hagberg, J. O. (2003). *Real power: Stages of personal power in organizations* (3rd ed.). Salem, WI: Sheffield Publishing Company. Reprinted by permission of Sheffield Publishing Co. © 2003 all rights reserved.

developing others' skills. Fourth-stage leaders focus on the mission of an organization. To become a great leader takes many years of hard work and movementn away from a focus on self.

Leaders who reach stages five and six of personal power seldom occupy leadership positions in organizations. We know these leaders because their bravery and generous work are archived iby history:Abraham Lincoln, Martin Luther King, Nelson Mandela, Mother Teresa, Jesus, Gandhi, Muhammad, Confucius, and Buddha are examples. Powerful nurse leaders include Florence Nightingale, Clara Barton, Hildegard Peplau, Martha Rogers, and Jean Watson.

Self-Awareness

Courage is an attitude successful DNP leaders embrace that can be learned through work on self, including reflection, goal setting, and seeking feedback. Fear is an attitude that prevents leaders from evolving to greatness. Overcoming fear requires trust in oneself, which leads to courage. How does the DNP leader develop trust in self that overcomes anxieties and fears? Realizing success in difficult projects helps build confidence. Allowing fear to limit the DNP-prepared nurse from accepting leadership roles on projects curtails personal development. Leading systems projects employs the same critical thinking as is used in providing care; however, the scope becomes more complex when considering the systems' impact, the need to include stakeholders, forming/organizing a team, and evaluating organizational outcomes.

Empowerment

Structural Empowerment

Kanter (1977, p. 166) defines *power* as "the ability to get things done, to mobilize resources, to get and use whatever it is that a person needs for the goals he or she is attempting to meet." Her definition of power moves the concept away from a hierarchical structure or formal position, which constrains the amount of power available to a few people at the top of organizations. Instead, her definition opens up the concept and is inclusive of more people having access to power to accomplish the work. She moved the definition of *power* from authhority or control that is held by a few to a strength held by many. She advances the definition of *power* to one of empowerment.

Empowerment can be thought of as a personal feeling that one's organization supports individuals in doing their jobs well. For staff to feel empowered, leaders ensure certain structural factors are in place (Spence Laschinger, 2008):

1. Access to information
2. Constructive feedback and guidance
3. Adequate resources, including personnel, supplies, and technology
4. Culture of personal growth and development.

In testing her Nursing Worklife Model, Spence Laschinger (2008) studied the relationships among structural empowerment, magnetic hospital characteristics, nurse satisfaction, and perceived quality patient care. Structural empowerment had a positive effect on quality of nursing leadership, nurse job satisfaction, and perceived patient care quality. In more recent studies, nurse researchers validated Laschinger's findings that structural empowerment is antecedent to psychological empowerment, which is positively related to job satisfaction (Cicolini, Comparcini, & Simonetti, 2014; Riley, Dearmon, Mestas, & Buckner, 2016).

DNP leaders provide staff *access to information* needed to perform their roles. This access includes data about the organization's mission, vision, values; how unit goals tie to the organization's strategic plan; finances of the organization and unit; ready access to evidence to inform practice; knowledge of the patient population, guidelines, and best practices; exquisite communication from leader meetings on reasons for operational and staffing decisions; and individual staff strengths. Increased emphasis on data transparency in healthcare is guiding emerging practices in leadership communication. Sharing quality metric data with all members of the team allows for ongoing input into improvement at every level (Oster & Braaten, 2016). Data transparency carries risks as well. Some leaders representing clinical agencies have taken advantage of data transparency by pursuing objectives that create value only for themselves. For example, a stakeholder may try to take advantage of big data more quickly and aggressively than his or her competitors, without regard to clinically proven outcomes. Advertising high-technology diagnostic equipment to patients in an underserved area can lead to unnecessary use of such equipment.

Constructive feedback and guidance are necessary for every individual to grow and develop. McCord (2017, p. 32) asked leaders to "practice radical honesty." She describes the high cost of not telling employees the truth. Leadership literature emphasizes not only the mechanisms for providing feedback, but the means by which a leader listens and gathers data. Often there is a significant gap between leader-level conversations and the reality of care at the front line (Reinertsen & Johnson, 2010). "Rounding to Influence" is an evidence-based leadership practice from the high-reliability literature that is enjoying increased adoption currently. Rounding to Influence can be used with any improvement practice for which a leader would like information; the practice places an emphasis on listening and gathering targeted data, rather than just being seen (Reinertsen & Johnson, 2010). Leaders' choices regarding how to provide timely, supportive, honest feedback as well as their listening practices are critical to leadership success.

Nurses need *adequate resources* to perform jobs at the highest level of scope, including adequate staffing, skill mix, trained staff, and access to interprofessional team members. Supplies include available quality medical/surgical products, capital equipment, and ergonomic workspace. Technology includes patient care systems, evidence/guidelines libraries and apps, and well-drafted policies and processes. Leaders provide necessary resources for staff to do their jobs. This support includes the right amount of staff to provide quality patient care. Evidence on safe staffing levels exists. Relying on financial officers to budget amount of nurses necessary is not the future of nursing administration. Nurse leaders monitor nurse-sensitive outcomes and usecreativity in observing data measuring nurses' unique contribution in various healthcare settings. Nurse leaders measure the value of nursing, defined as quality patient outcomes divided by cost (Pappas, 2013; Welton & Harper, 2016). See Figure 2.3 to see this equation.

Leaders create a *culture of personal growth and development*. They should understand the individual aspirations of each team member, including gathering a baseline assessment of strengths and areas for growth. The leader oversees a process in which realistic individual development plans guide each team member's growth. Supporting growth involves dedicating available time and resources for continuing education and pursuit of advanced degrees. Development plans are best discussed outside of the annual performance review, which is tied to merit increases (Coyle, 2018).

Empowerment presents a paradox. A leader must first have evolved personal power in order to empower others. Effective leadership always involves developing others. Effective empowerment requires intentional, relationship-focused leadership.

Relational Empowerment

Cummings et al. (2010) performed a systematic review of studies examining the relationships among leadership styles and nursing workforce/environment outcomes. The authors found that leaders with a relationship focus (transformational, resonant, high emotional intelligence) positively affect workplace outcomes better than those with a task focus (transactional, dissonant, laissez-faire, commanding). Intentionally embracing a relational style as a nurse leader can contribute to relational empowerment and have a positive impact on one's team. DNP leaders can learn relational leadership skills and become effective at positively influencing system, team, and patient outcomes. Relational empowerment focuses on taking time to build relationships and to understand the individual needs of team members, including backgrounds, learning styles, personalities, past challenges contributing to unconscious behavior, strengths, aspirations, areas of uncertainty, and frustrations.

Communication

Effective communication is the axis around which strong leadership operates. In our technology-driven world, communication is extremely complex with multiple platforms available to connect with others or spread

$$\frac{\text{Quality patient outcomes}}{\text{Cost}}$$

FIGURE 2.3 Nurse-value equation.

Source: From Pappas, S. H. (2013). Value, a nursing outcome. *Nursing Administration Quarterly, 37*(2), 122–128. doi:10.1097/NAQ.0b013e3182869dd9

information. Technology can both aid and hinder improvements in communication. The ease of use and rapid ability to spread information globally has transformed our world. The sheer volume of communication is daunting, however, and "information overload" is a common struggle in our modern work environments. Is information overload causing anxiety and inability to focus? Have our work cultures lost touch with human-to-human contact? Effective leaders make intentional decisions about the mix of modalities in their communication. Recent research suggests that team members generally prefer to receive information regarding new decisions, policies, events, or changes via email (Men, 2014). Leaders' use of face-to-face communication can provide some of the most profound support and is positively associated with employee satisfaction (Men, 2014). A nurse leader's decision on how to communicate with the team is often based on which modalities will offer the most efficient, timely, and clear communication. As no two microsystems have the same composition, an optimal combination is dependent on many microsystem-specific variables.

Effective communication is a core aspect of successful leadership and combines several levels, including intrapersonal, interpersonal, group, organizational, and mass communication. *Intrapersonal communication* forms the core of one's world schemata and is the conversation that occurs within an individual's own mind (Dainton & Zelley, 2015). One's internal conversation is shaped by values, experiences, family and other social structures, culture, media, education, and so on. Effective leaders develop self-awareness of their inner dialogue. Cognitive schemas formed from infancy forward provide building blocks for leaders to view the world, other humans, the workplace, society, gender, religion, success, disappointment, work ethics, amusement, and so on. DNP leaders must first understand their own values, and the cognitive schemas in their minds that contribute to the judgments and decisions they make every day. Strategies to increase one's self-awareness include engaging in reflective-practice activities, such as reflective journaling. *Interpersonal communication* occurs between two or more people and is the basis for a team's perception and understanding of a leader. *Group communication* is collaborative conversation that occurs within a team that has a specific aim, during which leaders of groups facilitate consensus decision-making. *Organizational communication* is systemic, occurs across multiple groups, and requires formal plans. *Mass communication* moves outside the organization to include community, state, country, and global conversations. Effective leaders work to develop all levels of communication in the service of developing and supporting cohesive, effective teams.

Innovation

Empowered individuals and teams are capable of innovating change (Masood & Afsar, 2017). Authors frequently express the need for innovation in nursing and healthcare. What is innovation? There are numerous definitions and an excellent nursing text containing comprehensive innovation resources is available (Porter-O'Grady & Malloch, 2018). McDermott described innovation as elemental, incremental, and monumental (McDermott & Sexton, 2004). Elemental innovation means everyone in the organization is involved every day to make the organization better. Incremental change involves small improvements in processes, service, and products that contribute to better outcomes. Monumental change is radical, transformative, and the rarest form of innovation.

Incremental Change

An innovative leader first focuses on incremental change. Effective leaders start with small changes to move a project forward, which ultimately contribute to large-scale changes. Starting small is often where the DNP leader focuses.

Change is inevitable and present every day. So many changes that occur are out of the leader's control. For instance, alterations in healthcare policy at the federal level create a need for leaders to respond within their own organizations. The leader may not be able to modify the enacted policy; however, leaders can influence how the organization will react to it. The shift from volume-based to value-based reimbursement for healthcare is an example of a radical policy change that affeced healthcare systems. Leaders proceeded by focusing effort on measuring quality patient care and innovating processes to improve less-than-optimal performance. The DNP leader has significant influence in moving quality metrics north. To do so, begin with developing a plan for improvement. Launch a blueprint for innovation by writing an aim statement and specifying how much the unit will improve in a specific area. Continue searching for best evidence on how to improve, involve key stakeholders, measure baseline data, implement best evidence, use change models to frame implementation, and evaluate outcomes. After following through on all steps and achieving the overall aim, create a plan to sustain the innovation. The point is, innovation is not connected to inventing the next device to save lives. Incremental innovation is always possible, and effective leaders identify the problem, include others, follow a systematic process, use data for measurement, and ultimately improve outcomes such as increasing leader-rounding rates.

Monumental Change

Innovation can be overwhelming for a nurse leader when considered in terms of monumental change. Grant (2016) studied highly original people and found they had anxieties, doubts, and fears about moving unconventional ideas forward. A quality of highly successful entrepreneurs is a propensity for action. Entrepreneurs move designs forward even when told they will never work or are not fundable. Effective leaders imagine solutions beyond the status quo and have the tenacity to move creative ideas forward.

Human-Centered Designs

Large-scale innovation will transform healthcare, whereas incremental steps are necessary to lead to the overall improvement. DNP nurse leaders can learn to develop the skills necessary for monumental innovation and to lead others to acquire innovation skills. Historically, healthcare systems have been slow to change because of their complexity. New approaches are necessary to change cultures in healthcare away from "the way we have always done it" to embracing innovation. Culture change begins with leaders identifying the competing needs for innovation.

Awareness of the culture in a microsystem and creating strategies to improve culture are important skills of an effective nurse leader. *Culture* is defined as "the product of individual and group values, attitudes and competencies and patterns of behavior that determine the commitment to and the style and proficiency of an organization's health" (Halligan & Zecevic, 2011, p. 339). In essence, workplace culture refers to "the way we do things around here," whereby the word "here" refers not to the hospital, but rather to a particular microsystem (Pronovost & Sexton, 2005). Microsystem culture can be difficult to assess as it is composed of the interplay between individual and collective beliefs that contribute to tacit norms and thus behaviors. A nurse leader's connection to culture is vital, as culture manifests itself in deep, often implicit levels of assumptions that can drive team behavior (Flin, 2007). Many nurse leaders in the acute care setting are actively involved in developing a strong culture around safety, often called *a safety culture*. Advances in healthcare quality and safety contribute to how leaders measure safety culture in relation to reducing errors (Nieva & Sorra, 2003; Pronovost & Sexton, 2005). Relational empowerment, a strong skill of a nurse leader, can contribute to an increasingly safe, relational, connected culture in a healthcare microsystem.

One approach leaders can use to contribute to relational empowerment is human-centered design (HCD). Tim Brown and Roger Martin created design thinking at IDEO and provide an online toolkit (IDEO, 2015). The mind-set of an innovative leader is that complex problems can be solved. Design thinking considers contextual needs of end users when creating solutions to complex problems. Innovative companies, such as Apple, use design thinking. HCD has been used to design products, but the methods and tools that allow cognitive structures to embrace change are moving into healthcare to improve operating room safety, assist with home care, redesign workspace, and improve public health (Criscitelli & Goodwin, 2017; Dijkstra, Sino, Heerdink, & Schuurmans, 2018; Doshi & Clay, 2017; Harte et al., 2017; Trail-Mahan, Heisler, & Katica, 2016; Vechakul, Shrimali, &

Sandhu, 2015). Key components of HCD are its focus on understanding the contextual needs of end users, generating creative solutions to meet needs, rapidly developing/testing prototypes, and learning from failures. A model for HCD includes need-finding, ideation, and experimentation (Figure 2.4).

An important component of HCD, *need-finding*, seeks to understand end-user needs and gain empathy and appreciation for the context of the user's lives. For instance, when DNP leaders innovates new models for patient care, they seek to comprehend both the needs of the patients and the nurses delivering care. An empathy map is a design tool used to guide comprehension of end-user needs. Figure 2.5 provides an example of an empathy map.

Leaders use the empathy map to organize themes from stories told by individuals within groups. Rapid collection of themes occurs in workshop settings. Scribes record the context of the story in the "say" and "do" sections, while writing underlying needs revealed in the "think" and "feel" shapes. Zuber and Moody (2018) used the tool to study innovators among 125 nurses in the Kaiser Permanente healthcare system (Zuber & Moody, 2018). The authors identified seven enablers to innovate change: (a) personal need for a solution, (b) challenges with meaningful purpose, (c) clarity of goal and control of resources, (d) active experimentation, (e) quick and visible progress, (f) positive encouragement and confidence, and (g) psychological safety. DNP leaders can use this knowledge to support nurses to innovate change incrementally, monumentally, and elementally. Leaders who develop a culture of elemental change in which innovation is embraced and practiced by all transform organizations.

Transforming Organizations

Examples of leaders with personal power who empower others to innovate change toward organizational transformation are described in the text that follows.

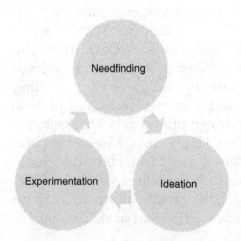

FIGURE 2.4 Components of HCD.
Source: Courtesy of Christi Dining Zuber, PhD, RN.

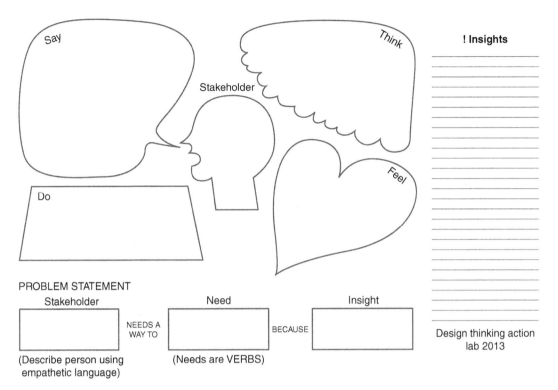

FIGURE 2.5 Example of an empathy map.
Source: Courtesy of DesignThinking Action Lab.

Academic Practice Partnership

The first case involves two exemplary nurse leaders: one from academia and one from practice, both working for the same healthcare system. In response to an AACN report on building transformative academic/practice partnerships (AACN, 2016), the leaders collaborated to integrate independently functioning nursing organizations. The leaders were not aiming for incremental change; rather their goal was monumental innovation leading to transformation of the system. "Relational leaders who thrive in collaborative and team-based cultures were identified as essential to transformation" (Pappas & McCauley, 2018, p. 55). The chief nursing officer and dean put together workgroups intentionally led by nurses with high emotional intelligence who could build trusting relationships and collaborate in teams to move work forward. True change occurred as workgroup leaders built trust; respected unique cultures; created structure inclusive of both cultures; and built partnership focused on excellence in education, practice, and research. Nurses uniquely positioned to break down silos are integrating new care models across the healthcare continuum. Nurse leaders are progressing with goals to provide quality, cost-effective, satisfactory patient care while providing joy-filled work across the multisystem enterprise. Both the academic and practice organizations involved are nationally ranked and strive for greater excellence.

Changing Culture

The second example comes from a small, Southwestern town in Texas led by another exemplary nurse, the senior vice president, chief operating officer, and chief nursing officer, Dr. Bob Dent (Tye & Dent, 2017). A few years back, this community gained a beautiful new hospital tower with state-of-the-art equipment and exquisite healing gardens. It was hoped that the new, esthetically pleasing environment would improve dismal patient-satisfaction scores. However, patient-satisfaction scores did not increase after the move to the new building. A consultant was hired who taught hospital leaders about the concept of *invisible architecture*. The consultant was Joe Tye, of Values Coach, Inc. Using a construction metaphor, Joe focused on core values as the foundation, organizational culture as the structural frame, and workplace attitude as the interior furnishings of the building. It is the invisible architecture and not the perceptible building that most influences staff and patient outcomes. Joe and Bob worked together to change the invisible architecture of the healthcare system. The focus was to convert to a values-driven, positive culture, in which employees exhibited behavior aligned with constructive attitudes. One example of a method used to change staff attitudes was the Pickle Pledge. A unifying metaphorical theme introduced was "Don't be a sour pickle." During the pickle challenge for charity in which staff contributed $0.25 every time they complained, the first week there were 4,000 complaints, so significant money was raised. This campaign was a fun way to work to change staff behavior from destructive to optimistic. In turn, activities, such as the Pickle Pledge, changed the organizational culture to one of personal accountability for success. Patient satisfaction increased from record lows to record highs. The staff turnover rate decreased. A theory underlying this cultural change is symbolic convergence theory (SCT; Dainton & Zelley, 2015). SCT uses fantasy themes, a device intended to dramatize a message to a group. The "sour pickle" fantasy theme offered a unifying message that included emotional revelations for staff at both a surface and deeper level. The fantasy chain, a similar reaction among group members in response to creative imagery or language, resulted in group cohesion or "symbolic convergence." The theme moved staff from individuals with selfish needs to a cohesive, identifiable group with a collective consciousness. DNP nurse leaders can use SCT to bring groups together using a fun, yet powerful approach.

To change culture, beliefs, values, and behaviors must shift. Building new towers, implementing progressive programs, and innovating new products does not improve negative culture. Improving culture is always about the human experience of working in a microsystem and attending to the values and beliefs of people who make up the work team.

Entrepreneurial and Intrapreneurial Nursing Initiatives—Practice Innovations

Opportunity exists for leaders to transform within healthcare systems (intrapreneurial) or externally (entrepreneurial). Rezvani (2010) described characteristics of an entrepreneur; here, her descriptions are applied to the DNP leader.

1. *Exceptional talent in some area.* DNP leaders have a strong clinical background, often in a specialty. Use of expertise to innovate new care models, focused on patient needs, is an effective approach for DNP leaders.

2. *A unique, competitive offering.* DNP leaders are creative and can imagine better healthcare systems in which patients thrive, families feel cared for, and nurses experience joy in providing care. Nurses are known for being creative members of the healthcare team and often have ideas to improve patient care or make better products. DNP nurse leaders create teams in which these ideas are freely shared and contribute to ongoing innovation.

3. *Optimism and confidence.* DNP leaders centered in love, hope, and compassion envision patient-focused care delivered by competent nurses.

4. *Risk tolerance.* DNP leaders take risks knowing one can learn from failure as well as success. Progressive clinical leaders do not let fear hold back movement away from the status quo and mediocrity toward achievement of dreams and goals. Innovative leaders avoid regret of what was not tried, not failure of attempted innovations.

5. *Passion.* DNP leaders bring excitement to begin important work and inspires others to find meaning, joy, and a sense of purpose in their work.

6. *Leadership guides, inspires, influences, and directs others.* DNP leaders have learned knowledge, skills, and attitudes and assembled a leadership toolkit used to bring out the best in themselves and others.

CONCLUSIONS

Effective leaders are vital to organizational improvement and success. Nurses who learn holistic, systemic, human-centered, integrated theory can become outstanding leaders through education, personal development, and practice. A model for leadership development, with personal power at its center to empower staff to innovate change and transform organizations, is useful for DNP leaders who seek to evolve to integrative, wise leaders. Healthcare systems desperately need bold leaders willing to take action to transform systems. Delivering high-quality, safe, satisfying patient care, in an environment that is joyful for nurses is an outcome that innovative leaders can achieve.

Case Study

R.B. is an adult–gerontology clinical nurse specialist (AGCNS) who has been a highly effective leader for a 32-bed neurology unit and 16-bed neuro ICU in an urban 400-bed hospital for 2 years. R.B. worked as a bedside nurse on the neuro unit for 12 years before going back to school to become an advanced practice nurse. She is currently enrolled in a DNP program. As an AGCNS whose practice has specialized in care of the neurologically compromised patient, R.B. has contributed to translation of best practices into the practice standards for both units and has developed continuing-education models for everyone on the care team (MDs, physician assistants [PAs], nurse practitioners [NPs], RNs, and certified nursing assistants [CNAs]). R.B. is a well-liked and trusted clinician, as well as an educator and a team leader. The care teams on both units often consult R.B. for both patient-specific decisions, as well as systems decisions that will affect the operations of the two units on which she practices.

The CNO has been tracking medication administration errors on both the neurology unit and neuro ICU and has been concerned about the ineffective leadership on both units in addressing recurring safety issues specific to medication administration. The CNO believes that a stronger clinical leader should oversee the operations of both units. She has approached R.B. about first taking over the leadership of the 32-bed neuro unit and 6 months later the 16-bed neuro ICU unit.

QUESTIONS

1. R.B. is a relatively new leader, having been an AGCNS for 2 years. R.B. assesses herself at stage two of personal power. What can R.B. do to embrace greater personal power in her emerging leadership work?
2. Most team members on the neuro unit and neuro ICU still see R.B. as a bedside nurse, who recently has a few extra skills. What can R.B. do to effectively communicate her new role as manager of the neuro unit to her team?
3. How might R.B. use structural empowerment and relational empowerment in her new leadership role to develop a strong safety culture on the neuro unit?
4. How will the CNO and R.B. know whether R.B. is successful in her new leadership work and is ready to assume managerial leadership for the neuro ICU?

REFERENCES

American Association of Colleges of Nursing. (2016). *Advancing healthcare transformation: A new era for academic nursing.* Washington, DC: Author.

Anderson, R. J., & Adams, W. A. (2016). *Mastering leadership: An integrated framework for breakthrough performance and extraordinary business results.* Hoboken, NJ: Wiley.

Cicolini, G., Comparcini, D., & Simonetti, V. (2014). Workplace empowerment and nurses' job satisfaction: A systematic literature review. *Journal of Nursing Management, 22*(7), 855–871. doi:10.1111/jonm.12028

Clavelle, J. T. (2012). Transformational leadership: Visibility, accessibility, and communication. *Journal of Nursing Administration, 42*(7–8), 345–346. doi:10.1097/NNA.0b013e31826193d2

Coyle, D. (2018). *The culture code: The secrets of highly successful groups.* New York, NY: Bantam.

Criscitelli, T., & Goodwin, W. (2017). Applying human-centered design thinking to enhance safety in the OR. *AORN Journal, 105*(4), 408–412. doi:10.1016/j.aorn.2017.02.004

Cummings, G. (2004). Investing relational energy: The hallmark of resonant leadership. *Nursing Leadership, 17*(4), 76–87.

Cummings, G. G., MacGregor, T., Davey, M., Lee, H., Wong, C. A., Lo, E., . . . Stafford, E. (2010). Leadership styles and outcome patterns for the nursing workforce and work environment: A systematic review. *International Journal of Nursing Studies, 47*(3), 363–385. doi:10.1016/j.ijnurstu.2009.08.006

Dainton, M., & Zelley, E. D. (2015). *Applying communication theory for professional life: A practical introduction* (3rd ed.). Thousand Oaks, CA: Sage.

Dijkstra, N. E., Sino, C. G. M., Heerdink, E. R., & Schuurmans, M. J. (2018). Development of eHOME, a mobile instrument for reporting, monitoring, and consulting drug-related problems in home care: Human-centered design study. *JMIR Human Factors, 5*(1), e10. doi:10.2196/humanfactors.8319

Dirik, H. F., & Seren Intepeler, S. (2017). The influence of authentic leadership on safety climate in nursing. *Journal of Nursing Management, 25*(5), 392–401. doi:10.1111/jonm.12480

Doshi, A., & Clay, C. (2017). Rethink space: (Re)designing a workspace using human-centered design to support flexibility, collaboration, and engagement among clinical and translational research support services. *Journal of Clinical and Translational Sciences, 1*(3), 160–166. doi:10.1017/cts.2017.5

Drath, W. H., McCauley, C. D., Palus, C. J., Van Velsor, E., O'Connor, P. M. G., & McGuire, J. B. (2008). Direction, alignment, commitment: Toward a more integrative ontology of leadership. *Leadership Quarterly, 19*(6), 635–653. doi:10.1016/j.leaqua.2008.09.003

Fischer, S. A. (2016). Transformational leadership in nursing: A concept analysis. *Journal of Advanced Nursing, 72*(11), 2644–2653. doi:10.1111/jan.13049

Flin, R. (2007). Measuring safety culture in healthcare: A case for accurate diagnosis. *Safety Science, 45*, 653–667. doi:10.1016/j.ssci.2007.04.003

Grant, A. (2016). *Originals: How non-conformists move the world.* New York, NY: Penquin.

Hagberg, J. O. (2003). *Real power: Stages of personal power in organizations* (3rd ed.). Salem, WI: Sheffield Publishing.

Halligan, M., & Zecevic, A. (2011). Safety culture in healthcare: A review of concepts, dimensions, measures and progress. *BMJ Quality & Safety, 20*(4), 338–343. doi:10.1136/bmjqs.2010.040964

Hanse, J. J., Harlin, U., Jarebrant, C., Ulin, K., & Winkel, J. (2016). The impact of servant leadership dimensions on leader–member exchange among health care professionals. *Journal of Nursing Management, 24*(2), 228–234. doi:10.1111/jonm.12304

Harte, R., Glynn, L., Rodriguez-Molinero, A., Baker, P. M., Scharf, T., Quinlan, L. R., & Gearóid, O. L. (2017). A human-centered design methodology to enhance the usability, human factors, and user experience of connected health systems: A three-phase methodology. *JMIR Human Factors, 4*(1), e8. doi:10.2196/humanfactors.5443

IDEO. (2015). *The field guide to human-centered design.* Retrieved from www.designkit.org/resources/1

Jarrin, O. F. (2012). The integrality of situated caring in nursing and the environment. *ANS: Advances in Nursing Science, 35*(1), 14–24. doi:10.1097/ANS.0b013e3182433b89

Kanter, R. M. (1977). *Men and women of the corporation.* New York, NY: Basic Books.

Laschinger, H. K., Wong, C. A., Cummings, G. G., & Grau, A. L. (2014). Resonant leadership and workplace empowerment: The value of positive organizational cultures in reducing workplace incivility. *Nursing Economics, 32*(1), 5–15, 44; quiz 16.

Mannix, J., Wilkes, L., & Daly, J. (2015). "Good ethics and moral standing": A qualitative study of aesthetic leadership in clinical nursing practice. *Journal of Clinical Nursing, 24*(11–12), 1603–1610. doi:10.1111/jocn.12761

Masood, M., & Afsar, B. (2017). Transformational leadership and innovative work behavior among nursing staff. *Nursing Inquiry, 24*(4), e12188. doi:10.1111/nin.12188

McCord, P. (2017). *Powerful: Building a culture of freedom and responsibility.* Jackson, TN: Publishers Group West/Silicon Guild.

McDermott, B., & Sexton, G. (2004). *Leading innovation: Creating workplaces where people excel so organizations thrive*. Canada: Nova Vista Publishing.

Men, L. R. (2014). Strategic internal communication: Transformational leadership, communication channels, and employee satisfaction. *Management Communication Quarterly, 28*(2), 264–284. doi:10.1177/0893318914524536

Nieva, V. F., & Sorra, J. (2003). Safety culture assessment: A tool for improving patient safety in healthcare organizations. *Quality & Safety in Healthcare, 12* (Suppl. 2): ii17–ii23. doi:10.1136/qhc.12.suppl_2.ii17

Oster, C., & Braaten, J. (2016). *High reliability organizations: A healthcare handbook for patient safety & quality*. Indianapolis, IN: Sigma Theta Tau International.

Pappas, S., & McCauley, L. (2018). Nursing integration and innovation across a multisystem enterprise: Priorities for nurse leaders. *Nursing Administration Quarterly, 42*(1), 54–61. doi:10.1097/naq.0000000000000265

Pappas, S. H. (2013). Value, a nursing outcome. *Nursing Administration Quarterly, 37*(2), 122–128. doi:10.1097/NAQ.0b013e3182869dd9

Pausch, R., & Zaslow, J. (2008). *The last lecture*. New York, NY: Hyperion.

Perry, S. M. (2017). The influence of authentic leadership on safety climate in nursing. *Journal of Nursing Management, 26*(4), 493. doi:10.1111/jonm.12557

Porter-O'Grady, T., & Malloch, K. (2018). *Quantum leadership: Creating sustainable value in health care* (5th ed.). Burlington, MA: Jones & Bartlett.

Pronovost, P., & Sexton, B. (2005). Assessing safety culture: Guidelines and recommendations. *Quality and Safety in Health Care, 14*(4), 231–233. doi:10.1136/qshc.2005.015180

Read, C. Y., Pino Betancourt, D. M., & Morrison, C. (2016). Social change: A framework for inclusive leadership development in nursing education. *Journal of Nursing Education, 55*(3), 164–167. doi:10.3928/01484834-20160216-08

Reinertsen, J. L., & Johnson, K. M. (2010). Rounding to influence. Leadership method helps executives answer the "hows" in patient safety initiatives. *Healthcare Executive, 25*(5), 72–75.

Rezvani, S. (2010). *The next generation of women leaders: What you need to lead but won't learn in business school*. Santa Barbara, CA: ABC-CLIO.

Riley, B. H., Dearmon, V., Mestas, L., & Buckner, E. B. (2016). Frontline nurse engagement and empowerment: Characteristics and processes for building leadership capacity. *Nursing Administration Quarterly, 40*(4), 325–333. doi:10.1097/naq.0000000000000186

Savel, R. H., & Munro, C. L. (2017). Servant leadership: The primacy of service. *American Journal of Critical Care, 26*(2), 97–99. doi:10.4037/ajcc2017356

Spano-Szekely, L., Quinn Griffin, M. T., Clavelle, J., & Fitzpatrick, J. J. (2016). Emotional intelligence and transformational leadership in nurse managers. *Journal of Nursing Administration, 46*(2), 101–108. doi:10.1097/nna.0000000000000303

Spence Laschinger, H. K. (2008). Effect of empowerment on professional practice environments, work satisfaction, and patient care quality: Further testing the Nursing Worklife Model. *Journal of Nursing Care Quality, 23*(4), 322–330. doi:10.1097/01.NCQ.0000318028.67910.6b

Trail-Mahan, T., Heisler, S., & Katica, M. (2016). Quality improvement project to improve patient satisfaction with pain management: Using human-centered design. *Journal of Nursing Care Quality, 31*(2), 105–112; quiz 113–104. doi:10.1097/ncq.0000000000000161

Tye, J., & Dent, B. (2017). *Building a culture of ownership in healthcare: The invisible architecture of core values, attitude, and self-empowerment*. Indianapolis, IN: Sigma Theta Tau International.

Vechakul, J., Shrimali, B. P., & Sandhu, J. S. (2015). Human-centered design as an approach for place-based innovation in public health: A case study from Oakland, California. *Maternal and Child Health Journal, 19*(12), 2552–2559. doi:10.1007/s10995-015-1787-x

Welton, J. M., & Harper, E. M. (2016). Measuring nursing care value. *Nursing Economics, 34*(1), 7–14; quiz 15.

Wilber, K. (2001). *The eye of spirit: An integral vision for a world gone slightly mad* (3rd ed.). Boston, MA: Shambhala.

Zuber, C. D., & Moody, L. (2018). Creativity and innovation in health care: Tapping into organizational enablers through human-centered design. *Nursing Administration Quarterly, 42*(1), 62–75. doi:10.1097/naq.0000000000000267

3

LEADERSHIP AND SYSTEMS THINKING

MARY A. DOLANSKY

This chapter addresses the following DNP American Association of Colleges of Nursing (AACN) Essentials:

II. Organizational and Systems Leadership for Quality Improvement and Systems Thinking
VI. Interprofessional Collaboration for Improving Patient and Population Health Outcomes

INTRODUCTION

Healthcare systems are complex. Healthcare teams deliver care in these complex systems and need to both understand and influence these complex systems to ensure safe, high-quality care. The target of safe, high-quality care is a Quadruple Aim: (a) enhancing the patient experience, (b) improving population health, (c) reducing the costs of care, and (d) improving the work life of healthcare providers and staff (Bodenheimer & Sinsky, 2014). Now more than ever, patients depend on healthcare professionals to deliver care congruent with these aims.

Many opportunities exist to achieve the quadruple aim. Compared to other developed and several developing nations, the United States ranks near the bottom (26th of 35 nations) in mortality and life expectancy, and exceeds other countries in health spending (World Health Organization [WHO], 2015). Medical errors are estimated to be the third leading cause of death, following cardiovascular disease and cancers (Makary & Daniel, 2016). Steady progress is being made in making healthcare systems more safe.

Hospitals report a significant reduction in hospital-acquired infections over the last 5years, although reduction targets have not been met (Tejal, Berwick, & Gandhi, 2016). In addition, large-scale projects like the Partnership for Patients (P4P) sponsored by the Centers for Medicaid & Medicare Services (CMS) focused on the quadruple aim (CMS, 2015; Gerhardt et al., 2013). The P4P demonstrated a reduction of 21 million hospital-acquired infections, estimated at saving 87,000 lives and $20 billion in costs. The project demonstrated that a focus on the systems of care delivery facilitates improvement.

Understanding and influencing the systems of care delivery are key to quality and safety. Current approaches to address quality and safety include system redesign to address broken processes of care, high-reliability efforts to ensure safe delivery of care, and frontline quality-improvement efforts to ensure care is safe, timely, efficient, equitable, effective, and patient centered (Institute of Medicine [IOM], 2000). Approaches aimed at systems improvement of care delivery require that healthcare professionals work in interprofessional teams, use a systems approach, and have an understanding of complex systems.

Nurses, as the largest population of professionals in healthcare today, are essential to ensure that care delivery is safe and of high quality. Florence Nightingale was the first nurse to demonstrate the capacity of nurses to influence quality and safety through use of a systems approach; she is referred to as one of the pioneers in quality and safety. Florence observed care delivery, collected data, and made changes in care to improve outcomes. Her polar-area diagrams, which displayed data on causes of death, are an example of her important contributions to quality (Nightingale, 1858).

Nurses take leadership roles in healthcare departments that influence quality and safety such as management, quality, risk management, legal, and professional developments that address systems issues. Nurses' roles in these efforts are important; however, we also need nurses at the front line of care to lead systems improvement. Expanding nurses' role from the delivery of patient care to changing the systems of care is a paradigm shift (Dolansky & Moore, 2013). Highlighting this shift is the American Nurses Association (ANA) definition of *nursing* as the protection, promotion, and optimization of health and abilities; prevention of illness and injury; alleviation of suffering through the diagnosis and treatment of human response; and advocacy in the care of individuals, families, communities, and populations (ANA, 2010). Expanding ANA's definition requires inclusion of care of the healthcare system. To address this need, the Quality and Safety Education for Nurses (QSEN) initiative suggests that the way to improve quality and safety is to expand nursing competencies from the traditional delivery of individualized care to attending to the systems of care (Figure 3.1).

The competencies required to improve systems are teamwork and collaboration, informatics, quality improvement, implementation of evidence-based practice, patient-centered care, and safety (Cronenwett et al., 2007; Sherwood

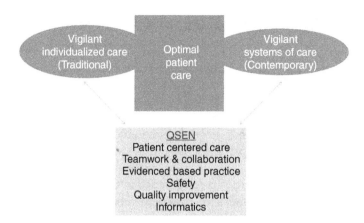

FIGURE 3.1 Key components of high-quality, safe patient care.

Source: From Dolansky, M. A., & Moore, S. M. (2013). Quality and Safety Education in Nursing: The key is systems thinking. *Online Journal of Issues in Nursing, 18*(3), 1.

& Barnsteiner, 2017). As Cronnenwett stated: "Our healthcare system has significant safety and quality problems. To fix that, we need to redesign what and how we teach the next generation of nurses and other healthcare professionals so that they understand what goes into ensuring good and safe care, and can identify and bridge the gaps between what is and what should be" (Linda Cronenwett, personal communication, February 26, 2009).

As nursing's role in healthcare expands, doctorally prepared nurses are needed for systems leadership to ensure that care delivery is of high quality. The AACN DNP Essentials reflect this role expansion, which addresses the system factors and emphasizes that DNP-prepared nurses must be competent in leadership and systems thinking (AACN, 2006). Box 3.1 displays the recommended DNP systems competencies.

LEADERSHIP

Leadership is a term widely used in healthcare that is often misunderstood. Recent nursing graduates believe leadership is the role of the nurse

BOX 3.1 AACN DNP Essentials

Essential II: Organizational and Systems Leadership for Quality Improvement and Systems Thinking
  The DNP program prepares the graduate to:

1. Develop and evaluate care delivery approaches that meet current and future needs of patient populations based on scientific findings in nursing and other clinical sciences, as well as organizational, political, and economic sciences.

(continued)

BOX 3.1 AACN DNP Essentials (*continued*)

2. Ensure accountability for quality of healthcare and patient safety for populations with whom they work.
   a. Use advanced communication skills/processes to lead quality-improvement and patient safety initiatives in healthcare systems.
   b. Employ principles of business, finance, economics, and health policy to develop and implement effective plans for practice-level and/or system-wide practice initiatives that will improve the quality of care delivery.
   c. Develop and/or monitor budgets for practice initiatives.
   d. Analyze the cost-effectiveness of practice initiatives accounting for risk and improvement of healthcare outcomes.
   e. Demonstrate sensitivity to diverse organizational cultures and populations, including patients and providers.
3. Develop and/or evaluate effective strategies for managing the ethical dilemmas inherent in patient care, the healthcare organization, and research.

Source: From American Association of Colleges of Nursing. (2006). AACN Essentials of the doctoral education for advanced nursing practice. Retrieved from http://www.aacnnursing.org/DNP/DNP-Essentials

manager and is not part of the role of the frontline nurse. Broadly defined, "leadership is a process of social influence which maximizes the efforts of others toward the achievement of a greater good" (Kruse, 2013).

> *If your actions inspire others to dream more,*
> *learn more, do more, become more, you are a leader.*
> —John Quincy Adams

Our current healthcare systems need nurses to be leaders who contribute to the improvement of the quality and safety of care. When an error is made, the nurse must report the error, participate in a group process about why the error was made (such as a root-cause analysis), follow up with the patient regarding the details of the error, and engage in system-improvement efforts to ensure that the error does not happen again (Dolansky, Helba, Drushel, & Courtney, 2012). These leadership skills are especially important in the role of the DNP-prepared leader who is charged with improving the systems of care delivery.

Leading Systems in Complex Healthcare

Current healthcare system models have been enhanced through increasing use of complex adaptive system models. Complex adaptive systems are often described as nonlinear, interactive systems that continuously adapt to changing environments through self-organization and by having many independent parts (Crowell, 2016). Evolving models based on complex adaptive systems contribute to an emerging understanding of how adaptive behavior and innovation emerge through these self-organizing systems, despite consistently shifting inputs into a system (Weberg, 2012). In complex systems leadership is conceptualized as a continuous process that stems from collaboration, complex systems thinking, and innovative mindsets (Weberg, 2012). When employing the lens of complexity, the leadership role moves away from providing answers or providing too much direction (e.g., initiating structure) to creating the conditions in which followers' behaviors can produce structure and innovation (Marion & Uhl-Bien, 2001).

The historical lack of appreciation for the complexity of healthcare systems has resulted in process fragmentation, such as the lack of structured transitions of care, which then result in communication errors and missed care. Processes that are unstandardized, such as handoffs, lead to uncoordinated care, replication of effort, and work-arounds. Hierarchical systems, such as top-down decision-making, lead to nondisclosure of errors and limited problem solving. In addition, an increased focus on attempts to simplify the measurement of outcomes has resulted in a lack of attention to the complex processes of care. An example of this is seen in the reduction in number of hospital-associated infections. Many measures track rates of specific kinds of infections (e.g., catheter-associated urinary tract infection, central-line associated bloodstream infection). However, measurement is lacking on adherence to bundles. Bundles are evidence-based strategies that are "bundled" together to reduce infections. Systems leaders must expand measurement strategies to include measuring the processes of care delivery, not just the outcomes.

The complex healthcare system includes various barriers to the delivery of high-quality care. Barriers include the tension between time constraints and the need for efficiency, attitudes that attending to systems issues are not a part of the role of the professional, activities that take on a higher priority, the inability to delegate care to assistive personnel, and the inability to work in interprofessional teams. For example, effective interprofessional teamwork requires trust and respect when giving and receiving feedback. Giving and receiving feedback in teams is essential in systems improvement, as these skills are operational, day-to-day skills used in collaboration. In contrast, many healthcare professions perceive that efforts to improve care are futile, so they adopt an attitude of "Why do we bother? These initiatives are just fads." An example is nurses' efforts to reduce falls. Healthcare improvement leaders have spent more than a decade researching how to prevent falls in the hospital, with minimal impact. Frontline nurses have initiated countless fall-prevention interventions, with few notable results, leading to a pervasive, professional attitude of hopelessness.

The DNP professional addresses these barriers and guides frontline professionals to bridge the evidence into practice and facilitates the delivery of high-quality care. They also provide essential leadership on integrating quality-related information to guide optimal care. The Institute for Healthcare Improvement (IHI) model for delivery of safe, reliable and effective care (Figure 3.2) is one framework that DNPs can use to guide systems leadership. The framework includes two components of the system: culture and learning. The DNP-prepared nurse who is a systems leader is aware that updated approaches, such as this framework, are needed to contribute to a culture of improvement.

SYSTEMS THINKING

Systems

Another model guiding systems leadership is the Learning Organization Model developed by Peter Senge in his book, *The Fifth Discipline: The Art and Science of the Learning Organization* (Senge, 2006). Senge proposed that what is needed to address the complexity in organizations is systems thinking.

Before defining *systems thinking*, it is important to understand levels of systems in the context of patient care. Systems are conceptualized at the micro, meso, and macro levels (Nelson et al., 2008). Figure 3.3 displays a visual representation of this framework. The patient and family are at the

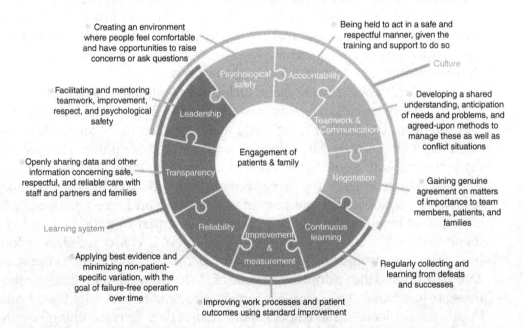

FIGURE 3.2 Framework for safe, reliable, and effective care with descriptive component detail.

Source: From Institute for Healthcare Improvement. (2018). Why do I feel too busy to work on culture? Retrieved from http://www.ihi.org/communities/blogs/why-do-i-feel-too-busy-to-work-on-culture. Reprinted from www.IHI.org with permission of the Institute for Healthcare Improvement, ©2018.

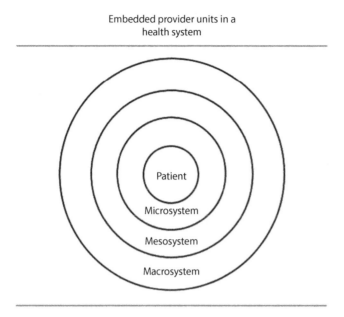

FIGURE 3.3 Levels of systems: Embedded provider units in a health system.

Source: From Nelson, E. C., Godfrey, M. M., Batalden, P. B., Berry, S. A., Bothe, A. E., McKinley, K. E., . . . Wasson, J. H. (2008). Clinical microsystems, Part 1. The building blocks of health systems. *The Joint Commission Journal on Quality and Patient Safety, 34*(7), 367–378. doi:10.1016/s1553-7250(08)34047-1

center and interact with their self-care system. Outside the patient and family system is the microsystem where the patient and the family join with providers and staff to form clinical microsystems. Examples of microsystems are hospital units or clinics. The collection of microsystems come together to form mesosystems, for example, clinical programs and centers that often are part of larger organizations. The mesosystem is held accountable by the macrosystem, such as a hospital or an integrated health system. The macrosystem operates with the microsystems and mesosystem to produce a seamless, satisfying journey for a patient and his or her family. Understanding various levels of system functioning is important for DNP nurse leaders, as identification of the correct level of a system in seeking the etiology of problems or exemplary practices is important.

Understanding Systems

The DNP-prepared nurse is charged with understanding systems and how they interact at all levels. Understanding interactions among and between systems facilitates the level of awareness of change that is required to achieve high-quality, safe care. Some helpful resources available to the DNP-prepared nurse to enhance understanding of systems are the Dartmouth Institute for Health Policy and Dartmouth College Clinical Practice at the Geisel School of Medicine. The online Knowledge Center has books, workbooks, videos, and assessment tools available to facilitate a systems approach (clinicalmicrosystem.org/knowledge). Some of the workbooks are specific to microsystems, such as primary care clinics, neonatal intensive care units, and inpatient units. Videos include details on microsystems, coaching, running effective meetings, and the Standards for Quality Improvement Reporting Excellence (SQUIRE) guidelines. A useful assessment tool, the Clinical Microsystem Assessment Tool, was developed by Dr. Julie Johnson, and can be found at the Institute for Healthcare Improvement website (www.ihi.org/resources/Pages/Tools/ClinicalMicrosystemAssessmentTool.aspx).

Understanding systems requires not only having an appreciation for levels of a system and how levels of systems function, but also the ability to use systems thinking skills. Systems thinking skills are essential for DNP leaders to continually drive improvement in quality and safety of healthcare delivery and achieving the quadruple aim.

Definition of Systems Thinking

In the discipline of management, *systems thinking* is defined as a "way of thinking about, and a language for describing and understanding the forces and interrelationships that shape the behavior of systems" (Senge, 2006, p. 69). Systems thinking "helps us to see how to change systems more effectively, and to act more in tune with the larger processes of the natural and economic world" (Senge, 2006, p. 69). Dolansky and Moore, who developed an instrument to measure systems thinking for healthcare professionals to advance the science of improvement, defined *systems thinking* as:

> The ability to recognize, understand, and synthesize the interactions, and interdependencies in a set of components designed for a specific purpose. This includes the ability to recognize patterns and repetitions in the interactions and an understanding of how actions and components can reinforce or counteract each other. These relationships and patterns occur at different dimensions: temporal, spatial, social, technical or cultural. (Dolansky & Moore, 2013)

Dolansky and Moore's definition was developed through an iterative process of obtaining responses from 10 international experts in quality improvement and systems thinking. The definition and responses from these experts were then used to develop an instrument to measure systems thinking (case.edu/nursing/research/research-studies-labs/systems-thinking/systems-thinking-scale-manual).

Systems thinking is also defined as a set of synergistic analytic skills that increases one's ability to appreciate the interactions among systems in order to identify appropriate action to produce desired outcomes (Arnold & Wade, 2015). The skill of systems thinking connects the environment with actions (Bleich, 2014) and is an essential skill in decision-making in order to achieve high-quality delivery of patient care. Nurses who use systems thinking recognize, understand, and synthesize interactions and interdependencies between their behavior and the complex, unpredicted events in the system in which they work (Moore, Dolansky, Singh, Palmieri, & Alemi, 2010). The science of systems thinking is emerging as leadership research further explores the connections of systems thinking to quality and safety outcomes (Hwang & Park, 2017; Stalter et al., 2017; Trbovich, 2014; Wieman & Wieman, 2004; Wiig et al., 2014).

A Systems Level Awareness Model was developed by Phillips, Stalter, Dolansky, and Lopez (2016) to guide the integration of systems thinking into RN-BSN curriculum (Figure 3.4). The model serves to guide educational strategies to enhance systems thinking skills.

Adding to our understanding of systems thinking, a concept analysis was published by Stalter and colleagues (Stalter et al., 2017). They defined *systems thinking* as a "process applied to individuals, teams and organizations to impact cause and effect where solutions to complex problems are accomplished through collaborative effort according to personal ability with respect to improving components and the greater whole (Stalter et al., 2017, p. 323). Four primary attributes were identified: dynamic system, holistic perspective, pattern identification, and transformation. The use of systems thinking facilitates decision-making in complex situations and serves as the link among a healthcare professional's environment, his or her behavior, and healthcare outcomes.

Systems Thinking Instrument

A Systems Thinking Scale is available to measure healthcare professionals' ability to understand the interdependencies encountered in efforts to improve care (Dolansky & Moore, 2013). The 20-item Systems Thinking Scale contributes to the science of healthcare quality and safety by increasing the understanding of one of the mechanisms (systems thinking) by which quality and safety processes achieve their results, and by improving the education efforts of future healthcare professionals. Other components for systems thinking measurement include personal effort and reliance on authority. Further testing of these components is underway.

The Systems Thinking Scale has been used in practice and education to demonstrate the effect of systems thinking on improving the quality and safety of healthcare systems (Trbovich, 2014). Practicing nurses who reported higher systems thinking also more frequently reported errors in practice (Hwang & Park, 2017). In medical education, medical students who attended education in systems thinking increased systems awareness

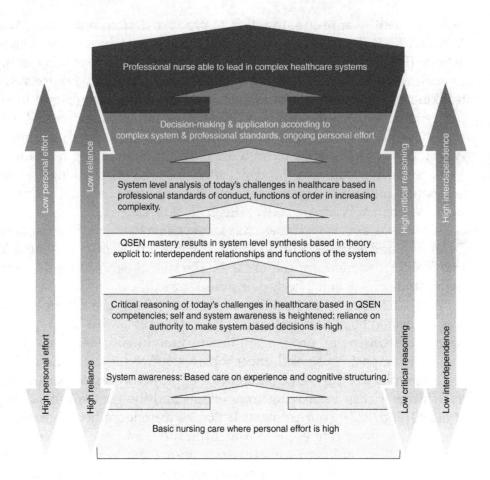

FIGURE 3.4 Systems Level Awareness Model.

QSEN, Quality and Safety Education for Nurses.

Source: From Phillips, J. M., Stalter, A. M., Dolansky, M. A., & Lopez, G. M. (2016). Fostering future leadership in quality and safety in health care through systems thinking. *Journal of Professional Nursing, 32*(1), 15–24. doi:10.1016/j.profnurs.2015.06.003

of safety knowledge as well as systems thinking (Aboumatar et al., 2012). And in nursing, students who participated in a 4-hour educational strategy using a systems approach on patient safety, delivery of care, and medication errors, demonstrated improved systems thinking (Fura & Wisser, 2017).

Elements of Systems Thinking

To enhance systems thinking, The Waters Foundation published, *The Habit-Forming Guide to Becoming a Systems Thinker* (Benson & Marlin, 2017). The book highlights 14 habits of a systems thinker that are applied to five systems: well-being, family, workplace, school, and community. Application of the 14 habits contributes to the better understanding of systems, and facilitates connections to produce meaningful change (Table 3.1).

TABLE 3.1 ELEMENTS OF SYSTEMS THINKING AND HOW THEY APPLY TO NURSING SYSTEMS LEADERS

Element of Systems Thinking*	Explanation	Nursing Systems Leadership Exemplar
Makes meaningful connections within and between systems	Continually make meaningful connections and weaves the connections together to form a clearer understanding	The systems leader identifies a pattern of increased satisfaction scores on a medical unit during the fall and spring; reflecting on the context of care, performing observations, and considering potential contributing factors, it was determined that the timing corresponded to when students were on the clinical unit
Seeks to understand the big picture	Builds a new perspective by moving to the broader view and balances the broader view with the details of the task	To increase satisfaction scores on the HCAPS, before implementing a teach-back intervention for heart failure patients prior to discharge, the systems leader interviews all stakeholders in the process and creates a process map to better understand the system
Changes perspectives to increase understanding	Constantly and intentionally seeks other perspectives by looking at the situation differently, seeking the views of others, and considering the context	Increasing the rates of pneumonia vaccine in the primary care clinic requires the involvement of staff, administrators, and patients; talking with all involved provides a deeper understanding of what components couldn't be enhanced
Considers how mental models affect current and future reality	Peoples' experiences shape their views and are incorporated into their mental models, assumptions, and beliefs; everyone has unique mental models	Working on a surgical unit that has an increased population of geriatric patients, the nursing staff are angry that the medical residents are reluctant to order adequate pain medications; the systems leader appreciates that the nursing staff and physicians have different mental models of the situation (one comfort and the other renal clearance of the opioid) and sets up a meeting to discuss these differences
Observes how elements within systems change over time, generating patterns and trends	Measure and focus on the change over time to increase understanding; userun charts and control charts and communicate results using this data	Working on fall reduction on the step-down unit, the systems leader shares the data displayed in a control chart with the staff; the staff work together to generate ideas as to why fall rates are increasing

(continued)

TABLE 3.1 ELEMENTS OF SYSTEMS THINKING AND HOW THEY APPLY TO NURSING SYSTEMS LEADERS *(continued)*

Element of Systems Thinking*	Explanation	Nursing Systems Leadership Exemplar
Surfaces and tests assumptions	Uses evidence to support or refute beliefs	The nurses on the unit believe that the current skin care processes are evidence based; the systems leader engages a group of nurses to search the literature and to inquire about best practices at other hospitals to support care practices
Recognizes that a system's structure generates its behavior	Takes into consideration the architectural and structural influences on the system	Transformation of primary care practices included team-based care, yet the systems leader observed that RNs were located down the hall from the clinic room; teamwork (communication and interventions) was enhanced by co-locating the physicians and nurses to the same area
Identifies the circular nature of complex cause-and-effect relationships	Appreciates the relationship of cause and effect is often circular in nature; uses causal loop diagrams to enhance this understanding	Observing the data trends of rehospitalizations on the unit, the system leader concludes that as the length of stay decreases, rehospitalization rates increase
Recognizes the impact of time delays when exploring cause-and-effect relationships	Appreciates that often cause and effect are mediated by time and the delay may not be expected	A handoff tool was implemented in obstetrical services to focus nurses on signs of hemorrhage; the impact of the handoff implementation was not observed until three quarters after the implementation; the systems leader recognizes that it took many PDSA cycless to fine tune the toll to ensure its use spread and was standardized
Considers short-term, long-term, and unintended consequences of actions	Takes the time to consider all aspects of the situation by thinking through all effects of a planned change	An improvement project was implemented to reduce CAUTI rates on the surgical floor. The systems leader anticipated that patients will be at higher risk of falls due to the early removal of Foley catheters and therefore implemented fall prevention as a part of the CAUTI reduction efforts

(continued)

TABLE 3.1 ELEMENTS OF SYSTEMS THINKING AND HOW THEY APPLY TO NURSING SYSTEMS LEADERS (continued)

Element of Systems Thinking*	Explanation	Nursing Systems Leadership Exemplar
Considers an issue fully and resists the urge to come to a quick conclusion	Takes the time to consider all aspects of a situation before making a decision	During quality-improvement project team meetings, the team stars suggesting solutions to address a high sepsis rate; he system leader reminds the team that more data are needed to understand the problem, so the team engages in building a cause–effect diagram
Pays attention to accumulations and their rates of change	Considers the changes that occur over time such as time to become competent in a skill or the time to change culture on a unit	On the medical unit, the staff nurses seem burned out and resistant to the change proposed by the DNP student; the DNP student investigated and found out that the unit was involved with 15 other QI projects and adding one more would not not be helpful
Uses understanding of system structure to identify possible areas for leverage	Takes the time to consider all aspects so as to identify the key factors required to make a change	The systems leader observes that the nurses are performing workarounds when medications are not available from pharmacy and realizes this poses a safety issue; a process map was constructed to identify possible solutions to reduce these workarounds
Checks results and changes actions if needed	Embraces change as an enduring process allowing constant strive for improvement	Integrating a primary care model brought major change to the unit; the systems leader knew that it would take several process changes (PDSAs), including testing and reviewing results before sustained change would be achieved

CAUTI, catheter-associated urinary tract infection; HCAPS, Hospital Consumer Assessment of Healthcare, Providers, and Systems; plan–do–study–act; QI, quality improvement.

Source: From Waters Foundation (n.d.). Elements of systems thinking and how they apply to nursing leadership. Retrieved from: www.watersfoundation.org

Why Systems Thinking Is Essential for Leadership to Improve Processes

As displayed in Table 3.1, the elements of systems thinking reflect key aspects of a systems leader. The systems leader is skilled in these elements and takes into consideration the complexity of the context of care. Appreciation of the complexity of care leads to development of critical aspects of leadership, including determination, the endurance to sustain one's efforts, the courage to try new solutions, and to respect the impact of interprofessional collaboration in addressing the quadruple aim.

Over the past 20 years, our colleagues in the medical profession have addressed the quadruple aim and implemented strategies to align care to achieve better quality and safer care. In 1993, Bataldin and colleagues published one of the first documents addressing systems of care (Batalden & Stoltz, 1993). In this innovative article, they proposed a systems-based framework for the continual improvement of healthcare. In 1999, the American College of Graduate Medical Education (ACGME) developed the Systems Based Practice and Practice-Based Learning and Improvement Competencies. These competencies focused on systems thinking to facilitate the development of physicians whose care extends beyond the individual approach to the treatment of disease to treatment of the system (Varkey, Karlapudi, Rose, Nelson, & Warner, 2009). Since the inception of the ACGME competencies, the American Medical Association has advocated for additional questions related to the competencies be added to their qualifying exams and published text books, such as *Health Systems Science* by Skochelak et al. (2016), on the subject. The discipline of medicine has aligned competencies throughout students' professional development from medical school certification maintenance to ensure that graduates and practicing physicians develop, strengthen, and maintain system-focused competencies. These shifts direct physicians to be aware and responsive to the larger context and system of healthcare to better achieve the quadruple aim. Acceleration of improvement will be achieved through the understanding of nurses' roles and the role of interprofessional collaborative efforts to enhance quality and patient safety.

CONCLUSIONS

Quality and Safety, Improving Process, Teachinging Organizations, Culture

Systems leadership is essential to improving healthcare quality and safety, as many barriers exist in our current healthcare system. The DNP, as a systems leader, needs to be aware of systems issues and approaches using frameworks such as the IHI's Framework for Safe, Reliable, and Effective Care (2018) and Senge's Learning Organization Model (2006). The effective DNP nurse leader has an appreciation of the levels of systems and works to close gaps to ensure that healthcare delivery is safe, timely, effective, equitable, efficient, and patient centered.

Case Study

A CASE STUDY HIGHLIGHTING SYSTEMS LEADERSHIP: SYSTEMS THINKING IN LONG TERM CARE

Created by Izabela Kanzana, DNP, RN

As an Advanced Practice Registered Nurse in a Long Term Care (LTC) facility you provide care to 10 residents on Unit A. Every time you are on that floor during lunch time the majority of residents are sitting in wheelchairs and eating their lunch at tables in the dining room. You have looked at several research studies that point to inactivity of residents as a major risk factor contributing to disability and the relationship between increased walking activity and higher functional performance and quality of life. You are curious whether those residents have severe physical limitations keeping them from walking. Your facility has a Walk to Dine program, led by the facility's restorative nurses. How many residents are able to walk? Is it safe for them to walk? When do they walk? Who assists them with walking? How far do they walk? You are motivated to engage in a project as you have identified an important practice problem. Because the evidence is strong that physical activity is the solution, you know that a QI project to implement the evidence into the process on your unit is the right way to go. The Medical director agrees with you that walking has potential benefits even in LTC.

QUESTIONS

1. Who would be on your QI team? Which members will be the most important to interview?
   You know that restorative nurses are in charge of Walk to Dine program for residents. You interview restorative nurses and they do not know how many residents are enrolled in Walk to Dine program. They do not know how often residents walk to meals and how far residents walk.
2. What would be helpful baseline data?
3. What might your goals be for your improvement project?

Searching the Literature

You searched the literature and found strong evidence that walking patients in LTC leads to better outcomes. You also find in the literature search evidence of key implementation strategies that support walking in LTC residents:

- Staff education (Galik et al., 2013; Slaughter & Estabrooks, 2013)
- Monitoring (Slaughter & Estabrooks, 2013)
- Mentoring and motivating (Galik et al., 2013; Taylor et al., 2015)

   You contacted your colleague in a different LTC facility and they successfully implemented a walking program designed by the Vanderbilt Center for Quality Aging (Schnelle & Simmons, 2013).

(continued)

Case Study (*continued*)

Context for the Improvement

You assess Unit A's readiness for a change using the organizational readiness to change survey. To understand the causes of the low participation in the Walk to Dine program, you collect information from all the stakeholders. The following data surfaces:

- Unit A is sometimes understaffed
- CNAs turnover is high
- There is no clear workflow process of walking a resident from an activity to a meal
- There are not enough walkers for residents who can ambulate with a walker
- A third manager was hired within last 2 months and is still getting oriented
- Family members request wheelchairs for residents to take residents to meals
- Many residents have dementia and they tell you they were assisted with walking even though you are told by staff they did not walk
- Two restorative nurses are in charge of the Walk to Dine program in the entire facility (230 beds)
- CNAs think that it is restorative staff function to provide walking activity to residents
- There is no log to track who walks to meals
- No one knows which residents are able to ambulate to meals
- There is no clear process for identification of residents who want to walk to meals
- There is no monitoring in how the residents that ambulate to meals tolerate the ambulation

4. Create a fishbone diagram using the data you discovered in exploring the context for the improvement. Use the following categories: people, policies, workflow process, equipment, measurement

   The QI team discusses the project aim thinking about feasibility and contextual barriers. It might be challenging, but your team plans to increase walking activity for eligible residents on Unit A to five times a week.

5. Write a SMART aim for this goal

   You and your team make a plan to evaluate the QI project. Patients would be screened and only eligible residents would be enrolled in the program. Each resident may have a different walking capacity. Markings on the walls would allow to measure the distance residents walk. CNAs will be educated about the Dine to Walk program and benefits of increased physical activity in LTC residents and consequences of immobility.

6. What data would you collect to evaluate the outcomes and sustainability of your QI project?

REFERENCES

Aboumatar, H. J., Thompson, D., Wu, A., Dawson, P., Colbert, J., Marsteller, J., . . . Pronovost, P. (2012). Development and evaluation of a 3-day patient safety curriculum to advance knowledge, self-efficacy and system thinking among medical students. *BMJ Quality & Safety*, 21(5), 416–422.

American Association of Colleges of Nursing. (2006). AACN Essentials of the Doctoral Education for Advanced Nursing Practice. Retrieved from http://www.aacnnursing.org/DNP/DNP-Essentials

American Nurses Association. (2010). *Nursing: Scope and standards of practice*. Silver Spring, MD: American Nurses Association Publishing.

Arnold, R. D., & Wade, J. P. (2015). A definition of systems thinking: a systems approach. *Procedia Computer Science, 44*, 669–678. doi:10.1016/j.procs.2015.03.050

Batalden, P. B., & Stoltz, P. K. (1993). A framework for the continual improvement of health care: Building and applying professional and improvement knowledge to test changes in daily work. *The Joint Commission Journal on Quality Improvement, 19*, 424–447. doi:10.1016/S1070-3241(16)30025-6

Benson, T., & Marlin, S. (2017). *The habit-forming guide to becoming a systems thinker*. Pittsburg, CA: Systems Thinking Group, Waters Foundation.

Bleich, M. R. (2014). Developing leaders as systems thinkers—Part II. *Journal of Continuing Education in Nursing, 45*(5), 201–202. doi:10.3928/00220124-20140424-13

Bodenheimer, T., & Sinsky, C. (2014). From triple aim to quadruple aim: Care of the patient requires the provider. *Annals of Family Medicine, 12*(6), 573–576. doi:10.1370/afm.1713

Centers for Medicare & Medicaid Innovation. (2015). Project eEvaluation activity support of partnership for patients. Interim evaluation report (contract No. GS-10F-0166R). Retrieved from https://downloads.cms.gov/files/cmmi/pfp-interimevalrpt.pdf

Cronenwett, L., Sherwood, G., Barnsteiner, J., Disch, J., Johnson, J., Mitchell, P., . . . Warren, J. (2007). Quality and Safety education for Nurses. *Nursing Outlook, 55*, 122–131. doi:10.1016/j.outlook.2007.02.006

Crowell, D. M. (2016). *Complexity leadership: Nursing's role in health-care delivery*. Philadelphia, PA: F.A. Davis Company.

Deming, W. E. (1993). *The new economics for industry, government, and education*. Boston: MA: MIT Press.

Dolansky, M. A., Helba, M., Druschel, K., & Courtney, K. (2012). Nursing student medication errors: A root cause analysis to develop a fair and just culture. *Journal of Professional Nursing, 29*(2), 102–108. doi:10.1016/j.profnurs.2012.12.010

Dolansky, M. A., & Moore, S. M. (2013). Quality and safety education in nursing: The key is systems thinking. *Online Journal of Issues in Nursing, 18*(3), 1.

Fura, L. A., & Wisser, K. Z. (2017). Development and evaluation of a systems thinking education strategy for baccalaureate nursing curriculum: A pilot study. *Nursing Education Perspectives, 38*(5), 270–271. doi:10.1097/01.NEP.0000000000000165

Galik, E., & Resnick, B. (2013). Psychotropic medication use and associations with physical and psychosocial outcomes in nursing home residents. *Journal of Psychiatric and Mental Health Nursing, 20*(3), 244–252. doi:10.1111/j.1365-2850.2012.01911.x

Gerhardt, G., Yemane, A., Hickman, P., Oelschlaeger, A., Rollins, E., & Brennan, N. (2013). Medicare readmission rates showed meaningful decline in 2012. *Medicare & Medicaid Research Review, 3*(2), E1–E12. doi:10.5600/mmrr.003.02.b01

Hwang, J. I., & Park, H. A. (2017). Nurses' systems thinking competency, medical error reporting, and the occurrence of adverse events: A cross-sectional study. *Contemporary Nurse, 1–11.*

Institute for Healthcare Improvement. (2018). Why do I feel too busy to work on culture? Retrieved from http://www.ihi.org/communities/blogs/why-do-i-feel-too-busy-to-work-on-culture

Institute of Medicine. (2000). *To err is human: Building a safer health system*. Washington, DC: National Academies Press.

Kruse, K. (2013, April 9). What is leadership? *Forbes*. Retrieved from https://www.forbes.com/sites/kevinkruse/2013/04/09/what-is-leadership/#3602ab855b90

Makary, M. A., & Daniel, M. (2016). Medical error: The 3rd leading cause of death in the US. *British Medical Journal, 353*, i2139. doi:10.1136/bmj.i2139

Marion, R., & Uhl-Bien, M. (2001). Leadership in complex organizations. *Leadership Quarterly, 12*(4), 389–418. doi:10.1016/S1048-9843(01)00092-3

Moore, S. M., Dolansky, M. A., Singh, M., Palmieri, P., & Alemi, F. (2010). *The systems thinking scale*. Retrieved from https://case.edu/nursing/sites/case.edu.nursing/files/2018-04/STS_Manual.pdf

Nelson, E. C., Godfrey, M. M., Batalden, P. B., Berry, S. A., Bothe, A. E., McKinley, K. E., . . . Wasson, J. H. (2008). Clinical Microsystems, Part 1. The Building Blocks of Health Systems. *The Joint Commission Journal on Quality and Patient Safety, 34*(7), 367–378. doi:10.1016/S1553-7250(08)34047-1

Nightingale, F. (1858). *Notes on matters affecting the health, efficiency and hospital administration of the British army.* Retrieved from https://archive.org/details/b20387118/page/n8

Phillips, J. M., Stalter, A. M., Dolansky, M. A., & Lopez, G. M. (2016). Fostering future leadership in quality and safety in health care through systems thinking. *Journal of Professional Nursing, 32*(1), 15–24. doi:10.1016/j.profnurs.2015.06.003

Schnelle, J. F., Rahman, A., Durkin, D. W., Beuscher, L., Choi, L., & Simmons, S. F. (2013). A controlled trial of an intervention to increase resident choice in long term care. *Journal of the American Medical Directors Association, 14*(5), 345–351. doi:10.1016/j.jamda.2012.11.013

Senge, P. (2006). *The fifth discipline* (rev. ed.). New York, NY: Currency Doubleday.

Sherwood, G., & Barnsteiner, J. (2017). *Quality and safety in nursing: A competency approach to improving outcomes* (2nd ed.). Hoboken, NJ: John Wiley.

Skochelak, S. E., Hawkins, R. E., Lawson, L. E., Starr, S. R., Borkan, J., & Gonzalo, J. D. (2016). *Health systems science e-book.* Elsevier Health Sciences. Philadelphia, PA: Elsevier Publishing.

Slaughter, S. E., & Estabrooks, C. A. (2013). Optimizing the mobility of residents with dementia: A pilot study promoting healthcare aide uptake of a simple mobility innovation in diverse nursing home settings. *BMC Geriatrics, 13*(110). doi10.1186/1471-2318-13-110

Stalter, A. M., Phillips, J. M., Ruggiero, J. S., Scardaville, D. L., Merriam, D., Dolansky, M. A., & Winegardner, S. (2017). A concept analysis of systems thinking. *Nursing Forum, 52*(4), 323–330. doi:10.1111/nuf.12196

Tejal, K., Berwick, D., & Gandhi, M. D. (2016). Patient safety at the crossroads. *Journal of the American Medical Association, 315*(7), 1829–1830. doi:10.1001/jama.2016.1759

Trbovich, P. (2014). Five ways to incorporate systems thinking into healthcare organizations. *Biomedical Instrumentation & Technology, 48*(s2), 31–36. doi:10.2345/0899-8205-48.s2.31

Varkey, P., Karlapudi, S., Rose, S., Nelson, R., & Warner, M. (2009). A systems approach for implementing practice-based learning and improvement and systems-based practice in graduate medical education. *Academic Medicine, 84,* 335–339. doi:10.1097/ACM.0b013e31819731fb

Waters Foundation (n.d.). Elements of systems thinking and how they apply to nursing leadership. Retrieved from www.watersfoundation.org

Weberg, D. (2012). Complexity leadership: A healthcare imperative. *Nursing Forum, 47*(4), 268–277. doi:10.1111/j.1744-6198.2012.00276.x

Wieman, T. J., & Wieman, E. A. (2004). A systems approach to error prevention in medicine. *Journal of Surgical Oncology, 88*(3), 115–121. doi:10.1002/jso.20121

Wiig, S., Robert, G., Anderson, J. E., Pietikainen, E., Reiman, T., Macchi, L., & Aase, K. (2014). Applying different quality and safety models in healthcare improvement work: Boundary objects and system thinking. *Reliability Engineering & System Safety, 125,* 134–144. doi:10.1016/j.ress.2014.01.008

4

QUALITY IMPROVEMENT: THE ESSENTIALS

SHARON SABLES-BAUS | GAIL E. ARMSTRONG

This chapter addresses the following DNP American Association of Colleges of Nursing (AACN) Essentials:

II. Organizational and Systems Leadership for Quality Improvement and Systems Thinking
VI. Interprofessional Collaboration for Improving Patient and Population Health Outcomes

INTRODUCTION

The DNP nurse leader is often identified as the clinical nurse leader who initiates and directs quality improvement (QI) work in healthcare (AACN, 2006). Understanding the scope and tools of QI is vital for DNP students and DNP graduates. Having a firm understanding of how QI moved from manufacturing models into healthcare enables the DNP nurse leader to appreciate the limitations and imminent growth of QI models. Similarly, DNP nurse leaders need to understand how to organize QI work, collect, and present QI data, and disseminate outcomes of QI work.

THE HISTORY OF QI IN HEALTHCARE

A wide variety of approaches have been used to improve the quality of healthcare. Two early attempts at QI are attributed to Ignaz Semmelweis, a nineteenth-century obstetrician who introduced hand washing to medical care, and Florence Nightingale, the English nurse who—in the second half of the nineteenth century—conceptualized the environmental theory that maintaining an environment that is favorable to healing and healthy living processes aids in the recovery process. Later came a QI forerunner, Ernest Amory Codman, an advocate for the creation of hospital standards and the study of medical outcomes. His work led to the formation of the American College of Surgeons' formation in 1919 of the Hospital Standardization Program–predecessor of The Joint Commission. There have been several notable QI efforts over the past halfcentury (Chassin & Loeb, 2013; Chun & Bafford, 2014; Colton, 2000; Marjoua & Bozic, 2012; Sheingold & Hahn, 2014).

Beginning in the mid-1920s, two physicists and an engineer, Walter A. Shewart, W. Edwards Deming, and Joseph M. Juran, laid the groundwork for modern QI. Their efforts focused on streamlining production processes while minimizing the opportunity for human error, forging important QI concepts like standardizing work processes, data-driven decision-making, and commitment from workers and managers to improving work practices (Marjoua & Bozic, 2012).

In the 1940s, during World War II, efforts to improve quality focused on statistics. Statistical sampling techniques were used to evaluate quality, and quality-control charts were used to monitor the production process. The formal pursuit and management of quality in the 20th century traces back to Walter Shewhart's statistical process-control models used in the 1920s and 1930s. Walter Shewhart, an American physicist and statistician, worked at Bell Labs during the 1920s and 1930s. He recognized that variability in the manufacturing process impacted the quality of products. He condoned using statistical quality control (SQC). SQC can be divided into three broad categories: (a) Descriptive statistics are used to describe quality characteristics and relationships. Included are statistics such as the mean, standard deviation, the range, and a measure of the distribution of data; (b) statistical process control (SPC), which involves inspecting a random sample of the output from a process and deciding whether the process is producing products with characteristics that fall within a predetermined range. SPC answers the question of whether the process is functioning properly or not; and (c) acceptance sampling—the process of randomly inspecting a sample of goods and deciding whether to accept the entire lot based on the results. Acceptance sampling determines whether a batch of goods should be accepted or rejected using SCQ. Shewhart demonstrated that employees could track variation in processes and product output on a chart, which allowed them to fine-tune work as it was completed. Such activities not only produced superior products, but also empowered employees to learn more about their work and be accountable for it. He is often referred to as the *grandfather of quality control* (Berwick, 1991). Figure 4.1 provides an example of a control chart.

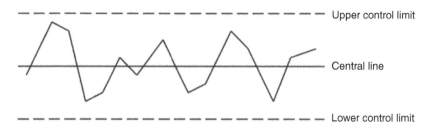

FIGURE 4.1 Shewhart's control chart showing evidence of controlled variation.

Source: From Berwick, D. M. (1991). Controlling variation in health care: A consultation from Walter Shewhart. *Medical Care, 29*(12), 1212–1225. doi:10.1097/00005650-199112000-00004

Shewhart is known as the *grandfather of quality control*, and W. Edwards Deming is known as the *father of quality control*. Deming was an American electrical engineer, statistician, and professor at New York University in the 1940s. After World War II, he worked with many Japanese companies to improve their efforts at improving quality. Deming's philosophy on quality control was a bit different from traditional notions. Historically, poor quality was blamed on the worker not doing a good job; Deming postulated that a large percentage or error was due to poor processes and systems. Therefore, it is up to management to improve the processes and systems so workers can do their jobs well (Colton, 2000).

According to Deming, the journey from the prevailing management style to one of quality requires an understanding of systems. To demonstrate this, Deming developed his Theory of Profound Knowledge, which is made up of four interrelated components: (a) appreciation of a system, (b) understanding variation, (c) the psychology of change, and (d) theory of knowledge. Understanding variation entails knowing about what he called *common cause variation*, which isvariation due to problems built into the system, such as defects, errors, mistakes, waste and rework; and *special cause variation*, variation that is a unique event that comes from outside the system, such as a natural disaster, and has to be managed in a different way. Reducing common cause variation and building stable systems is a key goal of effective system management. The psychology of change is about understanding what motivates people to do a good job. The theory of knowledge is based on the premise that management can predict what may happen from actual observation. The new knowledge is then reflected in the new theory of what action is needed to affect change. The Theory of Profound Knowledge is embodied in the Deming plan-do-study-act cycle—a systematic and dynamic process covering theory and application that helps gather knowledge, not simply data or information. It is a means of achieving a never-ending cycle of valuable learning for the continual improvement of a process or product.

Deming was convinced that quality is the result of use of a systematic process. He created the 14 Points for Management, or the Deming Model of Quality Management. These principles (points) were first presented in his book Out of the Crisis (Deming, 1986) and are a core concept in implementing Total Quality Management (TQM). Box 4.1 outlines Deming's 14 points. SoPK is the culmination of Dr. W. Edwards Deming's lifelong efforts to define a comprehensive theory of management that embraces his 14 Points for Management (deming.org/explore/so-pk).

It was the work of Shewhart and Deming that led to the concept of TQM. TQM is a management approach that originated in the 1950s. The term *TQM* was coined by the Naval Air Systems Command to describe its Japanese-style management approach to QI. TQM defines quality through the eyes of the customer. It is a data-driven approach that is mainly concerned with continuous improvement in all work, including improving processes, products, services, and the culture in the workplace (Chun & Bafford, 2014).

In the 1960s, with the help of so-called "quality gurus," the concept took on a broader meaning. Quality began to be viewed as something that encompassed the entire organization, not only the production process. Because all functions were responsible for product quality and all shared the costs of poor quality, quality was seen as an issue that affected the entire organization (Marjoua & Bozic, 2012).

The meaning of quality in business changed dramatically in the late 1970s. Before that time, quality was still viewed as something that

BOX 4.1 Deming's 14 Points for Management

Deming's 14 Points	
Create constancy of purpose toward improvement.	Drive out fear.
Adopt the new philosophy.	Break down barriers between departments.
Cease dependence on inspection.	Eliminate slogans.
Move toward a single supplier for any one item.	Eliminate management by objectives.
Improve constantly and forever.	Remove barriers to pride of workmanship.
Institute training on the job.	Institute education and self-improvement.
Institute leadership.	Transformation is everyone's job.

Source: From American Society for Quality (2019). W. Edwards Deming's 14 points for total quality management. Retrieved from http://asq.org/learn-about-quality/total-quality-management/overview/deming-points.htm

needed to be inspected and corrected. However, in the 1970s and 1980s many U.S. industries lost market share to foreign competition. In the auto industry, manufacturers, such as Toyota and Honda, became major players. In the consumer goods market, companies, such as Toshiba and Sony, led the way. These foreign competitors were producing lower priced products of considerably higher quality than American manufacturers could. To survive, American companies had to make major changes in their manufacturing programs. Many hired consultants and instituted quality training programs for employees. A new concept was emerging. One result was that quality began to have a strategic meaning. Today, successful companies understand that offering quality provides a competitive advantage. They put the customer first and define *quality work* as efforts that meet or exceed customer expectations (Chun & Bafford, 2014; Marjoua & Bozic, 2012).

With the introduction of Medicare and Medicaid in 1965, access to care was improved, but quality care outcomes were not well defined. The Health Services Research Section of the U.S. Public Health Service was created about 3 months after the Medicare and Medicaid programs were enacted. The goals of this organization, and health services research in general, were focused on access to healthcare and the costs of care, but also the delivery of high-quality care. Leaders from many health-related fields convened at a meeting in Chicago. These leaders considered the influence of social and economic research on public health, the organization of community health agencies, and the quality of health services. One of these experts, Avedis Donabedian, a professor of medical care organization at the University of Michigan School of Public Health, was commissioned to review the research on quality assessment (Chun & Bafford, 2014; Donabedian, 1966, 1988; Marjoua & Bozic, 2012).

Avedis Donabedian created the first conceptual framework for measuring healthcare quality. Assessing how clinical decision-making affects quality and analyzing the management and governance of healthcare systems and resources In his 1966 article "Evaluating the Quality of Medical Care," Donabedian first described what would later become known as the *Donabedian Model*. In this quality care model, he posits that improvements in the structure of care should lead to improvements in clinical processes, which in turn should improve patient outcomes. He defined *structure* as the settings, qualifications of providers, and administrative systems through which care takes place; *process* as the components of care delivered; and *outcome* as recovery, restoration of function, and survival. This model became the basis of an influential body of work on the theory and practice of quality assurance and the emerging field of health services research. These concepts remain the foundation of quality assessment today (Chun & Bafford, 2014; Donabedian, 1966; Donabedian, 1988; Hughes, 2008; Marjoua & Bozic, 2012).

The law that created Medicare also required hospitals to establish utilization review committees to assess quality, including medical necessity of admissions to the institution, duration of stays, and professional services. Unfortunately, these committees had no formal evaluation criteria to guide provider's decision-making and no way to adjust payment based on the quality of care. In 1983, the Medicare Utilization and Quality Control Peer Review Organization was formed. It was later renamed the QI Organization. The main emphasis of this program was to control costs by monitoring the use of services, as was ensuring or improving quality. It was during this time that the use of evidence-based clinical guidelines to improve the quality of care were established. In 1989, the Agency for Health Care Policy and Research was created. It was later renamed the Agency for Healthcare Research and Quality. Its initial intent was to focus on cost and quality (Hughes, 2008; Marjoua & Bozic, 2012).

The 1980s ushered in a new way of thinking about quality with an emphasis on building quality into process, identifying and correcting causes of quality problems, and focusing efforts on customer-driven quality. Dr. Joseph Juran, an electrical engineer who worked at General Electric, was a Japanese consultant tasked to find ways to improve their poor manufacturing quality. Although not as well-known as Shewhart and Deming, he is considered by many to have had the greatest impact on quality management. Whereas Deming stressed the need for an organizational "transformation," Juran believed that implementing quality initiatives should not require such a dramatic change and that quality management should be embedded in the organization. He is credited with defining *quality* as fitness for use by the customer rather than simply conformance to technical specifications. He is also credited with developing the concept of cost of quality, which allows us to measure quality in terms of dollars rather than on the basis of subjective evaluations. Dr. Juran's philosophy, formally published in 1986, is known as the *Quality Trilogy*; any organization taking up a journey in quality management will have to have three processes in place: (a) quality planning, (b) quality control, and (c) quality improvement (QI). *Quality planning* is defined as the activities that must be done to adhere to the vision, mission, and goals of the organization and to comply with customer needs. Planning activities should include an understanding of the customer, determining customer needs, defining the product or service, designing the product or service, and designing the processes necessary to accomplish these goals. Quality control now comes into play, processes and specifications for a particular product or service must be followed. Metrics are determined and measured and as audit results disseminated to ensure quality. The third and last process, QI, entails an examination of current processes and outcomes and devises innovative ways to achieve new targets and to implement them (Colton, 2000). A summary of the key leaders in the development of QI in healthcare can be found in Table 4.1.

TABLE 4.1 KEY LEADERS IN THE DEVELOPMENT OF QI IN HEALTHCARE

Walter A. Shewhart (1891–1967)	Contributed to understanding of process variability Developed concept of statistical control charts
W. Edwards Deming (1900–1993)	Stressed management's responsibility to quality Developed "14 Points" to guide companies in QI Developed the System of Profound Knowledge, which is grounded in systems theory and composed of four interrelated components: • Theory of Knowledge—prediction based on theory is requried • Respect for the system • Understanding variation • Psychology of change
Avedis Donabedian (1919–2000)	Donabedian's Quality Framework Structures of care (setting) Processes of care (care delivery and care coordination) leads to improved health outcomes
Joseph M. Juran (1904–2008)	Defined quality as "fitness for use." Developed the concept of cost of quality

CURRENT MODELS OF QI IN HEALTHCARE

The focus on QI in healthcare has dramatically intensified over the past two decades. More recent models around QI stem from the work done to standardize payment models, for example, in the development of diagnostic related groups (DRGs; Dolenc & Dougherty, 1985). DRG models explored whether quality of care could be improved through standardized payment models. Concurrently, quality-assurance departments were flourishing, where the emphasis of data collection focused on the measurement of characteristics of a healthcare product's conformity to identified standards (Bolmey, 2002; Bostick, Riggs, & Rantz, 2003). It was quickly ascertained that the evolving, complex processes involved in healthcare delivery make standardization close to impossible.

Continuous QI Model

By the late 1980s, hospitals and healthcare organizations began applying improvement methods that had worked in industry, such as continuous quality improvement (CQI). CQI is the systematic process of identifying, describing, and analyzing strengths and problems and then testing, implementing, learning from, and revising solutions. More simply, one can describe CQI as an ongoing cycle of collecting data and using it to make decisions that gradually improve program processes. The term *CQI* is often

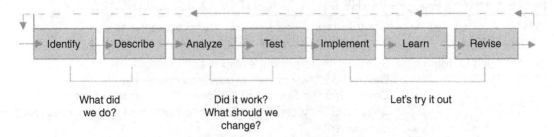

FIGURE 4.2 Steps of the CQI model.

CQI, continuous quality improvement.

used interchangeably with *TQM*. CQI is based on the principle that there is an opportunity for improvement in every process and on every occasion. The Joint Commission modified its hospital-accreditation process to focus on Donabedian's framework of structure, process, and outcome. This shift requires organizations to use evidence-based measures of performance as part of their QI programs (Berwick, Calkins, McCannon, & Hackbarth, 2006; Chassin, 1997; Hughes, 2008). Figure 4.2 outlines the steps of the CQI.

Plan-Do-Study-Act Cycles

QI in healthcare employs iterative cycles, completed in close proximity to one another, resulting in "rapid cycle change." To complete iterative cycles, the most common tool used is the plan-do-study-act (PDSA) tool. This approach employs a "trial learning" strategy in which a hypothesis or anticipated solution for improvement is made and repeatedly tested with slight adjustments in each cycle (Varkey, Reller, & Resar, 2007). These rapid cycles of change allow honing and modification of the improvement intervention until the desired outcome is achieved. The elements of the PDSA cycle are described in Table 4.2.

TABLE 4.2 ELEMENTS OF THE PDSA CYCLE

PDSA Element	Identified Work of Each Element
Plan	Identify objectives to improve work. Make predictions of improved outcomes. Develop a plan to carry out test cycles.
Do	Carry out the test. Document problems (expected/unexpected). Document relevant observations that will help in the next PDSA cycle.
Study	Summarize what was learned.
Act	Based on results of the cycle, determine what changes need to be made for the next cycle.

Source: Adapted from Varkey, P., Reller, M. K., & Resar, R. K. (2007). Basics of quality improvement in health care. *Mayo Clinic Proceedings, 82*(6), 735–739. doi:10.4065/82.6.735

The Model for Improvement

The Model for Improvement is widely used in many clinical settings to organize QI work in healthcare (Figure 4.3). This model was developed by associates in process improvement and consists of three fundamental questions that can be addressed in any order. The question, "What are we trying to accomplish?" facilitates team agreement on the main goal of the improvement. Teams must reach consensus on the overall goal of the improvement project at hand. This first question identifies the project's aim. The aim should identify the target patient population, the setting of the project, and use a SMART goal in its answer. *SMART* is an acronym for a goal that is specific, measurable, achievable, realistic, and time-specific (Institute for Healthcare Improvement [IHI], n.d.). The second question is often the most difficult to address: "How will we know that a change is an improvement?" The second question facilitates use of specific measures to quantify the identified outcome (IHI, n.d.). Through quantification, with every cycle of change the QI team can assess whether the improvement intervention is leading to actual improvement. The third question encourages the team to examine from where they will choose their change interventions. The QI literature may offer examples of changes made in similar contexts that have been successful. Or ideas for effective improvement may come from the QI team, who have the best understanding of the contextual factors impacting the clinical situation. The model for improvement also offers the most commonly used depiction of PDSA cycles for rapid cycle improvement (IHI, n.d.; Langley et al., 2009).

Tools for Measuring QI

A common aphorism in healthcare QI is, "You can only improve what you can measure." This saying highlights the important role of measurement

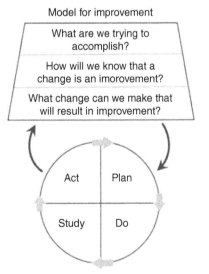

FIGURE 4.3 The Model for Improvement.

Source: From Langley, G. L., Moen, R., Nolan, K. M., Nolan, T. W., Norman, C. L., & Provost, L. P. (2009). *The improvement guide: A practical approach to enhancing organizational performance* (2nd ed.). San Francisco, CA: Jossey-Bass.

and data collection in effective QI. Effective data collection needs to be concerned about the quality of the data. Are the data valid? Do the data really measure the phenomenon that the QI team is most interested in? How will the data be collected? Can the data be mined from the electronic health record? Can the data be accessed in a timely manner? Are the data reliable (Finkelman, 2018)?

Close monitoring of selected data during each rapid cycle change is extremely important. Documentation provides the essence of what will eventually be reported as successful or unsuccessful QI. Data patterns over time can be displayed using a variety of tools. Demonstrating the fluctuation or progression of data over time provides a snapshot of the QI work. Common tools for QI data presentation are found in Table 4.3 IHI offers a robust toolkit on how to use the common QI presentation data tools (www.ihi.org/resources/Pages/Tools/Quality-Improvement-Essentials-Toolkit.aspx).

TABLE 4.3 QI TOOLS AND THEIR PRIMARY USES

QI Tool	Primary Use
Flowchart	Flowcharts describe a process in as much detail as possible by displaying all the steps in proper sequence. QI teams use flowcharts to identify areas of vulnerability, indicate areas for further improvement, and help explain and solve a problem. By flowcharting all steps in the care of a patient with a urinary catheter, the QI team may identify where common breaches of technique occur.
Check sheet	Check sheets help organize data by category. They show how many times each particular value occurs, and their information is increasingly helpful as more data are collected. Check sheets help clinicians identify problems. Using a check sheet for surveillance of a healthcare provider's adherence to proper hand hygiene helps identify where supportive processes are needed.
Pareto diagram	The Pareto diagram puts data in hierarchical order, allowing the most significant problems to be corrected first. Data are grouped in categories in order of frequency and a bar graph is created based on the results.
Cause-and-effect diagram	The cause-and-effect diagram is also known as a fishbone diagram because of its shape. It displays all contributing factors to an outcome needing QI, and shows their relationship to the outcome. These diagrams reflect the complexity of a problem and identify areas where further data should be collected and analyzed.
Histogram	The histogram plots data in a frequency distribution table. A histogram works best with small amounts of data that have a great deal of variation.
Control chart	Control charts display statistically determined upper and lower confidence limits drawn on either side of a mean.
Run chart	A run chart is a line graph of data points plotted over time. By mapping data over time you can find trends or patterns.

Source: Adapted from Hall, L., Moore, S., & Barnsteiner, J. (2008). Quality and nursing: Moving from a concept to a core competency. *Urological Nursing, 28*(6), 417–425.

Knowledge, Skills, and Attitudes of QI Competence

DNP nurse leaders may be responsible for the introduction of QI work in a microsystem. How does a leader know when members of a QI team are competent in the necessary knowledge, skills, and attitudes of QI? A national nursing initiative, Quality and Safety Education in Nursing (QSEN), developed operational definitions for competencies recommended for all members of the healthcare. The five competencies recommended for all health professions students (and therefore all health professionals) include patient-centered care, evidence-based practice, informatics, teamwork, and QI (Institute of Medicine [IOM], 2003). With funding from the Robert Wood Johnson Foundation, QSEN gathered thought leaders for each competency and developed requisite knowledge, skills, and attitudes (KSAs) for each Institute of Medicine competency. Table 4.4 outlines the requisite QI KSAs for the RN scope of care. Table 4.5 outlines the QSEN KSAs for advanced practice providers, applicable to DNP students and graduates.

Standards for QI Reporting Excellence

Many publication guidelines exist that provide a systematic approach to writing specific scientific papers. Consolidated Standards of Reporting Trials (CONSORT) guidelines address randomized trials. STrengthening the Reporting of OBservational studies in Epidemiology (STROBE) guidelines address observational studies. Preferred Reporting Items for Systematic Reviews and Meta-Analyses (PRISMA) guidelines address the writing of systematic reviews (all of these can be found at www.equator-network.org). The Standards for Quality Improvement Reporting Excellence (SQUIRE) guidelines were first published in 2008 to offer a standardized approach to reporting work aimed at improving the quality, safety, and value of healthcare. These guidelines were loosely modeled on the CONSORT guidelines and contained 19 items. The goals of the SQUIRE 1.0 guidelines included making published improvement papers more complete, accurate, and coherent to guide authors, editors, and peer reviewers in writing, judging, and editing improvement articles and to support development of a rigorous, scholarly improvement literature (Davidoff, 2012). Upon publication in 2005, SQUIRE 1.0 became the editorial policy of several journals that publish QI work.

Five years after publication of SQUIRE 1.0, the leadership of SQUIRE reevaluated the match between the intended use of the SQUIRE guidelines and end users' experience with them. Through focus groups and input from experts (e.g., editors, researchers, and improvers), the SQUIRE faculty received feedback that SQUIRE 1.0 helped in the planning of improvement, but not as much in the writing about the improvement. There were questions about what should be reported (e.g., should failed PDSA cycles be reported?). There were questions about some items, and noted redundancies in SQUIRE 1.0 (Davies, n.d.). In a unique approach, the leadership of

TABLE 4.4 QSEN QUALITY-IMPROVEMENT KNOWLEDGE, SKILLS, AND ATTITUDES FOR THE RN

Knowledge	Skills	Attitudes
Describe strategies for learning about the outcomes of care in the setting in which one is engaged in clinical practice.	Seek information about outcomes of care for populations served in the care setting. Seek information about QI projects in the care setting.	Appreciate that continuous QI is an essential part of the daily work of all health professionals.
Recognize that nursing and other health professions students are parts of systems of care and care processes that affect outcomes for patients and families. Give examples of the tension between professional autonomy and system functioning.	Use tools (such as flow charts, cause-effect diagrams) to make processes of care explicit. Participate in a root-cause analysis of a sentinel event.	Value own and others' contributions to outcomes of care in local care settings.
Explain the importance of variation and measurement in assessing quality of care.	Use quality measures to understand performance. Use tools (such as control charts and run charts) that are helpful for understanding variation. Identify gaps between local and best practice.	Appreciate how unwanted variation affects care. Value measurement and its role in good patient care.
Describe approaches for changing processes of care.	Design a small test of change in daily work (using an experiential learning method such as plan-do-study-act) Practice aligning the aims, measures, and changes involved in improving care. Use measures to evaluate the effect of change.	Value local change (in individual practice or team practice on a unit) and its role in creating joy in work. Appreciate the value of what individuals and teams can to do to improve care.

QI, quality improvement.

Source: From Cronenwett, L., Sherwood, G., Barnsteiner, J., Disch, J., Johnson, J., Mitchell, P., . . . Warren, J. (2007). Quality and Safety Education for Nurses. *Nursing Outlook, 55*(3), 122–131. doi:10.1016/j.outlook.2007.02.006

SQUIRE "road tested" its SQUIRE updates with 44 end users and received feedback about the updates included in SQUIRE 2.0 (Davies, Donnelly, Goodman, & Ogrinc, 2015). Significant updates to SQUIRE 2.0 include streamlining the language to make items more direct, an increased emphasis on description of the context of the improvement work, and increased clarity about how to study an intervention (Ogrinc et al., 2015).

TABLE 4.5 QSEN QUALITY-IMPROVEMENTKNOWLEDGE, SKILLS, ND ATTITUDES FOR ADVANCED PRACTICE PROVIDERS

Graduate-Level QSEN Competency: QI		
Knowledge	**Skills**	**Attitudes**
Describe strategies for improving outcomes at all points of care.	Translate aims for QI efforts. Align the aims, measures, and changes involved in improving care.	Commit to concepts of transparency, managing variability measurement and accountability.
Describe nationally accepted quality measures and benchmarks in the practice setting.	Use a variety of sources of information to review outcomes, compare benchmarks of care, and identify potential areas for improvement (e.g., National Database of Nursing Quality Indicators, Hospital Compare, Center for Medicare& Medicaid Services [CMS] indicators, The Joint Commission ORYX, National Public Health Performance Standards [NPHPS] and others). Participate in analysis of databases as sources of information for improving patient care. Use quality indicators and benchmarks for improving system processes and outcomes.	Commit to achieving the highest level of processes and outcomes of care. Inspire others to achieve benchmark performance. Model behaviors reflective of a commitment to high-quality outcomes.
Evaluate the relevance of quality indicators and their associated measurement strategies.	Identify useful measures that can be acted on to improve outcomes and processes.	Value the importance of the use of data in QI.
Explain variance and its common causes in patient care process and outcomes, including costs.	Select and use QI tools (e.g., run charts, control charts, root-cause analysis, flow diagrams and Gantt charts) to achieve best possible outcomes.	Commit to reducing unwarranted variation in care.
Analyze ethical issues associated with continuous QI.	Participate in the design and monitoring of ethical oversight of CQI projects. Maintain confidentiality of any patient information used in QI efforts.	Value ethical conduct in QI efforts. Value the roles of others, such as IRBs, in assessing ethical and patient rights/informed decision-making.

(continued)

TABLE 4.5 QSEN QI KSAS FOR ADVANCED PRACTICE PROVIDERS (*continued*)

Graduate-Level QSEN Competency: QI		
Knowledge	**Skills**	**Attitudes**
Understand principles of change management.	Apply change-management principles by using data to improve patient and systems outcomes.	Appreciate that all improvement is change. Demonstrate leadership in affecting the necessary change.
Evaluate the effect of planned change on outcomes.	Design, implement, and evaluate small tests of change in daily work (e.g., using an experiential learning method such as PDSA).	Value planned change.
Analyze the impact of linking payment to QI.	Use benchmarks that carry financial penalties (e.g., serious reportable events) to improve care.	Consistent with the National Quality Strategy, commit to achieving the highest quality of care in the practice setting (e.g., National Strategy's aims of Better Care, HealthyPeople.gov, Affordable Care Act).
Describe the intent and outcomes of public reporting.	Use public reporting information to advance QI efforts.	Appreciate that consumers will be more empowered to make decisions based on quality information. Value community engagement in QI decision-making.

IRB, institutional review board; KSAs, knowledge, skills, and attitudes; QSEN, Quality and Safety Education in Nursing.

Source: From American Association of Colleges of Nursing. (2012). Graduate-level QSEN competencies: Knowledge, skills and attitudes. Retrieved from http://www.aacnnursing.org/Portals/42/AcademicNursing/CurriculumGuidelines/Graduate-QSEN-Competencies.pdf

The SQUIRE guidelines provide an advantageous tool when DNP nurse leaders write up their improvement work. In addition, the guidelines are notably useful in planning improvement work. The organization of the SQUIRE guidelines is based on familiar and direct structures. SQUIRE retains the IMRaD (introduction, methods, results, and discussion) organization that is a recognizable part of most systematic investigations. SQUIRE also uses A. Bradford Hill's four fundamental questions for writing: Why did you start? What did you do? What did you find? And What does it mean (Huth, 1999)? Within each section of the SQUIRE guidelines are questions to guide planning of improvement work and to prepare the final output so the results will be ready for publication. Go to www. squire-statement.org to access the SQUIRE guidelines.

CONCLUSIONS

Because of the persistent need for ongoing improvement in processes and outcomes, QI is a quickly evolving area in healthcare. DNP nurse leaders are best equipped to adjust to the continual development of QI approaches by understanding the history of QI in healthcare, and staying abreast of the emerging QI literature. Use of standardized reporting guidelines, such as SQUIRE, in the planning stages of QI work positions a healthcare team to accomplish well-structured QI work that is appropriate for publication.

Case Study

J.B. is a DNP student whose scholarly project will focus on decreasing catheter-associated urinary tract infections (CAUTIs) on her 40 -bed med/surg unit.

QUESTIONS

1. What baseline data will J.B. want to collect before she plans her improvement work?
2. J.B. wants to compare the annual rate of CAUTIs atf her hospital to other hospitals. What national statistics will help her in this comparison?
3. Where might J.B. go to find evidence-based approaches to decreasing CAUTIs on a med/surg unit?
4. Which colleagues would be appropriate to invite to join J.B.'s CAUTI team?
5. What kind of data tools might J.B. use to analyze the cause of CAUTI on her unit and display CAUTI data over 6 months?

REFERENCES

American Association of Colleges of Nursing. (2006). The essentials of doctoral education for advanced nursing practice. Retrieved from http://www.aacnnursing.org/Portals/42/Publications/DNPEssentials.pdf

Berwick, D. M. (1991). Controlling variation in health care: A consultation from Walter Shewhart. *Medical Care, 29*(12), 1212–1225. doi:10.1097/00005650-199112000-00004

Berwick, D. M., Calkins, D. R., McCannon, C., & Hackbarth, A. D. (2006). The 100 000 lives campaign: Setting a goal and a deadline for improving health care quality. *Journal of the American Medical Association, 295*(3), 324–327. doi:10.1001/jama.295.3.324

Bolmey, A. L. (2002). Outcome measures in health-care industry: An elusive goal. *Obesity Research, 10*(Suppl. 1), 10S–13S. doi:10.1038/oby.2002.183

Bostick, J. E., Riggs, C. J., & Rantz, M. J. (2003). Quality measurement in nursing: An update of where we are now. *Journal of Nursing Care Quality, 18*(2), 94–104. doi:10.1097/00001786-200304000-00002

Chassin, M. R. (1997). Assessing strategies for quality improvement. *Health Affairs, 16*(3), 151–161. doi:10.1377/hlthaff.16.3.151

Chassin, M. R., & Loeb, J. M. (2013). High-reliability health care: Getting there from here. *Milbank Memorial Fund Quarterly, 91*(3), 459–490. doi:10.1111/1468-0009.12023

Chun, J., & Bafford, A. C. (2014). History and background of quality measurement. *Clinics in Colon and Rectal Surgery, 27*(1), 5–9. doi:10.1055/s-0034-1366912

Colton, D. (2000). Quality improvement in health care. Conceptual and historical foundations. *Evaluation & the Health Professions, 23*(1), 7–42. doi:10.1177/01632780022034462

Cronenwett, L., Sherwood, G., Barnsteiner, J., Disch, J., Johnson, J., Mitchell, P., . . . Warren, J. (2007). Quality and Safety Education for Nurses. *Nursing Outlook, 55*(3), 122–131. doi:10.1016/j.outlook.2007.02.006

Davidoff, F. (2012). Why SQUIRE? Standards for QUality Improvement Reporting Excellence. IHI Forum—Learning Lab 13. Retrieved from http://app.ihi.org/FacultyDocuments/ Events/Event-2206/Presentation-7265/Document-5993/L13_Presentation.pdf

Davies, L. (n.d.). From SQUIRE 1.0 to SQUIRE 2.0: A new way to evaluate and update publication guidelines. Retrieved from https://www.ebhcconference.org/previous_editions/2015/ presentations/PB.01_Davies_L.pdf

Davies, L., Donnelly, K. Z., Goodman, D. J., & Ogrinc, G. (2015). Findings from a novel approach to publication guideline revision: User road testing of a draft version of SQUIRE 2.0. *BMJ Quality & Safety, 25*(4). Retrieved from https://qualitysafety.bmj.com/content/ early/2015/08/11/bmjqs-2015-004117.full

Deming, W. E. (1986). *Out of the crisis.* Cambridge, MA: Massachusetts Institute of Technology, Center for Advanced Engineering Study.

Dolenc, D. A., & Dougherty, C. J. (1985). DRGs: The counterrevolution in financing health care. *The Hastings Center Report, 15*(3), 19–29. doi:10.2307/3560520

Donabedian, A. (1966). Evaluating the quality of medical care.*Milbank Memorial Fund Quarterly, 44*(3), 166–206. doi:10.2307/3348969

Donabedian, A. (1988). The quality of care. How can it be assessed? *Journal of the American Medical Association, 260*(12), 1743–1748. doi:10.1001/jama.1988.03410120089033

Finkelman, A. (2018). *Quality improvement: A guide for integration in nursing.* Burlington, MA: Jones & Bartlett Learning.

Hughes, R. (2008). *Patient safety and quality: An evidence-based handbook for nurses* (Vol. 3, pp. 1–39). Rockville, MD: Agency for Healthcare Research and Quality.

Huth, E. (1999). *Writing and publishing in medicine* (3rd ed.). Baltimore, MD: Williams and Wilkins.

Institute for Healthcare Improvement. (n.d.). Science of improvement: How to improve. Retrieved from http://www.ihi.org/resources/Pages/HowtoImprove/ScienceofImprovementHow toImprove.aspx

Institute of Medicine. (2003). *Health professions education: A bridge to quality.* Washington, DC: National Academies Press.

Langley, G. L., Moen, R., Nolan, K. M., Nolan, T. W., Norman, C. L., & Provost, L. P. (2009). *The improvement guide: A practical approach to enhancing organizational performance* (2nd ed.). San Francisco, CA: Jossey-Bass.

Marjoua, Y., & Bozic, K. J. (2012). Brief history of quality movement in US healthcare. *Current Reviews in Musculoskeletal Medicine, 5*(4), 265–273. doi:10.1007/s12178-012-9137-8

Ogrinc, G., Davies, L, Goodman, D., Batalden, P., Davidoff, F., & Stevens, D. (2015). SQUIRE 2.0 (Standards for QUality Improvement Reporting Excellence): Revised publication guidelines from a detailed consensus process. *BMJ Quality & Safety, 25*(12). Retrieved from https:// qualitysafety.bmj.com/content/25/12/986

Sheingold, B., & Hahn, J. (2014). The history of healthcare quality: The first 100 years 1860–1960. *International Journal of Africa Nursing Sciences, 1*, 18–22. doi:10.1016/j.ijans.2014.05.002

Varkey, P., Reller, M. K., & Resar, R. K. (2007). Basics of quality improvement in health care. *Mayo Clinic Proceedings, 82*(6), 735–739. doi:10.1016/S0025-6196(11)61194-4

LEADING PROCESS IMPROVEMENT

SARAH J. CAFFREY

This chapter addresses the following DNP American Association of Colleges of Nursing (AACN) Essentials:

II. Organizational and Systems Leadership for Quality Improvement and Systems Thinking
VI. Interprofessional Collaboration for Improving Patient and Population Health Outcomes

---

INTRODUCTION

Healthcare processes are highly variable, needlessly complex, and chaotic. This variability contributes to adverse outcomes, patient safety issues, and suboptimal healthcare quality. The mission of process improvement is to develop delivery systems that are reliable, predictable, and well managed. Processes that are more predictable should enable new advancements in care provision to be more quickly and easily brought into standard practice. Process improvement methods provide well-established, systematic approaches to improving processes. These methods are essential tools for nursing leaders in all healthcare settings.

Because today's leaders are walking into a healthcare system that is more costly, inefficient, and unsafe than it should be, posessing a process improvement mind-set is a fundamental component of every effective leader's job. This chapter reviews fundamental concepts of process improvement and connects process improvement to larger improvement work in healthcare.

Foci of this chapter include:

- Defining *process improvement*
- Identifying a DNP-prepared nurse's work in defining and achieving quality
- Identifying how to view the clinical world through the lens of process improvement
- Using approaches to quantifying quality
- Identifying steps for effective process improvement efforts

Improved systems of care contribute to quality, not just for patients, but also for the people who work in those systems. An effective leader is a catalyst for continuous improvement; one who leads it, nurtures it, and sustains it.

WHAT IS PROCESS IMPROVEMENT?

What is involved in process improvement? Does it differ from quality improvement? The Institute of Medicine proposes that quality care is safe, efficient, effective, patient/family centered, timely, and equitable (Committee on Quality Healthcare in America, Institute of Medicine, 2001). The definition is not a menu of options to select from; it is a cohesive set of criteria that jointly describe high-quality care. The aspirational goal of leaders in healthcare is to contribute to care delivery models that embody this definition of quality.

In healthcare, the notion that quality improvement and process improvement are somehow fundamentally different continues to be perpetuated. The goal of process improvement work *is* to improve quality. Variation in processes, or the quality of the inputs to those processes, results in an inability to predict whether the care process will result in a good or a bad outcome for the patient. Improved quality is achieved by understanding and eliminating (or minimizing) sources of variation that arise from poor processes or inputs so that the outcome can be predictably achieved. Process improvement techniques aide in achieving this aim. As a discipline, process improvement employs a keen focus on identifying root causes, redesigning key processes to increase the likelihood of good outcomes, and objectively measuring to see whether the interventions result in improvement. A *process* is defined as a series of steps taken to achieve an aim (Deming, 1986). Typically it requires multiple interrelated processes to produce a desired outcome, thus, process improvement must include gaining an understanding of how various processes interrelate to yield the outcomes achieved. Continual improvement of processes is essential to improving quality of care, and process improvement methodologies offer a systematic means to identify improvement opportunities, design effective interventions, and measure the improvement associated with those interventions.

Improved quality will lead to fewer errors and less redundancy, contributing to higher productivity and lower costs (Deming, 1986). The science of process improvement is based on four fundamental ideas:

- It is the **design of the processes** used when people work, not the people, that largely dictates the outcomes or results of those processes.
- To improve the outcome (the level of quality) one must understand and systematically **improve the processes** and inputs used to achieve it.
- People cannot reliably and consistently **overcome flaws in process design.**
- **High quality is more cost-effective** than mediocre or poor quality.

Understanding these fundamentals of process improvement contributes to a leader's effective use of process improvement methodologies in improvement work.

Design of Processes

A leader with a process improvement mind-set first looks to processes as a contributing source to problems and poor quality, not to the people who follow them. Well-designed processes are highly reliable processes, meaning that the processes, if executed as designed, minimize the likelihood of errors, rework, and missed steps. Well-designed processes produce consistent results that can be relied upon to achieve the identified aim of the process. They support the people who work in the process and do not strip the individual of the ability to apply critical thinking in a situation. In a work environment where processes are reliable, people adhere to standard work because doing so makes both the people and the outcomes more successful. Highly reliable processes allow people to focus on the intellectual components of the job, such as building rapport, handling unusual circumstances, and focusing on the patient. Poorly designed processes contribute to problems, errors, mistakes, absenteeism, rework, and, potentially, in the healthcare environment, adverse outcomes and death. Reliable processes free up leaders to plan proactively, instead of continuously responding reactively to poor outcomes. In an organization that has embraced process improvement as part of the microsystem culture, a manager's time can be spent monitoring the performance of key processes, engaging employees to make improvements, thinking strategically about the future needs of the department, and deciding which investments might be made in improvements to maintain a high standard of excellence.

Improve Processes for Better Results

Processes are usually part of a larger system. A **system** is a set of interrelated and interdependent processes that work together to achieve a common aim (Deming, 1993). When a nursing leader identifies a process that needs to be improved it is vital that this leader understands how the process fits into the overall system, or any improvement runs the risk of unintentionally creating suboptimal processes elsewhere in the system. The classic example of this phenomenon is a team that focuses on shortening length of stay on an inpatient unit only to realize later that readmissions have increased as a result of their efforts to facilitate quicker discharges. The goal is to improve processes and achieve better quality at lower costs. To accomplish this it is essential that processes are considered within the context of the whole system.

People Cannot Overcome Process Flaws

Human beings are remarkably resilient and innovative, especially in the context of inefficient processes and systems. People can overcome many obstacles in the course of a typical day at work. The question for leaders is, "Should they have to?" The time and effort required to overcome poorly designed processes would be better invested in the care of the patient. Inferior processes set people up for failure. Although vigilance is a part of any job, it cannot serve as the sole method for avoiding commonplace errors, especially in the context of complex healthcare systems. In addition, a reliance on inspection to catch errors is an insufficient method to use to create high-quality care. Inspecting for errors or mistakes means that the error or mistake has already happened by the time the mistake is identified (Deming, 1986). Although inspection might prevent the error from reaching the patient, this approach does not prevent the error from occurring again. Making changes that lead to redundancy of work or blaming individuals for process flaws are common leadership responses in healthcare. As a result, much of a leader's time might be spent tallying errors made by people, administering disciplinary action, and coping with high turnover rates. A focus on reliable processes frees healthcare leaders from the trap of this reactionary focus.

High Quality Is Low Cost

In a work environment where there is a culture that values high quality, reliable processes and associated costs are often much lower. Costs accrue each time something has to be fixed, done over, or thrown away. Inadequate processes contribute to a variety of waste. Poor quality does not just incur costs associated with rework, it also creates an environment of failure that can lead to absenteeism, high turnover rates, negative outcomes for patients, and poor quality ratings. In contrast, highly reliable processes achieve predictable outcomes much more consistently without the need for inspection, rework, and waste. Inherent in the process improvement mind-set is the concept that high quality contributes to cost-effectiveness.

COMMONLY USED METHODOLOGIES

Improvement leaders set the tone, foster a culture of continuous improvement, and sanction the use of time and resources to fix problems in healthcare. Without supportive and engaged leadership, most process improvement work will fail. Many healthcare organizations have process improvement teams that use one or more of the common improvement methodologies to aid the organization in improvement work. These teams of process improvement professionals may have a variety of backgrounds, training, and degrees. Most common is formal training attained by completing a certification program in Lean and/or Six Sigma or from completing coursework through the Institute for Healthcare Improvement (IHI). At the undergraduate level, degrees in industrial engineering are a more common preparation and at the graduate level, a master's in business administration with a focus on operations management may be the degree of choice for those in process improvement roles.

As a nurse leader, having some familiarity with process improvement methods is helpful in guiding your team. Three of the leading process improvement methodologies that are commonly employed in healthcare organizations are the Model for Improvement, Lean, and Six Sigma.

The Model for Improvement

The Model for Improvement was developed by Associates in Process Improvement and is espoused by IHI. This methodology focuses on answering three questions:

- What are we trying to accomplish?
- How will we know a change is an improvement?
- What change can we make that will result in an improvement(Berwick, 1996)?

Then, using the plan-do-study-act (PDSA), or Deming cycle, small tests of change are tried in the work setting (Deming, 1993). The results of each trial are studied and either accepted or refined to achieve better results. Small teams are typically built to analyze and address a specific problem. The team decides what the aim of the project will be, selects improvements to test, and measures the results of the improvement efforts on the outcome. Each PDSA cycle is typically undertaken on a small scale and then expanded if successful (Batalden & Stolz, 1993; Berwick, 1996).

This model is the cornerstone of all improvement work. PDSA cycles systematically contribute to increased clarity about which changes drive the desired improvement. Common pitfalls with this model include insufficient planning, failing to have measures that assist in understanding the efficacy of the changes, and losing sight of the intent of the improvements.

The Lean Method

The Lean method has its origins in the Toyota Production System. In the mid- to late 1980s Toyota embarked on a journey to improve quality and reduce costs of production by eliminating waste in the manufacturing process. Typical forms of waste in processes include rework, wait time, excess inventory, unnecessary motion by those doing the work, transportation, poor use of people, and so on. Teams using the Lean methodology systematically examine processes for evidence of waste. Waste reduction is achieved by improving flow and "mistake proofing." Mistake proofing focuses on including processes that prevent mistakes as well as processes that detect mistakes as soon as they occur. Lean encourages a more systemic view of the problem and requires that processes be examined more broadly than just at points where problems are experienced (Kimsey, 2010),

Leaders using the Lean approach participate in a rapid improvement, or Kaizen event. In a Kaizen event, people are brought together for an extended period of time—often 3 to 5 days—to work on a process. A facilitator will take the Kaizen team through a series of activities to understand the current process, identify waste, and create a new process with less waste. Teams try out their improvement ideas during the Kaizen event using PDSA cycles. After a Kaizen event, the facilitator may also act as a project manager to keep track of any completed tasks that were assigned to participants. Once the improvements are fully in place, the new process will be reevaluated to see whether it has achieved the desired target state.

Common pitfalls with Lean are not engaging the right stakeholders in the Kaizen event, failing to provide adequate resources to fully implement the changes, and a lack of support or visible endorsement from senior leadership to successfully sustain the changes over time.

Six Sigma Method

Six Sigma was invented by Motorola, Inc. in the mid-1980s in response to quality concerns from sales teams. Six Sigma has three fundamental components: An indexed quality-measurement system using a 6 sigma scale, a project management methodology, and a set of analytic tools used to drive decision-making (Fairbanks, 2007). Six Sigma focuses on reducing variation

TABLE 5.1 DIFFERENCES BETWEEN VARYING SIGMA LEVELS IN IMPROVEMENT

3.8 Sigma or "99% defect free"	6 Sigma or "99.99966%" defect free
20,000 articles of lost mail per hour	7 articles of lost mail per hour
5,000 incorrect surgical procedures per week	1.7 incorrect surgical procedures per week
Loss of electricity for approximately 7 hours each month	Loss of electricity for 1 hour every 34 years

Source: Adapted from General Electric Back Belt training manual. (1997). GE Capital Learning Services, GE Inc.

in business processes to achieve a reduction in defects (mistakes) produced by the process. Process performance is measured in "sigmas." Any process performance can be measured on this scale. To give you an idea of the different levels of quality achieved between a 3.8 sigma process and a 6 sigma process, a comparison can be found in Table 5.1.

In a Six Sigma organization, a certified project leader, typically called a Black Belt or Master Black Belt, leads a project through five phases and uses specific tools at each phase to allow a comprehensive understanding of the current process performance, identification of potential root causes, identification of potential improvements, implementation of those improvements, and implementation of sustainability measures (Fairbanks, 2007). These phases are commonly referred to as *DMAIC* (de-MAY-ick), an acronym that stands for **d**efine, **m**easure, **a**nalyze, **i**mprove, and **c**ontrol. In-depth attention is paid to measuring process performance with objective data both before and after any changes are made. An example of process performance data might be the wait time of patients in a primary care physician's office. A heavy emphasis is placed on making fact-based, data-driven decisions to improve performance.

As a leader in a Six Sigma organization, a DNP-prepared nurse might be asked to support or join a Six Sigma project team. Teams meet regularly to advance the project through the phases with the certified Six Sigma Black Belt acting as facilitator, project manager, analyst, and technical advisor. The team members provide subject matter expertise and ultimately agree to proceed with the changes recommended by the project team and/or the Black Belt. Leaders also support periodic reviews of the team's progress and are responsible for actively promoting the work of the project team to various stakeholders in the organization. Nurse leaders assist with monitoring the improved state to ensure improvements are sustained, and communicating changes in business priorities that might impact the team's work or decisions.

Some common pitfalls with Six Sigma include projects taking too long to complete and data being unavailable or difficult to get. Many organizations use a combination of Lean and Six Sigma to assist with shortening the project duration and decreasing the heavy reliance on data required in the Six Sigma methodology.

COMPLETING PROCESS IMPROVEMENT PROJECTS

How does an idea for improvement get implemented? How does a leader know the idea is going to be effective? Process improvement work follows a predictable series of phases from conception to completion. Identifying the work distinct to these phases contributes to strong organization of the work, facilitates effective communication with participating departments, and enables tracking of progress. These project phases are standard to professional project management practices and effective project management is essential to successful process improvement.

The five project phases are initiate, plan, execute, monitor, and close. Each phase has specific deliverables that are required for the next phase of the project. Skipping over phases will lead to rework and lost time later, so, as process improvement professionals like to say, "trust the process!"

The Initiate Phase

The initiate phase is where a project starts its journey. During this phase, leaders refine the project idea and receive support from the organization to use time, resources, and people to work on a specific problem. Some key questions to consider are:

- What is the problem you are trying to solve?
- How does this problem currently impact the organization?
- Is there a cost to the organization if this problem continues to occur?
- Does solving this problem contribute to the organization's achievement of its goals?
- From whom should you get permission or support to work on this project?

Often, when people initiate process improvement work, they start with an idea that they want to implement and give little thought to the problem this idea is intended to solve. Let us say that a nurse wants to hang whiteboards in each patient room on the unit. What is the underlying problem that this nurse is trying to solve? Why should hospital administration invest in purchasing and hanging whiteboards in every patient room? Asking "why" is an effective way to understand the intent of the improvement. One technique for reaching a better understanding of the underlying issues at stake is to use the "5 Whys" technique (Box 5.1). Iteratively asking "why" helps clarify the rationale for the improvement and may expose more efficacious options.

BOX 5.1 Example of 5 Whys Technique

5 WHYS

Idea: Hang whiteboards in each patient room

1. Why? To write easily visible information for the patient and family to see.
2. Why do we need to write down easily visible information? Patients and family members often can't remember their nurse's name or what time their next medication is due.
3. Why is it important for patients to know this sort of information? Patients and families don't have any other way to get this information so they ask nurses the same questions over and over again. Patient satisfaction is negatively impacted when this redundant communication occurs.
4. Why is higher patient satisfaction important? As nurses we want our patients to feel well cared for and comforted during their inpatient stay. Patients who are kept appraised of their care report higher satisfaction with their care.
5. Why is it important for patients to report higher satisfaction with their care? The hospital's reputation and reimbursement are impacted by the patient satisfaction scores. As nurses we want to work for a hospital that has a strong reputation for excellence in patient care.

The next step in the initiate phase is to estimate the potential impact of the problem to substantiate the need for the improvement project and gain support to use time and resources to complete it. Framing a justification for process improvement in terms of both the cost and risk of not addressing the problem as well as its opportunities will assist in the procurement of support. An effective way to present this analysis is to use a strengths/weaknesses, opportunities/threats (SWOT) analysis (Figure 5.1). The left side of the SWOT tool addresses the potential of improvement and the right side provides an assessment of the risks of maintaining the status quo.

The Planning Phase

There are multiple goals to achieve during the planning phase, as this phase builds the foundation of the improvement work. Some key questions to consider are:

- How can our team gain a solid understanding of the current state?
- How can the team define a target state or project aim?
- How will the team engage in an idea-generating process to formulate a hypothesis of what changes could be made to achieve the desired improvements?
- How will the team measure the impact of the process improvements?

SWOT analysis
Why this project, why now?

Strengths		Weaknesses	
	• Project attributes that align to the org? • What resonates with executives? • What resonates with your team?		• How dose the problem put the org at risk? • What about this project will be hard to do? Culturally, politically, structurally?
Opportunities		Threats	
	• Why this project and why now? • What will the potential benefits be?		• If we don't act, what is the impact?

FIGURE 5.1 SWOT analysis.

SWOT, strengths/weaknesses, opportunities/threats.

Source: From Hill, T., & Westbrook, R. (1997). SWOT analysis: It's time for a product recall. *Long Range Planning, 30*(1), 46–52. doi:10.1016/s0024-6301(96)00095-7

Using a combination of subjective and objective information, a hypothesis is developed about the root causes of the problem. Once a thorough understanding of why the problem occurs is achieved, improvement ideas can be formulated and attempted. It is also important to understand who the customers of this process are and to define a target state for improvement. Defining quality from the customer's perspective is essential to achieving a great project outcome.

Identifying the end user or "customer" is important. In healthcare, the patient and family are the recipients of the product or service provided and are generally considered healthcare's "customers." However, healthcare service that is provided involves a whole team, and so the term *customer* can be expanded to include team members who rely on each other to complete the work. Let us take an x-ray as an example. The patient getting the x-ray is certainly a customer, but is this patient the only customer? Other customers of this process might include the radiologist, the provider who ordered the x-ray, and the insurance company that will pay for the x-ray. Improvement of healthcare processes also affects the team carrying out the care. Looking at the provision of healthcare from a systems perspective facilitates accurate identification of the relevant "customers."

As stated earlier a system is a set of interrelated processes that work together to achieve a common aim (Deming, 1993). Inputs (e.g., data, raw materials, supplies) are fed into the process and yield outputs that are needed

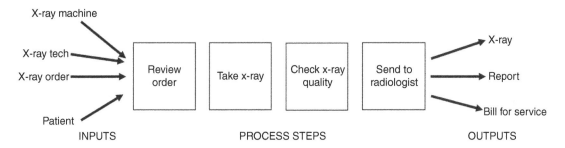

FIGURE 5.2 Example of inputs, process steps, and outputs.

by the customer. Provision of care as a set of processes is one important level of analysis that can provide significant insight into how to improve the quality of an outcome for the patient. Improving one's understanding of the inputs, processes, and outputs involved in a focal area of care is a well-established tool for achieving better quality. The process improvement tool for this work focuses on what elements contribute to the inputs, processes, and outputs. Using a diagram to depict the inputs, key process steps, and outputs assists in focusing process improvement work on the most relevant customers connected to the desired improvement. Figure 5.2 outlines the inputs, processes, and outputs in performing an x-ray.

The start of the process is an event or action that causes the process to begin. In this example, we could view the x-ray order as the starting point. The order triggers the x-ray to be performed. The outputs of our process would be an x-ray, a write-up of the interpretation that contributes to a diagnosis, and a bill.

How would the customers connected to the x-ray example define quality? Figure 5.3 (Kano model) provides a useful way to consider how customers might describe quality (Kano, Seraku, Takahashi, & Tsuji, 1984). The lower curve represents the minimal customer definition of quality. Basic customer expectations are often unspoken. When buying a new car, it would never occur to buyers to specify that they would like the new car to work, have functioning brakes, and a windshield. These are all expected attributes of a new car. Although it may take more than basic functioning to satisfy new-car buyers, the absence of any these would be immediately noticeable as poor quality.

The middle curve represents the characteristics that customers can articulate as critical to quality. These may be attributes that are commonly available or specialized. Again, an absence of them would leave a customer feeling dissatisfied but the presence of all of them only indicates your product or service is satisfactory to the customer. Satisfactory is fine but only adequate.

The top curve represents the level of achievement to aim for. This curve identifies attributes that will delight the customers. It is the highest, aspirational quality (Xu, 2009).

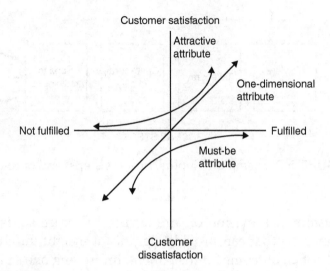

FIGURE 5.3 Kano model used to describing quality.

Source: From Lin, F-H., Tsai, S-B., Lee, Y-C., Hsiao, C-F., Zhou, J., Wang, J., . . . Shang, Z. (2017). Empirical research on Kano's model and customer satisfaction. *PLoS ONE, 12*(9), e0183888. doi:10.1371/journal.pone.0183888

Application of the Kano model to the x-ray example helps identify relevant customers and define various levels of quality. Table 5.2 explicates the various Kano elements in this clinical example, focusing on the process of an x-ray.

Although some aspirational attractive attributes, sometimes referred to as *customer delighters*, may not be able to be immediately realized, they are important to consider. As nurse leaders work to improve processes, they are faced with options of how best to do so. A clear vision of what the customer would consider to be highest quality facilitates selection of the improvements that are both feasible and come closest to delighting the

TABLE 5.2 KANO MODEL OF QUALITY ELEMENTS IN A CLINICAL EXAMPLE

Must-Be Attribute	One-Dimensional Attribute	Attractive Attribute
Clear order for x-ray	Easy to read report	No waiting
Good quality image	Timely results	Instant results, including
An accurate report	Reasonable cost	radiologist's notes and
Safe x-ray machine	Clean facility	diagnosis
	Friendly service	Mobile x-ray that comes to
	Convenient access	the patient
		No out-of-pocket expense
		Online reservation system
		Walk-in service at a grocery
		store or coffee shop
		Self-service kiosks

customer. Seeing healthcare delivery mechanisms as a process and understanding the customers' experience of quality is the first step to creating effective improvements.

In the planning phase it is also essential to have an adequate understanding of the current processes in place. A lack of clarity as to the underlying causes and the systems from which the improvements will be generated leads to suboptimal improvements, or *tampering*. Tampering arises when leaders seek to make quick fixes in response to surface-level, incomplete information. To prevent this deleterious approach to process improvement, it is important to make sense of the current state and find evidence to support the operational hypothesis of the problem and how the proposed improvements would effectively improve the current state. A good place to start is with a process map. A process map is an effective process improvement tool used to chart basic data about the current state of the process.

A process map depicts, *in detail*, the series of steps and decisions used in the process to produce a specific outcome. A process map is a visual diagram of the process steps involved in providing a service. Each step of the process is put into a box, and decision points in the process are placed in diamond-shaped boxes (see the key in Figure 5.4). The boxes are arranged from left to right in the order in which each step occurs. In applying this construct to the x-ray example, the process map might be similar to that in Figure 5.4.

Process maps are a commonly used, very effective process improvement tool. Useful outcomes of using process maps include clarifying a team's understanding of the current state, identifying measures of current performance, and exposing hidden complexity in processes that could be

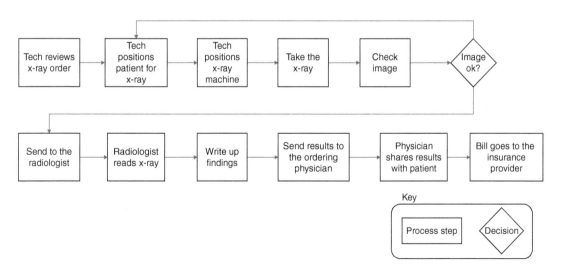

FIGURE 5.4 Example of a process map.

sources of poor performance. To be useful, a process map must be sufficiently detailed to depict what is useful or needed and what is wasteful about the process.

Similar to a process map, a time-motion study can reveal unappreciated steps in a complex process. The goal of a time-motion study is to assess inefficiencies in both time and motion. This tool breaks down a task or job into its component parts and measures the time needed and notes the necessary motion (physical activity) required for the parts. Often an objective observer is used to note both the motion and time required of either a healthcare team member or patient to complete an identified task. For even greater scrutiny, a task can be videotaped for repetitive review. The goal is to make processes more efficient by reducing both the time and motion required for certain tasks (Lopetegui et al., 2014).

The next step in the planning phase is to increase understanding of the current process' performance. Objective data must be gathered to understand the current performance of the process being analyzed. Data that indicate the frequency, duration, and/or magnitude of the problem will be useful to fully understanding current state. Analyzing available data will assist you in confirming or refining your hypothesis of what the root causes are. Data should relate back to the problem being solved. For example, if the challenge relates to delays in the current process, then the leader must confirm that the improvement idea will fix the identified delay. The case study described in Box 5.2 illustrates this concept of how data can shift understanding of the root causes of the problem and assist in selecting the most effective and most feasible ideas to solve it.

Once a clear understanding of the current state emerges and data have been used to measure the current state performance, the improvement team begins selecting specific improvements to try in the PDSA cycles. The execute and monitor phases follow.

The Execute and Monitor Phases

The transition between executing and monitoring during an improvement project can be indistinct so in this section we will consider these phases together. Some key questions to consider are:

- How will the team launch the targeted improvements?
- How will the team track and communicate the impact of the improvements?
- How will the team reinforce implementation of the prescribed changes?
- What has historically been effective in maintaining change over time in this microsystem?
- What ongoing support will the team need to support specific improvements over time?

BOX 5.2 Case Study: Patients Requiring Feeding-Tube Placement

A hospital identified patients who were being scheduled for feeding-tube placement who were experiencing delays in getting the feeding tubes placed. The prolonged malnourishment resulting from these delays was causing adverse health outcomes for these patients. The people who worked in this process believed that the delay was due to inefficient surgery-scheduling processes and a lack of surgery slots resulting in longer than desired wait times for the feeding-tube placement. A process map was created to depict the steps needed from the point when the physician recommended the feeding tube as a course of treatment, to the time that the feeding tube was placed in the patient and supplemental nutrition begun. Analysis of the process revealed that there were multiple points of potential delay. A chart review of patients who received feeding tubes was undertaken to tally both the count of delays and where those delays occurred. Analysis of this data revealed that the primary difference between effective and deleterious outcomes was whether or not the patient immediately agreed to the feeding-tube placement during the outpatient visit when it was first recommended, or if the patient and family wanted to think about this intervention. Patients who agreed quickly had better outcomes. The current process did not provide for timely or consistent follow-up with patients who were still deciding. This often resulted in weeks or months elapsing before these patients were placed on the surgery schedule. Had the team pursued its original hypothesis about where the source of the delays occurred, they would have seen only minimal improvements. By using the process map and looking at available data, they revealed a critical source of delay that they had not previously recognized. It is for this reason that understanding the current state and validating one's understanding of this current state with data is so critical for effective process improvements.

- How will the team know when to hold off on making any more new changes and focus instead on testing how effective the improvements are over time?

During the execute and monitor phases, the improvement trials are planned and implemented using PDSA cycles. Greater details about the composition of these steps can be found in Chapter 4. During implementation and monitoring of the process improvement of nursing leaders make decisions about how long to run the trial, how to collect the data to determine the impact of the trial, and what training is appropriate for members of the team. For each PDSA cycle, data and feedback are collected to learn about the effects of the improvements. Iterative interventions are attemptd until the desired effect is achieved.

As soon as a successful combination of interventions in the process have been identified, these should be maintained over a period of time to see how the process performs in the long run. This is the point at which the project transitions from the execute phase to the monitor phase. All processes vary with respect to time so it is important to collect data on how the new process is sustained over time to learn whether it will be sufficient to meet project goals.

Throughout both the execute and monitor phases, the team members who are conducting the PDSA cycles provide feedback on what is and what is not effective. Communicating on progress during the PDSA cycle is key to the success of the project. Progress and adjustments must be communicated frequently to the team involved in the improvement effort. Fostering opportunities for two-way communication, such as huddles and in-person meetings, facilitates effective involvement in the stages of improvement. Effective nurse leaders promote frequent open dialogue about how the processes being tested are working.

As previously stated, once the desired level of improvement is achieved the project officially moves into the monitoring phase. During this phase, steps are taken to sustain the improvements over time. Data and feedback continue to be collected to ensure that the improvements continue to achieve the desired outcome and also to learn how the improvements stand up over time. Documenting the improved process in a process map and establishing a clear way to monitor the new process and its performance over time are essential elements of this phase. Effective monitoring systems must be simple and easy to maintain so that the performance does not slip back to its prior state. Continuing to monitor and support adoption of new processes is necessary until the improvement is embedded in the microsystem culture and becomes the "new normal." More detail about how to sustain improvements over time can be found in Chapter 13.

Closing the Improvement Project

The goal of the closing phase is to celebrate success, acknowledge the hard work of those who partnered with you to make the changes, and to formally communicate the project's accomplishments. Some key questions to consider are:

- How will the organization know the impact of this improvement project?
- Could the resuts of this project be published?
- Would a change in leadership impact the sustainability of this improvement?
- Could the improvements be successfully spread to other aspects of the organization?

The close phase is a good time to consider publishing the process and outcomes of the process improvement work. The same key stakeholders who granted approval for the project in the initiate phase should be informed of the project's outcomes. A simple way to address these steps is through use of a project charter. A project charter serves to summarize the key points of the project so that others may learn from its successes and challenges. A project charter typically contains the following elements:

- A brief description of the problem a hand
- A project goal statement
- Measures of performance both before and after improvement
- A summary of the key interventions attempted
- Key insights learned in the course of working on the project
- Identification of the project lead and any project team members
- The date of the project's completion

In addition to the project charter, the new process should be documented in a process map, and any relevant documentation, such as policies or training manuals, should be updated to reflect the currently accepted practices. Accurate documentation of the process improvement work situates a team for more effective sustainment of the improvements as well as future improvement cycles.

CONCLUSIONS

Participating in and leading process improvement projects is both daunting and rewarding. As nursing leaders in healthcare, fostering a process improvement mind-set in your leadership will allow you to gain maximum engagement from your team, contribute to high-quality care, and pave the way for innovation in healthcare. Leveraging one of the many standard process improvement methodologies to facilitate improvement enables a DNP nurse leader to facilitate more effective and sustainable improvement results.

Case Study

Y.H. is a family nurse practitioner (FNP) pursing her DNP. She practices in a nurse-run primary care clinic. Y.H. has finished her coursework and is planning her DNP project. Y.H.'s primary care clinic has gathered patient-satisfaction data for approximately 24 months, and the clinic manager informs Y.H. that excessive waiting times in the waiting room and in the exam room before the FNP enters for the visit are a common cause of complaint among the clinic's patients. Y.H. decides to employ multiple process improvement approaches to address this patient dissatisfier.

(continued)

Case Study (*continued*)

QUESTIONS:

1. Who would be members of Y.H.'s ideal team to improve patient wait times in the FNP clinic?
2. What process improvement tools lend themselves to assessing the current state of waiting times at the FNP clinic?
3. What might be some processes occurring before the FNP begins the visit that might be contributing to long wait times?
4. What data would Y.H.'s team track to assess whether changes that were implemented were actual improvements?

REFERENCES

Batalden, P. B., & Stolz, P. K. (1993). A framework for the continual improvement of health care: Building and applying professional and improved knowledge to test changes in daily work. *The Joint Commission Journal on Quality Improvement, 19*(10), 424–447. doi:10.1016/S1070-3241(16)30025-6

Berwick, D. M. (1996). A primer on leading improvement of systems. *British Medical Journal, 312*, 619–622. doi:10.1136/bmj.312.7031.619

Committee on Quality Healthcare in America, Institute of Medicine. (2001). *Crossing the quality chasm: A new health system for the 21st century*. Washington, DC: National Academies Press.

Deming, W. E. (1986). *Out of the crisis*. Cambridge, MA: Massachusetts Institute of Technology, Center for Advanced Engineering Study.

Deming W. E. (1993). *The new economics for industry, government, education*. Cambridge, MA: Massachusetts Institute of Technology, Center for Advanced Engineering Study.

Fairbanks, C. B. (2007). Using Six Sigma and Lean methodologies to improve OR throughput. *AORN Journal, 86*(1), 73–82. doi:10.1016/j.aorn.2007.06.011

Kano, N., Seraku, N., Takahashi, F., & Tsuji, S. (1984). Attractive quality and must-be quality. *Journal of the Japanese Society for Quality Control, 14*(2), 39–48.

Kimsey, D. B. (2010). Lean methodology in healthcare. *AORN Journal, 92*(1), 53–60. doi:10.1016/j.aorn.2010.01.015

Lopetegui, M., Yen, P. Y., Lai, A., Jeffries, J., Embi, P., & Payne, P. (2014). Time motion studies: What are we talking about? *Journal of Biomedical Information, 49*, 292–299. doi:10.1016/j.jbi.2014.02.017

Xu, Q. (2009). An analytical Kano model for customer need analysis. *Design Studies, 30*(1), 87–110.

6

IMPROVEMENT, EVIDENCE-BASED PRACTICE, AND RESEARCH

MARY BETH FLYNN MAKIC

This chapter addresses the following DNP American Association of Colleges of Nursing (AACN) Essentials:

I.   Scientific Underpinnings for Practice
II: Organizational and Systems Leadership for Quality Improvement
III: Clinical Scholarship and Analytical Methods for EBP
VI. Inter-Professional Collaboration for Improving Patient and Population Health

INTRODUCTION

Research, evidence-based practice (EBP), and quality improvement (QI) are all distinct methods that can be used to improve practice, yet questions remain about how they are all connected. All three methods can be synergistic, but each has a distinct purpose. The intent of this chapter is to review the primary elements underpinning research and EBP and discuss how they are different yet complement each other in practice. QI methods are often required to effectively implement research and other forms of best evidence; thus, this approach to practice advancement is also discussed.

WHY IS EBP A PRACTICE FOCUS FOR THE DNP CLINICIAN?

In 2001 the Institute of Medicine (IOM), now referred to as the *National Academy of Medicine (NAM)*, sounded an alarm across the bow of healthcare with the influential publication, *Crossing the Quality Chasm: A New Health System for the 21st Century* (IOM (US) Committee on Quality of Health Care in America, 2001). This seminal publication listed six key principles to improve healthcare, stating that healthcare should be safe, effective, timely, efficient, equitable, and patientcentered (IOM(US) Committee on Quality of Health Care in America, 2001). This document also encouraged clinicians to embrace EBP to reach these goals. Now, almost two decades later, healthcare continues to strive to translate best evidence into practice to improve outcomes. Advancing practice requires the clinician to continually ask questions as to what constitutes best practice, seek answers to these questions, and then move the evidence into practice; reducing the unacceptable gap between what we know and how we care for patients (IOM (US) Committee on Quality of Health Care in America, 2001; Stevens, 2013).

Clinical practice guidelines continue to be developed, revised, and published. But implementing effective evidence-based clinical practice guidelines into practice is lacking. Clinical practice guidelines provide direction for care but stop short of facilitating "how" to move them into practice (Balas et al., 2018). The DNP clinician is perfectly poised to facilitate the movement of evidence-based guidelines into practice to improve outcomes. More pointed, DNP-prepared nurses are knowledgeable and skilled to facilitate the full implementation of science to achieve improvements in healthcare (AACN, 2017)

For EBP to be truly essential, implementing best evidence needs to be the underpinning for how nurses' practice; not a project that needs to be completed (Taylor, Priefer, & Alt-White, 2016). Ensuring nurses provide exceptional care requires continuous exploration of current evidence and application of the evidence in practice. Effectively impacting practice through EBP requires a fluid understanding of the differences and intersections of EBP, QI, and research. A pivotal role of the practice doctorate degree is for the nurse to develop skills to critically review the evidence, evaluate practice trends and data, and develop a process to effectively translate current best evidence in practice. The DNP nurse is in a position to lead EBP adoption that will facilitate meeting the goals of providing high-quality healthcare and thereby influence the healthcare system where they practice.

IMPROVING OUTCOMES THROUGH EBP ADOPTION

As healthcare continues to shift from volume metrics to value-based outcomes, embracing EBP as a foundation to guide practice culture is essential to meet the dynamic demands of the environment (Porter-O'Grady & Malloch, 2017; Shaw, Asomugha, Conway, & Rain, 2014). EBP should be the underpinning that guides how nurses practice, not an additional task for the nurse to complete. Achieving EBP as the foundation to practice requires a shift in culture and true adoption of evidence as the way to achieve patient-centered care.

EBP has been defined as a problem-solving process that incorporates current best evidence, clinician's expertise, and the patient's values and preferences in the delivery of care (Goode, Fink, Krugman, Oman, & Traditi, 2011; Ingersoll, 2000; Melnyk, Gallagher-Ford, Long, & Fineout-Overholt, 2014; Sackett, Rosenberg, Gray, Haynes, & Richardson, 1996) The review of evidence to answer clinical questions begins with a rigorous review of the research literature and expands from research evidence to other forms of evidence to inform practice. As efforts to improve and advance practice, the body of evidence used to inform practice also advances. For example, rigorous QI studies, benchmarking data, The Joint Commission documents, Institute for Healthcare Improvement bundles, and so on, become sources of evidence that impact practice.

Adoption of EBP as the overarching framework for practice requires the clinician to review and critique research evidence, examine EBP clinical practice guidelines, and explore the findings from QI and program evaluation efforts (Figure 6.1).

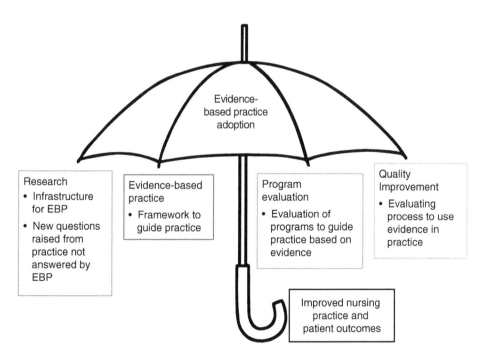

FIGURE 6.1 Evidence-based practice adoption.

EBP, evidence-based practice.

Reviewing research and evidence-based clinical practice guidelines should be the first sources explored to answer clinical questions. Then, seeking insights into how others successfully implemented EBP changes, the clinician should review QI and program evaluation literature. However, research is the foundation of practice science and should be the starting point when seeking answers to clinical inquiries (Goode et al., 2011). The DNP clinician provides the knowledge and skills to ask the clinical questions and then critically evaluate the evidence to improve practice through EBP adoption.

WHAT CONSTITUTES RESEARCH?

Research is defined as a systematic investigation intended to develop or contribute to generalizable knowledge (National Institutes of Health, 2018). The AACN expounds on this definition, stating that nursing research provides a significant body of knowledge to advance nursing practice, shape health policy, and impact the health of people and the quality of professional nursing practice (AACN, 2006). Nursing research provides the scientific knowledge to inform practice.

What separates researchfrom EBP, QI, and program evaluation is the purpose or intent of the study. The purpose of research is to generate new knowledge that may be generalized and must adhere to federal regulations that protect the rights of subjects (The National Commission for the Protection of Human Subjects of Biomedical and Behavioral Research, 1979; Newhouse, Pettit, Poe, & Rocco, 2006; Shirey et al., 2011). Researchers seek to answer questions that remain unclear, validate knowledge, or explore new knowledge (Groves, Burns, & Gray, 2013). The scope of nursing research is vast and inclusive of clinical research, education focused, health systems, and outcomes research. Clinical research provides an understanding of the biobehavioral dynamics of patient care; education-focused research provides answers to improve instruction and training of clinicians; and health systems and outcomes research provides understanding as to the quality, cost, and optimal methods used to improve care (AACN, 2006). It is essential for all clinicians to understand research as a first step to EBP. However, conducting research requires an understanding of theoretical frameworks, research methods, analysis, and human subject protection and oversight. Research conduction follows a plan of study defined a priori. Reports by investigators may be required to be conveyed back to the oversight entity or funding body. Last, the risks and burdens of the proposed study must be fully disclosed to the subjects and consent obtained. Research is disciplined and is conducted along a well-structured plan that does not deviate from the proposed study protocol(s). Although at all academic levels

TABLE 6.1 AACN RESEARCH EDUCATION AND TRAINING EXPECTATIONS AND COMPETENCIES OF NURSING GRADUATES

Baccalaureate programs	• Basic understanding of the process of research • Understand and apply research findings • May collaborate on a research team
Masters programs	• Evaluate research findings to develop and implement them into practice • Identify practice gaps that require scientific exploration • Collaborate with researchers to build nursing science
Practice-focused doctorate (i.e., DNP)	• Integrate and translate scientific knowledge into practice • Lead implementation of complex interventions based on science to improve patient outcomes • Collaborate with researchers to identify and explore gaps in practice and current science • Practice expertise includes the evaluation and use of research rather than the conduct of research
Research-focused doctorate (i.e., PhD)	• Conduct independent research for the intent of generating knowledge that is generalizable • Develop, plan, and implement a program of research to advance knowledge and the profession of nursing • Engage others in the conduct of research

Source: From American Association of Colleges of Nursing. (2006, March). Nursing research. Retrieved from https://www.aacnnursing.org/Portals/42/News/Position-Statements/Nursing-Research.pdf

nurses receive instruction on research concepts and review of common research methods, specific, rigorous training in research conduction is usually provided during doctoral education. The AACN offers guidance as to the expectations and competencies of nursing graduates with regard to research education and training. Table 6.1 provides a summary of AACN's (2006) stated expectations and competencies.

Generating science to guide practice through nursing research is essential to the advancement of the profession. However, if the science is not applied to practice, the gap between knowledge and practice will persist. As practice doctorates translate evidence into practice, gaps in knowledge may be uncovered. In this event, practice and research doctorates have an opportunity to collaborate to advance nursing practice through research led by the research-focused doctorate.

EBP MODELS

Numerous EBP models are available in the literature. A study by Mitchell, Fisher, Hastings, Silverman, and Wallen (2010) found 47 prominent models for translating evidence into practice. Analysis of the models results in four thematic areas: (a) EBP, research utilization, and knowledge transformation processes; (b) strategic/organizational change theory to promote uptake and adoption of new knowledge; (c) knowledge exchange and synthesis for application and inquiry; and (d) designing and interpreting dissemination research (Mitchell et al., 2010). Understanding the theoretical underpinning of the model used to drive practice change is an important decision to be made by the DNP clinicians to optimize best practice adoption. Models provide road maps that can be conceptual, iterative, or stepwise. Several EBP models that may be explored include ACE Star Model (Stevens, 2004); Advancing Research and Clinical Practice Through Close Collaboration (ARCC) Model (Melnyk, Fineout-Overholt, Gallagher-Ford, & Stillwell, 2011); The Colorado Model (Goode et al., 2011); The Iowa Model (Iowa Model Collaborative et al., 2017); and the John Hopkins Model (Dang & Dearholt, 2018). Regardless of the model chosen, the benefit of using an EBP model allows for a comprehensive approach to translate evidence into practice.

Commonalities are present within most models. All EBP models start with asking the clinical question, searching and appraising the evidence, developing teams and a strategy to implement the evidence, and evaluating the patient outcome success. A process referred to as the 5A's: ask, acquire, appraise, apply, and assess has been in the literature dating back to early discussions of EBP (Goode et al., 2011; Sackett et al., 1996). DNP clinicians develop the essential knowledge and skill to apply the 5A's and lead efforts to improve practice. Once a clinical question is identified, the DNP nurse applies clinical inquiry skills to develop a clear and articulate clinical question to allow for a rigorous review of the literature (Box 6.1).

Rigorous DNP led practice projects may require the clinician to develop several PICO(T) questions to effectively search the evidence for interventions to improve practice outcomes. Common types of clinical questions include therapy/treatment, prevention, diagnostic, prognosis, etiology, meaning/understanding the patient experience (Groves et al., 2013). The

BOX 6.1 The PICO(T) Question Format

PICO(T) question format is used to develop a clinical question to facilitate a review of the literature:

P = Population
I = Intervention of interest
C = Comparison intervention of interest or current practice
O = Outcome
T = Time frame

clinical question may have many PICO(T) statements to allow for a rigorous yet focused search of the evidence.

Next, using the PICO(T) format, a search of the evidence is completed. Several search engines are available to facilitate finding the best knowledge. When feasible, the Cochrane Collaboration and Joanna Briggs Institute both provide systematic reviews of the literature and meta-analyses to answer clinical questions. Search engines, such as PubMed CINHAL (Cumulative Index of Nursing and Allied Health Literature), Ovid, Clinical Key, and so on, provide access to larger, more diverse bodies of evidence that include the highest level of evidence by research method design (i.e., systematic review and meta-analysis), to other forms of research (e.g., randomized control trials [RCT], cohort studies, qualitative studies, etc.), clinical articles, editorials, and clinical practice guidelines. Other sites, such as UpToDate and DynaMed Plus, provide a synthesis of best practice knowledge based on current evidence. Clinical practice guidelines may be published in journals, at key organizational websites—such as CHEST, American Academy of Family Physicians (AAFP), Guideline Central, U.S. Preventative Services Task Force (USPSTF), and so forth. Google Scholar may also be used as a general search engine in the event full access to a health science library is not available.

Clinical practice guidelines (CPG) provide important summaries of the evidence on specific topics. As the need for synthesis of best evidence to guide practice continues to grow, more and more CPGs have been developed, but questions began to arise as to the rigor and quality of the CPG. In 2011, the IOM published a document outlining minimum expectations for CPG to guide practice. The IOM framework stipulates that as healthcare clinicians we should expect certain elements of rigor in the development of a CPG. These elements include that CPGs are developed based on a rigorous systematic review of the evidence; critically critiqued by a team of knowledgeable, interprofessional experts who are free of bias and conflict of interest and who provide clear explanation, rationales, rating of the quality and strength of the evidence supporting the suggested interventions; and the process needs to be transparent and open to external review with continued review and revision of the CPG (IOM, 2011).

The DNP clinician should critically review a CPG to ensure rigor in the creation of the document. The Appraisal of Guidelines for Research and Evaluation II (AGREE II) is an instrument that was developed to critically appraise CPGs (Brouwers et al., 2010; Brouwers, Kerkvliet, Spithoff, & on behalf of the AGREE Next Steps Consortium, 2016). The AGREE II appraisal tool allows for critical examination of the CPG along six domains consistent with the IOM guidelines (www.agreetrust.org).

On the other hand, care bundles are not CPGs. Rather, the concept of care bundles was introduced by the Institute of Healthcare Improvement (IHI) to enhance the reliability of care leading to improved patient outcomes by bundling small sets of interventions together (Resar, Griffin, Haraden, &

Nolan, 2012). Bundles combine three to five evidence-based care interventions to be applied together, but this does not constitute a CPG. That said, care bundles have been found to be an effective way to move evidence-base interventions toward more successful adoption of best practice (Borgert, Binnekade, Paulus, Goossens, & Dongelmans, 2017).

Once the evidence is acquired, the DNP nurse leads the process of critically appraising the evidence for both quality and strength. Reliance on evidence hierarchy tables based on research methods alone fail to critically examine the strength of the study. Along with the value of the study informing practice decisions, relevant questions as to the strength and weakness of the studies should be identified (Duffy, 2005). The practice doctorate clinician has honed the skills essential to critically appraise a rigorous evidence review to ensure EBP adoption decisions are appropriate for the intended patient population and practice environment. To inform practice decisions, this clinician may synthesize the evidence into a table to organize the review and allow a visual understanding of the multiple forms of evidence involved, study summaries, the impact of the intervention, and overall strength of the study.

Once the evidence is reviewed, steps to take to apply evidence into practice are developed. At this stage of the process, factors concerning unit culture, policy updates, available equipment, and process-focused interventions need to be considered. EBP adoption may require a QI methodology to "hardwire" the practice change. Metrics to assess the effectiveness of the EBP adoption should be developed, tracked, and disseminated.

EBP: FIRST STEP TO QI INITIATIVES

Nationally and internationally, EBP guidelines are often developed by groups of experts using rigorous methods to review and evaluate science to guide practice. However, the impact of EBP clinical practice guidelines are not appreciated by the patients, nor are practice outcomes improved unless there is a process to effectively move evidence into practice (Balas et al., 2018). Within the context of care, EBP requires a vehicle for the best practice evidence to be used consistently, reducing practice variation that can optimize outcomes. Rigorous QI methods that are framed in EBP facilitate adoption of best practices to improve outcomes and reduce healthcare costs (Balas et al., 2018; Newhouse et al., 2006; Stevens, 2013).

As practice evolves, practice routines or habits need to be challenged. Makic and Rauen (2016) evaluated 30 practice traditions that continue despite evidence that suggests the practice tradition is not evidence based. For example, nurses report comparing blood pressure readings obtained from noninvasive, oscillatory blood pressure cuffs to readings obtained from invasive arterial lines, despite evidence stating these two measures should not be compared as brachial and radial measures are not the same nor are the two measurement techniques comparable (i.e., noninvasive compared to invasive; McGhee & Bridges, 2002; Rauen, Chulay, Bridges, Vollman, & Arbour, 2008). Equally important, the position of the arm correctly aligned horizontal to heart level is essential to obtain accurate blood pressure readings that may be treated by the nurse based on the value obtained (Netea, Bijlstra, Lenders, Smits, & Thien, 1998; Rauen et al., 2008). Yet nurses frequently do not prop a pillow under a patient's arm or position the arm in a manner to ensure it is at heart level while obtaining blood pressure measurements. Removing practice habits and adopting EBP norms are essential to improving practice outcomes. Knowledge of these practice traditions alone will not result in EBP adoption unless there is process to move the evidence into practice effectively and efficiently.

Similarly, the movement of evidence-based deimplementation is gaining momentum in which processes are necessary to stop practices (i.e., deimplement) that are no longer evidence based (Prasad & Ioannidis, 2014). The Choosing Wisely campaign was launched in 2012 to encourage providers to reevaluate unnecessary tests or procedures that are not evidence based. (American Board of Internal Medicine Foundation, 2018; van Bodegom-Vos, Davidoff, & Marang-ven de Mheen, 2017) The list of low-value practices has continued to grow and there are more than 25 nursing-specific interventions identified that should be "deimplemented" or challenged in practice based on the evidence (American Academy of Nursing, 2015). Identifying low-value practices that are not evidence-based provides a jumping-off point for DNP clinicians to question practice, deimplement potentially harmful nursing actions, and introduce evidence-based practice interventions. "De-implementing practices reflects a recommitment to evidence-based healthcare" (Prasad & Ioannidis, 2014, p. 4).

Practice doctorate nurses are the pivotal clinicians to facilitate ongoing critical reviews of practice, challenge practice traditions, deimplement interventions that are no longer evidence based, and elevate practice so it is based on current best evidence. The DNP has mastery of the skills essential to identify a clinical problem, critically review and evaluate the evidence, and develop a process to move the evidence into practice that will be sustained and can be evaluated.

RESEARCH/EBP/QI INTERSECTION

Evidence-based practice is the explicit use of evidence, clinician expertise, and patient preferences to guide practice decisions. When EBP is the foundation of practice, variation is reduced, outcomes are improved, and healthcare savings are appreciated. EBP relies on scientific evidence (i.e., research) along with methods to translate the evidence into practice in a consistent process (i.e., QI). But the purpose of each concept drives the actions of the nurse. The purpose of research is to generate new knowledge and findings that are generalizable and that can be translate d into practice by the DNP. The purpose of EBP is to move evidence into practice by reducing variation and improving outcomes. The purpose of QI initiatives is to enhance processes so that evidence can be used effectively in practice and efficiencies in care, along with improved patient outcomes and cost-efficiencies, are achieved.

The DNP should be leading healthcare efforts to move evidence into practice and enhance processes of care. Several institutional review boards (IRB) provide decision trees to help determine the difference in the intent of a study to ensure a rigorous QI project is not misunderstood to be research and vice versa. Nurses are encouraged to use IRB resources if questions arise as to the nature of the study being considered to improve practice. Table 6.2 provides questions that may be asked to determine the nature of the study.

TABLE 6.2 POSSIBLE INSTITUTIONAL REVIEW BOARD QUESTIONS REGARDING THE NATURE OF A STUDY

	Research	EBP	Quality Improvement
Intent/ purpose	Generate new knowledge that is generalizable	Translate current best evidence into practice	Improve a practice process within a specific organization or unit
Who will benefit	Scientific community; possibly subjects	Patients, staff, providers	Patients, staff, providers, organization
Scope of study	Determined by research question; population determined by research question	Unit/organization	Unit/organization
Burdens or risk	Disclosed to subjects and consent required; harm cannot outweigh benefits	None	None
Time frame	Controlled, measured process for implementing and following the study protocol	Variable	Variable with rapid-cycle measures to allow for changes to protocol to improve process(es)
Data collection	Tightly controlled; data is protected	No patient-level data; outcome measures in aggregate are reported	No patient-level data; process and outcome measures in aggregate reported
Regulated	IRB, organization, federal law	Organization	Organization
Dissemination	Generalizable knowledge gained	Localized knowledge gained	Localized knowledge gained

IRB, institutional review board.

Differences among research, QI, and EBP studies are not always immediately clear. Thus, necessary steps are required to ensure the intent of the study is clearly understood by the entire team and appropriate human and financial resources are available to advance practice improvement.

CONCLUSIONS

Innovative practice leaders are always grounded in the evidence to foster meaningful change in practice (Porter-O'Grady & Malloch, 2017). Understanding and optimizing the intersection of research, EBP, and QI facilitates a practice environment based on current best evidence as the norm, or way of practice. DNP clinicians are essential to the effective translation of evidence into practice. It is time to close the chasm in the quality of patient care.

Case Study

James is an adult gerontology clinical nurse specialist working in a small rural hospital. He recently completed his DNP and has been evaluating different practice policies and protocols within the hospital. The chief nursing officer asked James to evaluate the current fall-prevention practices as the fall rate for the hospital has been consistently higher than national benchmarks for hospitals of similar size, according to the National Database for Nursing Quality Indicators (NDNQI). James obtained fall-rate data for the past year from the chief quality officer. He stratified the fall data by unit and age groups and noticed that patients over the age of 65 experienced the greatest number of falls. James reviewed the policies, protocols, and electronic health record (EHR). The policy and EHR corresponded in terms of guiding nursing practice expectations. The organization was using a valid and reliable fall-risk assessment tool and instructed nurses to identify patients at high risk of falls with yellow socks and armbands, bed alarms, and door labels. James conducted a brief audit of patients identified as at high risk for falls and found that indeed the nurses were following policy. He then talked with nurses on different units to ask about how they implemented the fall-prevention policy. Conversations with the staff revealed that because of the fear of falls older patients are frequently placed on bed and chair alarms and sometimes in soft restraints to restrict independent mobility. James spoke with a few older patients who conveyed frustration with the restricted mobility while hospitalized. He had a conversation with the nursing leadership, who suggested James conduct a research study as to the difference in falls in older patients and use of restraints within the hospital. James sent an email to his college research professor asking for for guidance and to partner in developing and conducting a research study. The research professor suggested James conduct a thorough review of the literature on older patients, falls, and immobility. James reviewed the literature and in his search found a Choosing Wisely® statement which identified that older adults should not lay in bed or have restricted mobility while hospitalized. The statement

(continued)

Case Study (*continued*)

went on to say that mobility during hospitalization was critical to maintaining functional abilities of the older adult postdischarge. James reflected on the comments from the nurses and patients. The policy and protocol were evidence based, but fear of falling had the nurses restricting mobility of older patients rather than providing interventions that fostered patient ambulation. James realized he had an opportunity to deimplement a practice habit that was restricting older patients' mobility, thereby increasing the fall risk during hospitalization (American Academy of Nursing, 2014; Creditor 1993; Padula, Hughes, & Baumhover, 2009; Pashikanti & Von, 2012). James determined a research study was not needed but rather he had an opportunity to deimplement a practice standard that was not evidence based and to lead an EBP initiative to improve the use of evidence to prevent falls in the older adults by implementing an evidence-based mobility protocol.

James reported back to the nursing leadership and chief nursing officer that indeed the policy for falls was evidence based but that the organization lacked an evidence-based mobility protocol to prevent deconditioning of older patients, which was increasing this populations' fall risk. He reviewed the fall-data stratification, comments from nurses and patients, and provided an evidence table that summarized his review of the literature that informed the recommendation for practice change. He requested permission to form an interprofessional task force to develop and implement an evidence-based mobility protocol. The chief quality office suggested he review the protocol with the hospital IRB and gain provider approval prior to initiating the task force. The chief nursing officer asked whether the protocol would increase the nurses' workload and require more staff. James suggested he would generate a business plan but that deimplementing a practice that was not evidence based and moving to an evidence-based practice would provide improved care and optimally reduce falls, which is a substantial cost saver and ultimately results in improved patient care outcomes.

QUESTIONS:

1. What DNP essentials are evident and/or missing from this project?
2. Did the DNP adequately involve key stakeholders in the review of the clinical practice problem?
3. Should the DNP clinician have pursued a research study testing the effectiveness of a mobility protocol to reduce falls in older adults?
4. What metrics should be tracked to evaluate the deimplementation of a practice tradition and impact of the evidence-based mobility protocol?

REFERENCES

American Academy of Nursing. (2014). Choosing Wisely: Don't let older adults lie in bed or only get up to a chair during their hospital stay. Retrieved fromhttp://www.choosingwisely.org/clinician-lists/american-academy-nursing-walking-for-older-adults-during-hospital-stays
American Academy of Nursing. (2015). Choosing Wisely: Twenty-Five things nurses and patients should question. Retrieved from http://www.choosingwisely.org

American Association of Colleges of Nursing. (2006, March). Nursing research. https://www.aacnnursing.org/Portals/42/News/Position-Statements/Nursing-Research.pdf

American Association of Colleges of Nursing. (J, 2017, June). DNP fact-sheet. Retrieved from https://www.aacnnursing.org/DNP/Fact-Sheet

American Board of Internal Medicine Foundation. (2018). Choosing Wisely. Retrieved from http://www.choosingwisely.org

Balas, M. C., Weinhouse, G. L., Denehy, L., Chanques, G., Rochwerg, B., Misak, C.J., . . . Fraser, G. L. (2018). Interpreting and implementing the 2018 pain, agitation/sedation, delirium, immobility, and sleep disruption clinical practice guideline. *Critical Care Medicine, 46*(9), 1464–1470. doi:10.1097/CCM.0000000000003307

Borgert, M., Binnekade, J., Paulus, F., Goossens, A., & Dongelmans, D. (2017). A flowchart for building evidence-based care bundles in intensive care: Based on a systematic review. *International Journal for Quality in Health Care, 29*(2), 163–175. doi:10.1093/intqhc/mzx009

Brouwers, M., Kho, M. E., Borwman, G. P., Burgers, J. S., Cluzeau, F., Feder, G., . . . for the AGREE Next Steps Consortium. (2010). AGREE II: Advancing guideline development, reporting and evaluation in healthcare. *Canadian Medical Association Journal, 182*, 839–842. doi:10.1503/cmaj.090449

Brouwers, M.C., Kerkvliet, K., Spithoff, K., & on behalf of the AGREE Next Steps Consortium. (2016). The AGREE Reporting Checklist: A tool to improve reporting of clinical practice guidelines. *British Medical Journal, 352*(3), e1–e2. doi:10.1136.bmj.i1152

Creditor, C. M. (1993). Hazards of hospitalization in the elderly. *Annals of Internal Medicine, 118*, 219–223. doi:10.7326/0003-4819-118-3-199302010-00011

Dang, D., & Dearholt, S. L. (2018). *Johns Hopkins nursing evidence-based practice: Model and guidelines* (3rd ed.). Indianapolis, IN: Sigma Theta Tau International.

Duffy, J. R. (2005). Critically appraising quantitative research. *Nursing & Health Sciences, 7*, 281–283. doi:10.1111/j.1442-2018.2005.00248.x

Goode, C. J., Fink, R. M., Krugman, M., Oman, K. S., & Traditi, L. K. (2011). The Colorado patient-centered interprofessional evidence-based practice model: A framework for transformation. *Worldviews on Evidence-Based Nursing, 8*(2), 96–105. doi:10.1111/j.1741-6787.2010.00208.x

Groves, S. K., Burns, N., & Gray, J. R. (2013). Discovering the world of nursing research. In S. K. Groves, N. Burns, & J. R. Gray (Eds.), *The practice of nursing research: Appraisal, synthesis, and generation of evidence* (pp. 1–11). St. Louis, MO: Elsevier.

Ingersoll, G. L. (2000). Evidence-based nursing: What it is and what it isn't. *Nursing Outlook, 48*(4), 151–152. doi:10.1067/mno.2000.107690

Institute of Medicine (US) Committee on Quality of Health Care in America. (2001). *Crossing the quality chasm: A new health system for the 21st century*. Washington, DC: National Academies Press. Retrieved from https://www.ncbi.nlm.nih.gov/books/NBK222274

Institute of Medicine. (2011). *Clinical practice guidelines we can trust*. Washington, DC: National Academies Press. Retrieved from http://www.nationalacademies.org/hmd/Reports/2011/Clinical-Practice-Guidelines-We-Can-Trust.aspx

Iowa Model Collaborative, Buckwalter, K. C., Cullen, L., Hanrahan, K., Kleiber, C., McCarthy, A. M., . . . Authored on behalf of the Iowa Model Collaborative. (2017). Iowa Model of Evidence-based practice: Revisions and validation. *Worldviews on Evidence-Based Nursing, 14*(3), 175–182. doi:10.1111/wvn.12223

Makic, M. B. F., & Rauen, C. A. (2016). Maintaining your momentum: Moving evidence into practice. *Critical Care Nurse, 36*(2), 13–18. doi:10.4037/ccn2016568

McGhee, B. H., & Bridges, E. J. (2002). Monitoring arterial blood pressure: What you may not know. *Critical Care Nurse, 22*(2), 60–70.

Melnyk, B. M., Fineout-Overholt, E., Gallagher-Ford, L., & Stillwell, S. (2011). Evidence-based practice step by step: Sustaining evidence-based practice through organizational policies and in innovative model. *American Journal of Nursing, 111*(9), 57–60. doi:10.1097/01.NAJ.0000405063.97774.0e

Melnyk, B. M., Gallagher-Ford, L., Long, L. E., & Fineout-Overholt, E. (2014). The establishment of evidence-based practice competencies for practicing registered nurses and advanced practices nurses in real-world clinical settings. *Worldviews on Evidence-Based Nursing, 11*(1), 5–15. doi:10.1111/wvn.12021

Mitchell, S. A., Fisher, C. A., Hastings, C. E., Silverman, L. B., & Wallen, G. R. (2010). A thematic analysis of theoretical models for translational science in nursing: Mapping the field. *Nursing Outlook, 58*(6), 287–300. doi:10.1016/j.outlook.2010.07.001

The National Commission for the Protection of Human Subjects of Biomedical and Behavioral Research. (1979). The Belmont report (DHEW Publication no. (OS) 78-0013). Washington, DC: Department of Health, Education and Welfare. Retrieved from https://www.hhs.gov/ohrp/sites/default/files/the-belmont-report-508c_FINAL.pdf

National Institutes of Health. (2018, March). Glossary. Retrieved from https://humansubjects.nih.gov/glossary#systematic-investigation

Netea, R. T., Bijlstra, P. J., Lenders, J. W., Smits, P., & Thien, T. (1998). Influence of the arm position on intra-arterial blood pressure measurement. *Journal of Human Hypertension, 12*(3), 157–160. doi:10.1038/sj.jhh.1000479

Newhouse, R. P., Pettit, J. C., Poe, S., & Rocco, L. (2006). The slippery slope: Differentiating between quality improvement and research. *Journal of Nursing Administration, 36*(4), 211–219. doi:10.1097/00005110-200604000-00011

Padula, P., Hughes, C., & Baumhover, L. (2009). Impact of a nurse-driven mobility protocol on functional decline in hospitalized older adults. *Journal of Nursing Care Quality, 24*(4), 325–331. doi:10.1097/NCQ.0b013e3181a4f79b

Pashikanti, L., & Von, A. D. (2012). Impact of early mobilization protocol on medical-surgical inpatient population. *Clinical Nurse Specialist, 26*(2), 87–91. doi:10.1097/NUR.0b013e31824590e6

Porter-O'Grady, T., & Malloch, K. (2017). Evidence-based practice and the innovation paradigm: A model for the continuum of practice excellence. In S. Davidson, D. Weberg, T. Porter-O'Grady, & K. Malloch (Eds.), *Leadership for evidence-based innovation in nursing and health professions* (pp. 3–42). Burlington, MA: Jones & Bartlett Learning.

Prasad, V., & Ioannidis, J. P. A. (2014). Evidence-based de-implementation of contradicted, unproven, and aspiring healthcare practices. *Implementation Science, 9*, 1–5. Retrieved from https://implementationscience.biomedcentral.com/articles/10.1186/1748-5908-9-1

Rauen, C. A., Chulay, M., Bridges, J., Vollman, K., & Arbour, R. (2008). Seven evidence-based practice habits: Putting some sacred cows out to pasture. *Critical Care Nurse, 28*(2), 98–124.

Resar, R., Griffin, F. A., Haraden, C., & Nolan, T. W. (2012). *Using care bundles to improve health care quality.* IHI Innovation Series White Paper. Cambridge, MA: Institute for Healthcare Improvement. Retrieved from www.ihi.org/resources/Pages/IHIWhitePapers/UsingCareBundles.aspx

Sackett, D. L., Rosenberg, W. M. C., Gray, J. A. M., Haynes, R. B., & Richardson, W. S. (1996). Evidence-based medicine: What it is and what it isn't. *BMJ, 312*, 71–73. doi:10.1136/bmj.312.7023.71

Shaw, F., Asomugha, C., Conway, P. H., & Rain, A. (2014). The Patient Protection and Affordable Care Act: Opportunities for prevention and public health. *Lancet, 384*(9937), 75–82. doi:10.1016/S0140-6736(14)60259-2

Shirey, M. R., Hauck, S. L., Embree, J. L., Kinner, T. J., Schaar, G. L., Phillips, L. A., . . . McCool, I. A. (2011). Showcasing difference between quality improvement, evidence-based practice, and research. *Journal of Continuing Education in Nursing, 42*(2), 57–68. doi:10.3928/00220124-20100701-01

Stevens, K. (2013, May). The impact of evidence-based practice in nursing and the next big ideas. *OJIN, 18*(2), Manuscript 4. Retrieved from http://ojin.nursingworld.org/MainMenuCategories/ANAMarketplace/ANAPeriodicals/OJIN/TableofContents/Vol-18-2013/No2-May-2013/Impact-of-Evidence-Based-Practice.html

Stevens, K. R. (2004). ACE Star Model of EBP: Knowledge transformation. Academic Center for Evidence-based Practice. The University of Texas Health Science Center at San Antonio. www.acestar.uthscsa.edu

Taylor, M. B., Priefer, B. A., & Alt-White, A. C. (2016). Evidence-based practice: Embracing integration. *Nursing Outlook, 64*(6), 575–582. doi:10.1016/j.outlook.2016.04.004

van Bodegom-Vos, L., Davidoff, F., & Marang-van de Mheen, P. J. (2017). Implementation and de-implementation: Two sides of the same coin? *BMJ Quality & Safety, 26*, 495–501. doi:10.1136/bmjqs-2016-005473

7

LEADING WITH QUALITY METRICS

GAIL E. ARMSTRONG | JENNIFER DISABATO | SCOTT HARPIN | KIM PAXTON | LAURA ROSENTHAL

This chapter addresses the following DNP American Association of Colleges of Nursing (AACN) Essentials:

II. Organizational and Systems Leadership for Quality Improvement and Systems Thinking
III. Clinical Scholarship and Analytical Methods for Evidence-Based Practice
VI. Interprofessional Collaboration for Improving Patient and Population Health Outcomes
VII. Clinical Prevention and Population Health for Improving the Nation's Health
VIII. Advanced Nursing Practice

INTRODUCTION

Since the Institute of Medicine's (IOM) report, "To Err Is Human," there has been widespread agreement that the quality and safety of healthcare must be improved (IOM], 2000). Measuring quality of care can be difficult because of all of the subjective, patient-specific, and care-specific variables. Quality of care can be defined as, "the degree to which health services for individuals and populations increase the likelihood of desired health outcomes and are consistent with current professional knowledge" (Lohr, 1990, p. 4).

Quality metrics serve as outcome targets for quality-improvement (QI) work (Bonow et al., 2008). The complexity of healthcare systems contributes to the challenge of identifying standardized quality metrics. Clinical outcomes that might indicate high quality in cardiac care will probably have minimal relevance in identifying high-quality neurologic care. Similarly, the setting of healthcare is important to consider when identifying quality metrics. Quality metrics important to the acute care setting will have limited application to outpatient settings. Due to the individual specificity of quality metrics related to area of care and setting of care, DNP students should familiarize themselves with the quality metrics specific to their clinical focus.

Within the expanding QI literature, there are many terms used synonymously for *quality metric* (e.g., *quality outcomes, quality indicators, performance measures, nurse-sensitive indicators*). The American College of Cardiology (ACA) and the American Heart Association (AHA) have differentiated the operational definitions of performance measures from quality metrics, emphasizing that performance metrics are for clinical reporting to the public (Bonow et al., 2008). "Performance measures are those process, structure, efficiency or outcome measures that have been . . . specifically . . . intended not only for clinical quality improvement but also may be considered for purposes of public reporting or other forms of accountability" (Bonow et al., 2008, p. 2664). "Quality metrics are those measures that have been developed to support self-assessment and quality improvement at the provider, hospital and/or healthcare system level" (Bonow et al., 2008, p. 2664).

Within this chapter, quality metrics specific to the acute care setting, pediatric care, geriatric care, public health, and the ambulatory setting will be considered.

ACUTE CARE QUALITY METRICS: BACKGROUND

In 2001, The Joint Commission (TJC) released the first four core measurements to assist in the standardized process for accreditation of hospitals. The original measures included acute myocardial infarction (AMI), heart failure (HF), pneumonia (PN), and pregnancy and related conditions (PR). The Joint Commission developed these measures in alignment with the Centers for Medicare & Medicaid Services (CMS) as well as with numerous stakeholders, including state hospital associations, care providers, consumers, and performance measurement experts.

The first reporting database for the core measures within TJC was the ORYX Performance Measurement program. Many people mistake ORYX for an acronym, but in actuality, the program was named after the animal species, oryx, meaning a "swiftly moving and graceful gazelle" (TJC, n.d). Throughout the following decade, TJC refined these core measures, eventually reclassifying (or retiring) them based on input from CMS and data collected on these core measures since 2003. TJC believes that retiring core measures and moving to reporting on electronic clinical quality measures and chart-abstracted measures through the ORYX system can improve healthcare delivery and outcomes (TJC, n.d.).

Significance

The Joint Commission uses electronic clinical quality measures within its accreditation process. All hospitals with an average daily census of more than 10 inpatients accredited through TJC are required to report specific, chosen, individual measures on a quarterly basis. TJC created a standards-based expectation for minimum performance on all electronic clinical quality measures (eCQMs). These minimum performance standards are integrated into TJC's survey of every facility and its requirements for improvement generated from that survey. A hospital-specific eCQM feedback report is supplied to all organizations that submit data to the ORYXsystem. This allows hospitals to actively engage in QI efforts.

Electronic Clinical Quality Measures

Currently there are 15 eCQMs supported by the CMS that provide data on provider-level (hospital) performance. TJC recognizes 13 of these eCQMs and requires hospital reporting on four of the 13 measures (Table 7.1). Quality measures are obtained automatically through the electronic

TABLE 7.1 INPATIENT ELECTRONIC CLINICAL QUALITY MEASURES SUPPORTED BY THE JOINT COMMISSION

ED-1 Median Time from ED Arrival to ED Departure for Admitted ED Patients
ED-2 Median Admit Decision Time to ED Departure Time for Admitted Patients
STK-2 Discharged on Antithrombotic Therapy
STK-3 Anticoagulation Therapy for Atrial Fibrillation/Flutter
STK-5 Antithrombotic Therapy by End of Hospital Day 2
STK-6 Discharged on Statin Medication
STK-10 Assessed for Rehabilitation
AMI-8a Primary PCI Received Within 90 Minutes of Hospital Arrival
VTE-1 Venous Thromboembolism Prophylaxis
VTE-2 Intensive Care Unit Venous Thromboembolism Prophylaxis
PC-01 Elective Delivery
PC-05 Exclusive Breast Milk Feeding
CAC-3 Home Management Plan of Care Document Given to Patient/Caregiver
EHDI-1a Hearing Screening Prior to Hospital Discharge

AMI, acute myocardial infarction; CAC, children's asthma care; ED, emergency department; EHDI, early hearing, detection, and intervention; PC, perinatal care; STK, stroke; VTE, venous thromboembolism.

Source: Electronic Clinical Quality Improvement Resource Center (n.d.). Inpatient electronic clinical quality measures supported by The Joint Commission. Retrieved from https://ecqi.healthit.gov/eligible-hospital/critical-access-hospital-ecqms

medical record through the use of software that uses specific data coding. Descriptions and definitions of each measurement are available (ecqi.healthit.gov/eligible-hospital-critical-access-hospital-ecqms).

Chart-Abstracted Measures

TJC also reviews chart-abstracted measures. These differ from eCQMs, in that the data is manually collected in a narrative manner from each chart, not obtained through the electronic medical record (EMR) automatically in a structured, codified manner with specific software. Hospitals are required to report on all five measures (Table 7.2).

Data Reporting

TJC requires that all data reporting proceed through a TJC-certified vendor listed on the ORYX‾certified website. Direct data submission is a new option for hospitals that choose to upload directly to TJC. All measures are also reported by TJC on Quality Check. Quality Check is a website where consumers can learn about the performance of their hospital. A patient may obtain data by entering an organization name, type, and/or location.

Resources for Acute Care Quality Metrics

1. CMS eCQI Resource Center: ecqi.healthit.gov/ecqms
2. Quality Check: www.qualitycheck.org
3. QualityNet: www.qualitynet.org/dcs/ContentServer?c=Page&pagename=QnetPublic%2FPage%2FQnetHomepage&cid=1120143435383

PEDIATRIC QUALITY METRICS: BACKGROUND

Measuring and reporting healthcare quality is now standard across the U.S. healthcare system, driven in part by the passage of the Patient

TABLE 7.2 TJC CHART-ABSTRACTED MEASURES

ED-1 Median Time from ED Arrival to ED Departure for Admitted ED Patients
ED-2 Median Admit Decision Time to ED Departure Time for Admitted Patients
PC-1 Elective Delivery
VTE-6 Hospital Acquired Potentially-Preventable Venous Thromboembolism
IMM-2 Influenza Immunization

ED, emergencydepartment; IMM, immunizations; PC, perinatal care;TJC, The Joint Commission; VTE, venous thromboembolism.

Source: From Eligible Hospital / Critical Access Hospital eCQMs. Retrieved from https://ecqi.healthit.gov/eligible-hospital/critical-access-hospital-ecqms

Protection and Affordable Care Act (ACA), and in pediatrics, the Children's Health Insurance Program Reauthorization Act (CHIPRA). Gaps between care expected and care delivered based on quality reporting requirements put forth by health plans or federal agencies like the Child Health Insurance Program can impact payment for services and are also tracked on publicly available dashboards. Indicators, or measures of quality care in pediatrics, are developed by varied entities, including federal agencies and healthcare professional organizations (National Academies [U.S.] Committee on Pediatric Health and Health Care Quality Measures, 2011).

Identifying the important elements of care to measure includes a rigorous review of the current available evidence that applies to the population. Input from experts in the field and others who have a stake in the outcomes of care delivered is also sought. This can include healthcare professionals, parents, the public and/or other invested groups, like large healthcare associations or foundations (CMS, 2018). Agencies that publish quality measures develop several key focus areas and update the measures, revising and adding new indicators in regular intervals based on progress, and new developments or healthcare challenges (American Academy of Pediatrics, 2018; House, Coon, Schroeder, & Ralston, 2017).

National quality indicators in pediatric healthcare encompass a broad range of care delivery settings, including the primary care medical home (Sternberg, Co, & Homer, 2011), inpatient hospitals (Stang, Straus, Crotts, Johnson, & Guttmann, 2013), and home or community care settings (CMS, 2018). In addition, over the past several years, quality indicators have been identified for a number of specific pediatric populations. Some examples include children with special healthcare needs, those requiring complex care (Barnert et al., 2018; Chen, Schrager, & Mangione-Smith, 2012), those in foster care (Deans et al., 2018), and adolescents in transition from pediatric to adult care settings (Fair et al., 2015). Less common patient populations, including children who are ventilator dependent (González et al., 2017), or receiving palliative care services (Thienprayoon, San Julian Mark, & Grossoehme, 2018), also have established metrics for quality care. This section highlights broader national pediatric specific quality metrics.

Healthcare Effectiveness Data and Information Set Pediatric Measures

The National Committee for Quality Assurance (NCQA) developed the Healthcare Effectiveness Data and Information Set (HEDIS) measures and describes them as widely used performance-improvement tools. The NCQA also has accreditation for health plans and recognition of patient-centered medical homes. The 2018 key pediatric measures for primary care include frequency of well-child visits (6 by 15 months) and and an adolescent well-child visit. Screening measures include weight assessment counseling for nutrition and physical activity once in the adolescent years and laboratory screening for lead exposure by 2 years of age. Other measures include follow-up care for children prescribed medication for attention deficit hyperactivity disorder (ADHD) both within 30 days of initiation and for ongoing care. Appropriate testing for pharyngitis and medication management for children with asthma and appropriate time frames for childhood immunizations (by age 2 years) and adolescent immunization for meningococcal disease are other key measures to report.

American Academy of Pediatric Measures for Pediatric Populations

According to the American Academy of Pediatrics (AAP), quality measurement in pediatrics should have impact at the patient and practice level and children and families should remain the central focus of relevant and meaningful measures that are scientifically sound and easily integrated into practice (AAP, 2018). House et al. (2017) published a summary categorization of national pediatric quality measures, identifying 257 unique measures. The review encompassed national metrics and those from databases of leading quality organizations. The authors categorized the measures by disease, with measures related to asthma and depression being the most frequent. Some conditions with high prevalence, like upper respiratory infections, had fewer metrics; they identified some areas lacking in measures, like childhood injury which, is a common reason for healthcare encounters in pediatrics, as well as medically complex care, which uses disproportionate healthcare resources.

The authors note that process measures make up the majority of the quality metrics, but outcome measures related to discouraging excessive use of antibiotics, specifically eight unique measures related to immunizations (House et al., 2017). The CMS has an established incentive program for meaningful use of the electronic health record (EHR) that includes nine measures spanning use of asthma medications, screening for chlamydia, appropriate treatment for upper respiratory infections, and assessment for dental decay or caries in children under 20 months of age (CMSs, 2014).

Pediatric Mental Healthcare

In 2013, Zima and colleagues published national quality measures for mental healthcare in children based on an extensive review of the indicators placed by the U.S. Department of Health and Human Services through CHIPRA, and those from the National Quality Forum, a private nonprofit group that promotes healthcare quality through measurement. Nine measures were identified covering a broad range of mental health issues that impact children across the developmental spectrum. Included were measures related to management of ADHD care in primary care settings, developmental screening prior to the age of 3 years, followup after hospitalization for mental illness within 30 days, administration of the pediatric symptom checklist to assess psychological well-being between the ages of 4 to 16 years, depression screening at various ages, use of the Common Risky Behaviors Checklist, and a suicide risk assessment for children diagnosed with major depressive disorder (Zima et al., 2013).

Agency for Healthcare Research and Quality Pediatric Quality Measures Program

The Agency for Healthcare Research and Quality (AHRQ) Pediatric Quality Measures Program (PQMP) has metrics developed through chosen Centers of Excellence grantees and includes measures in eight specific areas: perinatal care, child clinical preventive services, management of acute conditions, management of chronic conditions, patient reported outcomes, duration of enrollment and coverage, availability of services, and medication reconciliation. Within each of these areas exist multiple and varied measures. For example, in the acute conditions section there is a measure for nutrition screening within the first 24 hours of admission to the pediatric intensive care unit, lower respiratory readmission rates, and overuse of imaging in children with a simple febrile seizure.

Using Pediatric Quality Measures in a DNP Project

Practice doctorate students leading change in healthcare systems through a team-based project should investigate the specific quality metrics being tracked by the organization prior to choosing an area or population of focus for improvement or program evaluation. Organizational challenges in adhering to specific measures are potential areas for conceptualizing a DNP project. For example, in a pediatric primary care setting the HEDIS measure noted previously related to ongoing follow-up for patients prescribed medication for ADHD may be an area of inconsistency and poor outcomes. Establishing baseline data on follow-ups occurring, and determining processes that impact poor adherence, leading a team to plan and implement interventions, then measuring success is an example of how using a quality measure as a focus of a project can lead to improved patient outcomes.

GERIATRIC QUALITY METRICS: BACKGROUND

DNP-prepared geriatric advanced practice nurse practitioners play an expanded role in the delivery of care, the development of care standards, and in evaluating outcomes for a growing population of adults 70 to 75 years of age and older. The broad generalized outcomes associated with geriatric care have historically been categorized as "the five Ds": death, disease, disability, discomfort, and dissatisfaction (emotional reactions; Mainz, 2003). More recent geriatric-focused outcomes refer to the "individual, family, population state, behavior, or perception that are measured along a continuum in response to an intervention" (Moorhead, Johnson, Mass, & Swanson. 2018, p. 2) specific to chronological advanced age or combined with multiple comorbid disease processes. Quality indicators (QIs) associated with geriatric care are "evidence based and are used to identify variations in the quality of care provided on both an inpatient and outpatient basis" (Farquhar, 2008, pp. 3–41). Geriatric DNPs play a key role in assessing delivery of geriatric care as it relates to continuity of care across multiply providers and ensuring care delivered is age, health, and health-status appropriate (Rand Health, 2004).

QIs associated with geriatric care have several foci, including home care, primary care, emergent care, acute care, frailty, general medical conditions, pharmacologic management, neurocognitive alterations, safety, and palliative/hospice care (Akpan et al., 2018). These care locations, or types of care delivery, can be seen to have a topical association within the AHRQ. The AHRQ indicators have three distinct domains of care quality assessment: prevention quality indicators (PQIs), inpatient quality indicators (IQIs), and patient safety indicators (PSIs;Farquhar, 2008, pp. 3–41). Although the AHRQ indicators refer to outcomes and quality of inpatient care, the intrinsic domain associations of care location or care delivery, prevention. and patient safety form the foundation of care quality assessment that extends beyond the inpatient setting. This foundation demonstrates outcome association to domain-of-care location/care delivery foci and how the specific indicators they are composed of are interdependent with each other, which, in turn, spurs care improvement.

Any project that investigates the relationships between indicators and outcomes is based on continual process improvement through use of quality indicators linked to outcomes (Ingraham et al., 2017). Important to remember is that a quality outcome is more patient centered than a process improvement indicator, and thus harder to identify and link with a specific treatment or intervention (Chin, 2014). If investigating or testing an outcome as part of a project, it is important to "ensure that reliable and valid clinical indicators are used and that they must be designed, defined, and implemented with scientific rigor" (Mainz, 2003, p. 529).

Geriatric practice and care recommendations typically have been investigated with the view of providing if/, then associations of the indicators underlying the assessed outcome. The Society for Academic Emergency Medicine (SAEM) Geriatric Task Force states that:

> Quality indicators involve operational definitions to assess
> whether care is delivered well or poorly. Unlike practice guidelines
> that strive to characterize the nuances of best possible care, quality

indicators set a minimum standard for the care expected from
clinicians and health systems. (Terrell et al., 2009, p. 422)

The care associated with the geriatric patient can be complex, involving
multiple physical, behavioral, environmental, and fiscal factors competing against the optimization of their health. The geriatric DNP is uniquely
positioned to manage and analyze clinical, financial, and health outcomes
that are reported relationally between medical interventions and health
outcomes (Edwards, Coddington, Erler, & Kirkpatrick, 2018). The process by which understanding and determining what quality indicators are
influencers of outcome(s) comprising geriatric syndromes is a fundamental
aspect of the geriatric DNP leadership role. The use of data obtained from
the outcome indicators provides a foundation from which the geriatric
DNP is able to engage in the process of evaluation to determine the need
for quality- standard changes.

For the geriatric population ideal outcome indicators capture the effect
of care processes influencing their health and well-being. These in turn
are integrated into resultant guidelines that strive to reduce variations of
practice among providers (Ingraham et al., 2017). These geriatric indicators allow for process benchmarking and assist in identifying opportunities
to address areas of care deficiencies. Part of the DNP-prepared geriatric
advanced practice nurse's role is to explore, test, evaluate, and revise current geriatric quality indicators and associated outcomes of care delivery as
well as design new innovative models of care (Edwards et al., 2018).

General Geriatric Care Quality

Age (65 years or more) in conjunction with the severity of a comorbid health
deficit or multiple comorbid health deficits, influences whether a person
is or becomes a geriatric patient requiring geriatric care (Healthy Aging,
n.d.). This defining element is important to understand as it underlies the
constructs associated with the development of quality indicators and outcomes for geriatric care and preventative practices. In general, *quality of care*
is defined as "the degree to which health services for individuals and populations increase the likelihood of desired health outcomes and are consistent
with current professional knowledge" (Maniz, 2003, p. 523). In the geriatric
population this definition is viewed through the lens of management and
prevention as effective management and preventive strategies can reduce
the deterioration in physiological capacity due to the aging process and lack
of physical stimulation (Jahan, 2016).

In 2012 the International Consortium for Health Outcomes Measurement
(ICHOM) was founded to compose global consensus-based measurement tools and documentation for different conditions and populations,
including that of older persons (65–70 years of age; Akpan et al., 2018). The

TABLE 7.3 GENERAL GERIATRIC CARE INDICATORS

Domains of Indicators	Indicators
Tier 1 *Overall survival* *Place of death* *Frailty*	***General category*** Health status, quality of life, mortality, independence, remaining at home, caregiver health, autonomy, physical health, functional status, symptom occurrence, sleep, harm, frailty stage, nutrition, weight loss
Tier 2 *Polypharmacy* *Falls* *Participation in decision-making* *Time spent in hospital*	***Mental and psychological health*** Cognition, mood, and loneliness
	Social and community Social network, support, and isolation
Tier 3 *Loneliness and isolation* *ADL* *Pain* *Mood and emotional health* *Autonomy and control* *Carer burden*	***Healthcare utilization*** Length of stay, care coordination, and discharge to place of choice
	Experience/process category Dignity, shared decision-making, access to information and advice

ADL, activities of daily living.

Source: Adapted from Akpan, A., Roberts, C., Bandeen-Roche, K., Batty, B., Bausewein, C., Bell, C., . . . Banerjee, J. (2018). Standard set of health outcome measures for older persons. *BMC Geriatrics, 18*(36), 4–10.

ICHOM developed multiple global outcome measures for older persons and consists of the following categories: general, physical health, mental and psychological, social and community, healthcare utilization and experience/process category (Akpan et al., 2018). These categories are further delineated into three tiers of outcomes based on the identified indicators of each of the categories (Table 7.3). Akpan et al. (2018) utilized the framework of Porter's outcome hierarchy to derive the outcomes of the older person for the ICHOM and explain the tiers as follows:

> Tier 1 is the most important with the outcome being survival or the best possible state achieved for a condition. Tier 2 outcomes are the issues related to achieving tier 1 outcomes such as the time to recovery from a flare up of a chronic disease or recovery from an acute disease. Included in this tier 2 are all the harms associated with investigations and treatment. Tier 3 outcomes relate to long term health status. (p. 4)

In the primary care setting, the focus of care tends to utilize assessing for geriatric syndromes versus addressing singly all of the components found in the multimorbidity of aging (Ferris et al., 2018). The decision-making and care options associated with primary care versus that of a geriatric specialty clinic, may not reflect the patient's priorities but more those of the providers, families, and or caregiver's needs (Ferris et al., 2018). In geriatric specialty clinics, clinician–patient partnerships strive to promote patients knowing their health goals and clinicians knowing how to achieve these goals (Ferris et al., 2018). This nuance is an important element to understand as it correlates with the differences observed in the foci of outcomes and indicators observed in the different types of associated primary care settings.

Geriatric Home Care

As healthcare continues to shift from an inpatient focus to an outpatient focus, the home and the use of the home as the center for care delivery is becoming synonymous with geriatric care. Home care typically includes "independent living facilities, independent living at home or living at home with supports and/or modifications to enhance health and independence" (Boland et al., 2017, para 6). Home care quality indicators (HCQIs) were first developed in 2004 by an international research network known as the International Resident Assessment Instrument (interRAI), which was a multinational effort between Canada and the United States to develop HCQIs and associated risk adjusters for the Minimum Data Set—Home Care (MDS-HC; Hirdes et al., 2004). The HCQIs developed from this initiative remain the standard by which geriatric home care outcomes are measured (Table 7.4). According to Hirdes et al. (2004) "these indicators can provide high-quality evidence on performance of plans of care, however, the ability to actually improve quality also depends on successful communication of those findings to the appropriate target audiences" (p. 679).

TABLE 7.4 HOME-CARE INDICATORS

Domains of Indicators	Indicators
Nutrition, medication, incontinence, ulcers, physical function, cognitive function, pain, safety/ environment, other	**Prevalence HCQIs** Inadequate meals, weight loss, dehydration, not receiving medication review by MD, difficulty with locomotion and no assistive device, ADL/rehab potential and no therapies, falls, social isolation and distress, delirium, negative mood, disruptive/ intense daily pain, inadequate pain control, neglect or abuse, any injuries, no flu vaccination, and any hospitalization
	Failure to improve/incidence of HCQIs Bladder incontinence, skin ulcers, ADL impairment, impaired locomotion in home, cognitive function and difficulty communicating

ADL, activities of dailing living; HCQI, home care quality indicators.

Source: Adapted from Hirdes, J., Fries, B., Morris, J., Ikegami, N., Zimmerman, D., Dalby, D., . . . Jones, R. (2004). Home Care Quality Indicators (HCQIs) based on the MDS-HC. *The Gerontologist, 44*(5), 665–679.

Geriatric Emergency Care

Care of the complex unhealthy geriatric patient requires an interprofessional team approach for the patient and support for their families and other caregivers. This is especially important when working with older adults, many of whom have multiple chronic conditions and challenging healthcare needs such as occurs with emergent care. "The Society for Academic Emergency Medicine (SAEM) and the American College of Emergency Physicians (ACEP) created the SAEM Geriatric Task Force" (Terrell et al., 2009, p. 442). This task force developed special specific outcomes for emergent impatient care focusing on outcomes associated with readmission, length of stay, complications, morbidity, and mortality (Ingraham et al., 2017; Terrell et al., 2009).

The SAEM Geriatric Task Force utilized the Assessing Care of Vulnerable Elderly (ACOVE) quality indicators as a framework for the development of their outcomes and associated indicators. This methodology approach originated in 2000 and utilized an if/then clinical phrasing that covered general medical and geriatric conditions, including comorbidities (Askari et al., 2011). From this framework, the SAEM Geriatric Task Force identified three quality gaps in care: cognitive assessment, pain management, and transitional care (Terrell et al., 2009). These, in turn, became the outcomes domains and their associated indicators of general geriatric emergent care (Table 7.5).

TABLE 7.5 EMERGENT GERIATRIC GENERAL CARE INDICATORS

Emergent Geriatric General Care	Outcome Domains	Indicators
	Cognitive assessment Pain management Transitional care	Cognitive assessment 1. Assessment of Patients with Cognitive Impairment in the ED 2. Support in the home environment to manage the patient's care 3. A plan for medical follow-up 4. Detecting whether cognitive abnormalities were previously recognized 5. ED care of patients with baseline abnormal mental status who are discharged to home Pain management 1. Assessment for the presence of acute pain should be documented within 1 hour of arrival to the ED 2. If an older adult remains in the ED for more than 6 hours, then a second pain assessment should be documented within 6 hours of arrival in the ED

(continued)

TABLE 7.5 EMERGENT GERIATRIC GENERAL CARE INDICATORS (*continued*)

Emergent Geriatric General Care	Outcome Domains	Indicators
		3. If an older adult receives pain treatment while in the ED, then a pain reassessment should be documented prior to discharge home from the ED 4. If an older adult presents to the ED and has moderate to severe pain (i.e., a numerical rating scale score of 4 or higher out of 10), then pain treatment should be initiated (or the provider should document why treatment was not initiated) 5. If an older adult receives analgesic medication while in the ED, then meperidine should be avoided Transitions of care Patient transferred to the ED nursing home or facility needs to send: 1. Reason for transfer 2. Code status (i.e., resuscitation status) 3. Medication allergies 4. Contact information for the nursing home, the primary care or on-call physician, and the resident's legal healthcare representative or closest family member 5. Medication list from care facility 6. Tests requested by nursing home providers: Need, results, done or not done Patient transferred back to care facility 7. Communication between nursing home and ED providers: Patient discharged back to care facility 8. ED diagnosis 9. Tests performed with results (and tests with pending results) 10. Provider follow-up recommended: The patient should receive the follow-up (or the medical record should indicate why the follow-up did not occur) 11. ED provider prescribes or recommends a medication: The nursing home should administer the medication (or document in the medical record why the medication was not administered)

ED, emergency department.

Source: Adapted from Terrell, K. M., Hustey, F. M., Hwang, U., Gerson, L. W., Wenger, N. S., Miller, D. K., & on behalf of the Society for Academic Emergency Medicine Geriatric Task Force. (2009). Quality indicators for geriatric emergency care. *Academic Emergency Medicine, 16*(5), 441–449.

Geriatric Safety

Geriatric safety and the associated elements that impact outcomes are divided into inpatient and outpatient settings. AHRQ patient safety indicators reflect the inpatient assessment of care outcomes for all patients, including those of the geriatric population, which is a subset of the adult population. Although the literature has identified that the geriatric population has unique inpatient care needs (Brand et al., 2011; Ingraham et al., 2017; Terrell et al., 2009), the AHRQ patient safety indicators do not currently address monitoring of specific geriatric care such as those associated with geriatric syndromes or geriatric prone complications.

Although AHRQ does not define specific geriatric inpatient care indicators, geriatric comanagement programs are emerging as collaboratives that identify inpatient quality indicators. The intent of these collaborative programs is to focus on the prevention and management of geriatric syndromes and geriatric complications in the acute care setting (Van Grootven et al., 2018) thus reflecting an extension of the AHRQ patient safety indicators. According to Van Grootven et al. (2018), the quality indicators for in-hospital comanagement programs incorporate three types of indicators, which are explained as:

> Structure indicators which refer to health system characteristics that affect the system's ability to meet the healthcare needs of individual patients or a community. Process indicators refer to what the provider did for the patient and how well it was done and outcome indicators refer to states of health or events that follow care and that may be affected by healthcare. (Van Grootven et al., 2018, p. 2)

Within each of these indicator domains specific indicators are clearly defined (Table 7.6). The structure domain has eight indicators that identify who is part of the collaborative team, their roles, and responsibilities; how evidence-based practice will be used and how order sets are integrated. The process domain has seven indicators that identify patient care team timing interactions, ongoing team communication requisites, patient preference documentation, and discharge planning initiation. The outcomes domain indicator incorporates sixteen indicators that more closely mirror AHRQ inpatient safety indicators related to the hospitalization, readmission, patient/caregiver satisfaction, discharge type, and mortality. This indicator domain also addresses assessing for geriatric syndrome advancement and hospitalization complications, specifically those affecting the geriatric patient more prevalently.

Outpatient quality safety outcomes and indicators for geriatric patients tend to be based on processes of care delivery and management of associated care, which indirectly reflect back to patient safety. Within ICHOM tier two,

TABLE 7.6 GERIATRIC SAFETY COLLABORATIVE MANAGEMENT INDICATORS

Geriatric Safety Collaborative Management	Domains of Indicators	Indicators
	Structure Process Outcome	**Structure Indicators** 1. Collaborative team: A geriatrician, PCP, RN, NP PT, OT, social worker, case manager 2. Daily team availability 3. Annual team indicator evaluation meeting 4. New-member orientation, annual education meeting 5. Multidisciplinary pathway for roles and responsibilities 6. Use EB geriatric screening tools 7. Use EB protocols for prevention and management of geriatric syndromes and complications 8. Use standard geriatric order sets
		Process indicators 1. Care instituted within 24 hours of patient admission 2. Daily patient rounds by a team member 3. Collaborative care management meetings at min 2 times per week 4. Tracking (by %) of patients who were screened using an EB tool associated with specified geriatric syndrome problems 5. Tracking (by %) of patients who had personal care preferences documented 6. Tracking (by %) of patients who had a discharge plan documented in record 7. Tracking (by %) of patients' summary of their hospital care and postdischarge instructions sent to their PCP and/or care facility
		Outcome indicators 1. Mean length of stay in the hospital 2. Mean time spent in the ED 3. Mean time from hospital admission to surgery 4. Readmission rate within 30 days and 3 months of hospital discgarge 5. Patient satisfaction with hospital care 6. Caregiver satisfaction with hospital care provided for patients included in the geriatric comanagement program 7. Percentage of time restraints used during admission 8. In-hospital mortality rate Percentage of patients admitted to rehab/nursing home at discharge 9. Percentage of patients who declined in functional status between hospital admission and hospital discharge 10. Percentage of patients who developed delirium

(continued)

TABLE 7.6 GERIATRIC SAFETY COLLABORATIVE MANAGEMENT
INDICATORS (*continued*)

Geriatric Safety Collaborative Management	Domains of Indicators	Indicators
		11. Percentage of patients who developed a urinary tract infection
		12. Percentage of patients who developed a wound infection
		13. Percentage of patients who developed pneumonia
		14. Percentage of patients who developed sepsis
		15. Percentage of patients who developed pressure ulcers

EB, evidence based; OT, occupational therapy; PCP, primary care provider; PT, physical therapy.

Source: Adapted from Van Grootven, B., McNicoll, L., Mendelson, D., Friedman, S., Fagard, K., Flamaing, J., & Deschodt, M. (2018). Quality indicators for in-hospital geriatric co-management programmes: A systematic literature review and international Delphi study. *BMJ Open, 8,* e020617. doi:10.1136/bmjopen-2017-020617

polypharmacy and falls are the main safety-focus domains. Polypharmacy is identified as an indicator of probability for drug-related problems occurring in the geriatric population as well as a means to determine the need for medication evaluation for potential reduction (Gustafsson et al., 2015). According to Levy (2017), the Beers Criteria (developed by the American Geriatrics Society), the Screening Tool of Older Persons' potentially inappropriate Prescriptions (STOPP; Gallagher et al., 2008), and the Screening Tool to Alert doctors to the Right Treatment (START; Gallagher et al., 2008), although not technically termed *quality indicators*, do provide identification of risk and need for evaluation or intervention from a provider to ascertain safe continuation of a patient's current medication regimen.

PUBLIC HEALTH QUALITY METRICS: BACKGROUND

The U.S. public health system has a long history of measuring and disseminating population quality metrics, tbeginning in the early 20th century as the nation's public health tiered infrastructure was taking hold (Starr, 1982). Evaluation of *quality* in public health is as multifactorial and multifaceted as the public health system itself, encompassing metrics being tracked and collated at the federal level as much as they are compiled and reported by local health departments. *Public health quality metrics* are as diverse as the epidemiological data of disease burden in the United States, which might include citizen's satisfaction with public health services in their community, or time-trend data tracked on a specific primary-prevention initiative (Derose, Schuster, Fielding, & Asch, 2002). This diversity of quality metric types can make it difficult for the beginning advanced public health nurse (APHN) clinician to identify the best data to report in change projects. In this section, we discuss how quality metrics are defined in public health systems, the developing arena of public health quality improvement, and applications of quality metrics for clinical doctorate projects having a public health focus.

Public Health Quality Metrics Defined

Those working in the U.S. public health system have long struggled with how best to measure *health*, in addition to defining the value of public health as well as defining quality (Turnock, 2004). Over the years, morbidity and mortality data have remained constant benchmarks for the health of the United States as well as how state and local health departments assess well-being of its citizenry. Such measures as *total life expectancy, health status index, years of healthy life, years of potential life lost, quality-adjusted life years,* and *disability-adjusted life years* indeed describe "quality of life" from a population standpoint, but are much harder to track as an indicator for program evaluation projects desiring short-term results.

Since the initiation of the Affordable Care Act initiatives, there has been more attention paid to the term *population health* and its related metrics (Stoto, 2013), which, in turn, has shifted more focus to primary prevention initiatives long administered by the public health system (IOM, 2014). For public health practitioners working in that arena, *population-focused care* and population health defines the groups of people or communities that public health systems serve (Kindig & Stoddart, 2003; McGinnis, Williams-Russo, & Knickman, 2002). Because the ACA redefined aspects of health payment systems and the economics of care (Geruso & McGuire, 2016), health plans, primary care systems, and acute care facilities have embraced population health when identifying at-risk care groups and costly patient populations for new care initiatives (American Hospital Association, 2014). The metrics used in these settings tend to be the same epidemiological data for illness and disease that public health systems might use, only with the population denominator of the organization or agency. And still emerging from this shift in more widespread use of the term *population health* is how primary prevention initiatives are being realized (or not) in these alternative settings. Advanced practice clinicians of all stripes would do well to watch for these trends in redefining population health and care of those most in need over the next decade.

An accreditation coalition of national public health agencies worked together in the late 2000s to define public health quality metrics and quality improvement in order to build on the IOM's *Future of Public Health* report (IOM, 1988) and to support quality initiatives occurring in other areas of the U.S. healthcare constellation. From these expert panel meetings, the *Consensus Statement on Quality in the Public Health System* (US Department of Health and Human Services [USDHHS], 2008) was written to serve as the unanimous voice for defining quality in public health.

Public Health Quality Improvement

Only in the past decade have public health systems and practitioners turned an eye to public health quality improvement and its potential to improve program delivery (Riley et al., 2010). As these landmark white papers have made their way to administrators and frontline practitioners of public health, it has forced a re-visioning of how programs and agencies are evaluated and by what indicators. Public health systems began to apply principles of "Big QI" and "small qi," as described by Riley et al. (2010), to address organizational infrastructure and individual projects, respectively, for a more holistic approach to systems change. Traditional public health planning models like Mobilizing Action for Community Health (MATCH; https://uwphi.pophealth.wisc.edu/match) then underscored the need for clear quality metrics in logic model outcomes (Pestronk, 2010).

Another watershed moment for public health quality improvement came about in tandem with these other national movements, when the Public Health Accreditation Board incorporated in 2007 and public health standards for accreditation launched in 2011 (Public Health Accreditation Board [PHAB], 2019). Standard 9 of the Public Health Accreditation Standards (PHAB, 2013) focuses on continuous quality improvement of health departments and ensuring that process management includes quality metrics. As a result of these changes in public health system infrastructure, APHNs now find themselves leaders of QI initiatives in their local and state public health departments andas such need to develop advanced skills in QI processes and quality metric interpretations for their organizations.

Application of Quality Metrics in Clinical Doctorate Programs

APHN education has long featured graduate educational preparation in community needs assessment, health need prioritization, program planning, development, implementation, and evaluation. The few DNP programs nationally that feature community/public health degree options have tended to embrace such change projects to create new programs from scratch as scholarship for the terminal degree. With the advent of public health quality improvement as a developing methodology, APHNs must develop skills in QI and consider change projects in health departments akin to clinical peers in acute or primary care settings.

For the clinical doctoral APHN, epidemiological data must frame change projects as they would any DNP project. But students considering quality metrics for population-focused projects should be cautioned not to get lost in the many levels of potential impacts of new programs and to carefully match metrics to their logic models in order to stay focused on project outcomes. Because APHN graduate students often walk "two worlds" integrating the disciplinary perspectives of both public health and nursing, they can sometimes lose sight of project scope and outcomes without clear advising and mentorship. Another common pitfall relates to the timeline of doctoral change projects and public health projects that can take much more of the time needed to implement and see tangible outcomes.

There are incredible resources for the APHN graduate student to rely on to frame public health change projects and track quality metrics. The Public Health Quality Improvement Exchange (www.phqix.org), supported by the Robert Wood Johnson Foundation, has emerged as a top resource to support public health practitioners . The Public Health Improvement Resource Center (www.phf.org/improvement), powered by the Public Health Foundation, has proven another incredible tool to collate knowledge on facets of public health QI accreditation, and public health essential services. A number of program planning models such as Mobilizing Action Toward Community Health (MATCH), Assessment Protocol for Excellence in Public Health (APEX-PH), and Mobilizing for Action through Planning and Partnerships (MAPP) highlight how to best develop public health metrics and reasonable outcomes for program evaluation. Finally, the *Guidebook for Performance Measurement* (Lichiello & Turnock, 1999) is an incredible resource to guide readers through performance metric development and its application to projects.

In summary, the U.S. public health system has embraced metrics and quality in program delivery for the past 80 years. APHNs have been leaders in public health systems since that time and contribute a great deal to how quality is measured in their communities. Population health demands value and QIs to support the critical work happening in local and state health departments, with the important end goal of meeting the World Health Organization's (WHO) definition of health as "a state of complete physical, mental and social well-being, and not merely the absence of disease or infirmity" (WHO, n.d.).

QUALITY METRICS FOR AMBULATORY CARE: BACKGROUND

Increasing the amount of care has moved away from the inpatient setting and into ambulatory care. With the variation of clinical foci in ambulatory care, it is difficult to identify common quality metrics to use for assessment of quality of care. In January of 2014 the American Nurses Association (ANA) held an Ambulatory Care Summit, which included members of the American Academy of Ambulatory Care Nursing (AAACN; Martinez, Battaglia, Start, Mastal, & Matlock, 2015). After an iterative process of considering a variety of quality metrics for ambulatory care, the group proposed the following indicators: readmissions, pain assessment and follow-up, hypertension, depression screening, and medication reconciliation (Martinez et al., 2015). Further work the following year added additional measures of falls, body mass index (BMI), nurse demographics, and patient satisfaction. Table 7.7 describes these various measures.

TABLE 7.7 AAACN NURSE-SENSITIVE INDICATORS TASK FORCE-PROPOSED INDICATORS FOR DEVELOPMENT OF AMBULATORY CARE NURSE-SENSITIVE INDICATORS

Measure Name	Measure Description
Hospital Readmission	Risk-adjusted percentage of accountable care organization (ACO)-assigned beneficiaries who were hospitalized and readmitted to a hospital within 30 days following discharge from the hospital for the index admission
Pain Assessment and Follow-Up	Percentage of patients of all ages with documentation of a pain assessment through discussion with the patient, including the use of a standardized tool(s) on each visit and documentation of a follow-up plan when pain is present
Hypertension and Follow-Up Care	Percentage of patients of all ages seen during the measurement period who are screened for high blood pressure and a recommended follow-up plan is documented based on the current blood pressure reading as indicated
Depression Screening and Follow-Up	Percentage of patients in one of the identified populations who received a depression screening during a visit encounter Percentage of patients in one of the identified populations who screened positive and have a follow-up plan of care for depression
Falls in the Institution	All documented falls, with our without injury, experienced by patients on eligible unit types in a calendar quarter; reported as total falls per 1,000 patient visits and unassisted falls per 1,000 patient visits
Screening for BMI	Percentage of patients with a calculated BMI in the past 6 months or during the current visit documented in the medical record and if the most recent BMI is outside of normal parameters, a follow-up plan is documented within the past 6 months or during the current visit
Ambulatory Care Nurse RN Demographics	• % diploma RN FTE • % associate's degree RN FTE • % bachelor's of science degree RN FTE • % master's of science degree RN FTE • % doctorate in nursing degree RN FTE • % certified RN FTE • % certified RN in specialty field FTE • % turnover RN by FTE • % vacancy RN by FTE
Nurse Patient Satisfaction	The percentage of surveys that were returned within a defined period and of questions that are nursing specific and answered by the patient as "always"

BMI, body mass index; FTE, full-time equivalent.

Source: Adapted from Start, R., Matlock, A.M., & Mastal, P. (2016). *Ambulatory care nurse-sensitive indicator industry report: Meaningful measurement of nursing in the ambulatory patient care environment.* Pitman, NJ: American Academy of Ambulatory Care Nurses.

AAACN has recently partnered with the Collaborative Alliance for Nursing Outcomes (CALNOC) to further define quality metrics for ambulatory care settings. CALNOC is advancing this work through delineation of ambulatory care quality indicators for various service lines, including surgery and procedure centers, cancer centers, and urgent care centers (CALNOC, n.d.). Use of consistent measures across ambulatory service lines will facilitate the adoption of evidence-based practice and best practices, and contribute to more reliable measures of quality of ambulatory care.

CONCLUSIONS

Clinical specialties often identify quality metrics specific to the care provided in that care area. Having well-targeted, relevant quality metrics facilitates the honing of quality-improvement work to impact care that is meaningful and significant. As DNP leaders work to improve healthcare systems, it is important that they are familiar with the quality metrics specific to their clinical area and their clinical setting. The increased standardization of quality metrics facilitates effective comparison of matched outcomes across similar settings. Being able to benchmark performance compared to similar practices provides helpful data for systems leaders to target their improvement work.

Case Study

Exemplar Hospital (EH) is a small, 40-bed care facility located within Rural town, a small town within the United States. EH has one of the only emergency departments (ED) within a 60-mile radius. A recent survey was conducted by The Joint Commission, in conjunction with evaluation of electronic clinical quality measures (eCQM) data supplied by EH. It was determined that emergency wait times at EH were longer than at other facilities within the state and compared to national statistics. In order to provide improved access to care for patients coming through this busy emergency department, the ED director wants to examine the wait time at their facility. A DNP student has been recruited to assist with this project in the ED at EH.

QUESTIONS

1. What two databases are available for the DNP student to evaluate EH emergency department wait times?
2. What eCQMs are pertinent to this project?
3. What other data provided by TJC would be useful in helping the DNP student set goals for the emergency department wait times?

REFERENCES

Akpan, A., Roberts, C., Bandeen-Roche, K., Batty, B., Bausewein, C., Bell, C., . . . Banerjee, J. (2018). Standard set of health outcome measures for older persons. *BMC Geriatrics, 18*(36). 4–10. doi:10.1186/s12877-017-0701-3

American Academy of Pediatrics. (2018). Pediatric quality measurement. Retrieved from https://www.aap.org/en-us/professional-resources/quality-improvement/Pages/Pediatric-Quality-Measurement.aspx

American Hospital Association. (2014). Population health definition. Retrieved from https://www.aha.org/infographics/2014-11-12-population-health-definition

Askari, M., Wierenga, P. C., Eslami, S., Medlock, S., de Rooij, S. E., & Abu-Hanna, A. (2011). Assessing quality of care of elderly patients using the ACOVE quality indicator set: A Systematic Review. *PLoS ONE, 6*(12), e28631. doi:10.1371/journal.pone.0028631

Barnert, E. S., Coller, R. J., Nelson, B. B., Thompson, L. R., Klitzner, T. S., Szilagyi, M., . . . Chung, P. J. (2018). A healthy life for a child with medical complexity: 10 domains for conceptualizing health. *Pediatrics, 142*(3), e20180779. doi:10.1542/peds.2018-0779

Boland, L., Légaré, F., Becerra Perez, M., Menear, M., Garvelink, M., McIsaac, D., . . . Stacey, D. (2017). Impact of home care versus alternative locations of care on elder health outcomes: An overview of systematic reviews. *BMC Geriatrics 17*(1), 1–15. doi:10.1186/s12877-016-0395-y

Bonow, R. O., Masoudi, F. A., Rumsfeld, J. S., DeLong, E., Estes, N. A., Goff, D. C., . . . Shahian, D. M. (2008). ACC/AHA classification of care metrics: Performance measures and quality metrics. *Circulation, 118*, 2662–2666. doi:10.1161/CIRCULATIONAHA.108.191107

Brand, C., Martin-Khan, M., Wright, O., Jones, R. N., Morris, J., Travers, C., . . . Gray, L. (2011). Development of quality indicators for monitoring outcomes of frail elderly hospitalized in acute care health settings: Study Protocol. *BMC Health Services Research, 11*(281), 1–8. Retrieved from http://www.biomedcentral.com/1472-6963/11/281

Center for Medicare & Medicaid Services. (2014). *2014 clinical quality measures: Pediatric recommended core measures*. Bethesda, MD: CMS Publications.

Centers for Medicare & Medicaid Services. (2018). Childrens health care quality measures. Retrieved from https://www.medicaid.gov/medicaid/quality-of-care/performance-measurement/child-core-set/index.html

Chen, A. Y., Schrager, S. M., & Mangione-Smith, R. (2012). Quality measures for primary care of complex pediatric patients. *Pediatrics, 129*(3), 433–445. doi:10.1542/peds.2011-0026

Chin, M. H. (2014). How to achieve health equity. *New England Journal of Medicine, 371*(24), 2331–2332. doi:10.1056/NEJMe1412264

Collaborative Alliance for Nursing Outcomes. (n.d.). CALNOC ambulatory service lines and measures. Retrieved from https://www.aaacn.org/sites/default/files/documents/misc-docs/CALNOCAmbulatoryBrochure.pdf

Deans, K. J., Minneci, P. C., Nacion, K. M., Leonhart, K., Cooper, J. N., Scholle, S. H., & Kelleher, K. J. (2018). Health care quality measures for children and adolescents in Foster Care: Feasibility testing in electronic records. *BMC Pediatrics, 18*(1), 79. doi:10.1186/s12887-018-1064-4

DeRose, S. F., Schuster, M. A., Fielding, J. E., & Asch, S. M. (2002). Public health quality measurement: concepts and challenges. *Annual Review of Public Health, 23*(1), 1–21. doi:10.1146/annurev.publhealth.23.092601.095644

Edwards, N., Coddington, J., Erler, C., & Kirkpatrick, J. (2018). The impact of the role of doctor of nursing practice nurses on healthcare and leadership. *Medical Research Archives, 6*(4). Retrieved from https://journals.ke-i.org/index.php/mra/article/view/1734

Electronic Clinical Quality Improvement Resource Center. (n.d.). Inpatient electronic clinical quality measures supported by The Joint Commission. Retrieved from https://ecqi.healthit.gov/eligible-hospital/critical-access-hospital-ecqms

Fair, C., Cuttance, J., Sharma, N., Maslow, G., Weiner, L., Betz, C., . . . for the International and Interdisciplinary Health Care Transition Research Consortium. (2015). International and interdisciplinary identification of healthcare transition outcomes. *JAMA Pediatrics, 170*(3), 205. doi:10.1001/jamapediatrics.2015.3168

Farquhar, M. (2008). AHRQ quality indicators. In R. G. Hughes (Ed.), *Patient safety and quality: An evidence-based handbook for nurses* (pp. 3-41–3-67). Rockville, MD: Agency for Healthcare Research and Quality. Retrieved from https://www.ncbi.nlm.nih.gov/books/NBK2664/pdf/Bookshelf_NBK2664.pdf

Ferris, R., Blaum, C., Kiwak, E., Austin, J., Esterson, J., Harkless, G., . . . Tinetti, M. (2018). Perspectives of patients, clinicians, and health system leaders on changes needed to improve the health care and outcomes of older adults with multiple chronic conditions. *Journal of Aging and Health, 30*(5), 778–799. doi:10.1177/0898264317691166

Gallagher, P., Ryan, C., & Byrne, S. (2008). STOPP (Screening Tool of Older Persons' Prescriptions) and START (Screening Tool to Alert Doctors to Right Treatment): consensus validation. *International Journal of Clinical Pharmacology, 46*, 72–83.

Geruso, M., & McGuire, T. G. (2016). Tradeoffs in the design of health plan payment systems: Fit, power and balance. *Journal of Health Economics, 47*, 1–19. doi:10.1016/j.jhealeco.2016.01.007

González, R., Bustinza, A., Fernandez, S. N., García, M., Rodriguez, S., García-Teresa, M., . . . López-Herce, J. (2017). Quality of life in home-ventilated children and their families. *European Journal of Pediatrics, 176*(10), 1307–1317. doi:10.1007/s00431-017-2983-z

Gustafsson, M., Sandman, P. O., Karlsson, S., Isaksson, U., Schneede, J., Sjölander, M., & Lövheim, H. (2015). Reduction in the use of potentially inappropriate drugs among old people living in geriatric care units between 2007 and 2013. *European Journal of Clinical Pharmacology, 71*(4), 507–515. doi:10.1007/s00228-015-1825-z

Healthy Aging. (n.d.). Aging & health A to Z: Geriatrics: Basic facts and information. Retrieved from https://www.healthinaging.org/a-z-topic/geriatrics/basic-facts

Hirdes, J., Fries, B., Morris, J., Ikegami, N., Zimmerman, D., Dalby, D., . . . Jones, R. (2004). Home care quality indicators (HCQIs) based on the MDS-HC. *The Gerontologist, 44*(5), 665–679. doi:10.1093/geront/44.5.665

House, S. A., Coon, E. R., Schroeder, A. R., & Ralston, S. L. (2017). Categorization of national pediatric quality measures. *Pediatrics, 139*(4), e20163269. doi:10.1542/peds.2016-3269

Ingraham, A., Nathens, A., Peitzman, A., Bode, A., Dorlac, G., Dorlac, W., . . . Bilimoria, K. (2017). Assessment of emergency general surgery care based on formally developed quality indicators. *Surgery, 162*(2), 397–407. doi:10.1016/j.surg.2017.03.025

Institute of Medicine. (1988). *The future of the public's health in the 21st century.* Washington, DC: National Academies Press.

Institute of Medicine. (2000). *To err is human: Building a safer health system.* Washington, DC: National Academies Press.

Institute of Medicine. (2014). *Population health implications of the Affordable Care Act: Workshop summary.* Roundtable on Population Health Improvement; Board on Population Health and Public Health Practice. Washington, DC: National Academies Press. Retrieved from https://www.ncbi.nlm.nih.gov/books/NBK268842

Jahan, F. (2016). The role of primary care physician in geriatric care. *Diversity and Equality in Health Care, 13*(3), 245. Retrieved from http://diversityhealthcare.imedpub.com/the-role-of-primary-care-physician-in-geriatric-care.pdf

Kindig, D., & Stoddart, G. (2003). What is population health? *American Journal of Public Health, 93*(3), 380–383. doi:10.2105/AJPH.93.3.380

Levy, H. B. (2017). Polypharmacy reduction strategies. *Clinics in Geriatric Medicine, 33*(2), 177–187. doi:10.1016/j.cger.2017.01.007

Lichiello, P., & Turnock, B. J. (1999). *Guidebook for performance measurement.* Turning Point Resources on Performance Management. Retrieved from http://www.phf.org/resources tools/Documents/PMCguidebook.pdf

Lohr, K. N. (1990). Medicare: A strategy for quality assurance. Vols I and II. Washington, DC: National Academies Press. Retrieved from https://www.nap.edu/catalog/1547/medicare-a-strategy-for-quality-assurance-volume-i

Mainz, J. (2003). Defining and classifying clinical indicators for quality improvement. *International Journal for Quality in Healthcare, 15*(6), 523–530.

Martinez, K., Battaglia, R., Start, R., Mastal, M. F., & Matlock, A. M. (2015). Nursing-sensitive indicators in ambulatory care. *Nursing Economics, 33*(1), 59–66.

McGinnis, J. M., Williams-Russo, P., & Knickman, J. R. (2002). The case for more active policy attention to health promotion. *Health Affairs, 21*(2), 78–93. doi:10.1377/hlthaff.21.2.78

Moorhead, S., Johnson, M., Maas, M. L., & Swanson, E. (2018). *Nursing outcomes classification (NOC) E-book: Measurement of health outcomes.* St Louis, MI: Elsevier.

National Academies (U.S.) Committee on Pediatric Health and Health Care Quality Measures. (2011). *Child and adolescent health and health care quality: Measuring what matters.* Washington, DC: National Academies Press.

Pestronk, R. M. (2010). Using metrics to improve population health. *Preventing Chronic Disease, 7*(4). Retrieved from https://journals.ke-i.org/index.php/mra/article/view/1734

Public Health Accreditation Board. (2013). Public Health Accreditation Board standards & Measures (Version 1.5). Retrieved from http://www.phaboard.org/wp-content/uploads/PHABSM_WEB_LR1.pdf

Public Health Accreditation Board. (2019). Public health department accreditation background (online). Retrieved from https://www.phaboard.org/accreditation-background/

Rand Health. (2004). Developing quality of care indicators for the vulnerable Eelderly: The ACOVE project. Retrieved from https://pdfs.semanticscholar.org/19a7/9fd70bb7caf98d981644525bf23ec49a2a9a.pdf

Riley, W. J., Moran, J. W., Corso, L. C., Beitsch, L. M., Bialek, R., & Cofsky, A. (2010). Defining quality improvement in public health. *Journal of Public Health Management and Practice, 16*(1), 5–7. doi:10.1097/PHH.0b013e3181bedb49

Stang, A. S., Straus, S. E., Crotts, J., Johnson, D. W., & Guttmann, A. (2013). Quality indicators for high acuity pediatric conditions. *Pediatrics, 132*(4), 752–762. doi:10.1542/peds.2013-0854

Starr, P. (1982). *The social transformation of American medicine.* New York, NY: Basic Books.

Sternberg, S. B., Co, J. P., & Homer, C. J. (2011). Review of quality measures of the most integrated health care settings for children and the need for improved measures: Recommendations for initial core measurement set for CHIPRA. *Academic Pediatrics, 11*(3 Suppl.), S49–S58.e43. doi:10.1016/j.acap.2011.02.006

Stoto, M. A. (2013). *Population health in the Affordable Care Act era* (Vol. 1). Washington, DC: Academy Health.

Terrell, K. M., Hustey, F. M., Hwang, U., Gerson, L. W., Wenger, N. S., Miller, D. K., & on behalf of the Society for Academic Emergency Medicine Geriatric Task Force. (2009). Quality indicators for geriatric emergency care. *Academic Emergency Medicine, 16*(5). 441–449. doi:10.1111/j.1553-2712.2009.00382.x

The Joint Commission. (n.d). Facts about ORYX for hospitals (national hospital quality measures). Retrieved from https://www.jointcommission.org/facts_about_oryx_for_hospitals

Thienprayoon, R., San Julian Mark, M., & Grossoehme, D. (2018). Provider-prioritized domains of quality in pediatric home-based hospice and palliative care: A study of the Ohio pediatric palliative care and end-of-life network. *Journal of Palliative Medicine, 21*(3), 290–296. doi:10.1089/jpm.2017.0333

Turnock, B. J. (2004). *Public health: What it is and how it works* (3rd ed.). Sudbury, MA: Jones & Bartlett.

U.S. Department of Health and Human Services. (2008). *Consensus statement on quality in the public health system.* Washington, DC: Author.

Van Grootven, B., McNicoll, L., Mendelson, D., Friedman, S., Fagard, K., Flamaing, J., & Deschodt, M. (2018). Quality indicators for in-hospital geriatric co-management programmes: A systematic literature review and international Delphi study. *BMJ Open, 8*, e020617. doi:10.1136/bmjopen-2017-020617

World Health Organization. (n.d.). World Health Organization Constitution. Retrieved from https://www.who.int/about/who-we-are/constitution.

Zima, B. T., Murphy, J. M., Scholle, S. H., Hoagwood, K. E., Sachdeva, R. C., Mangione-Smith, R., . . . Jellinek, M. (2013). National quality measures for child mental health care: Background, progress, and next steps. *Pediatrics, 131*(Suppl. 1), S38–S49. doi:10.1542/peds.2012-1427e

8

LEADERSHIP AND TEAM SCIENCE

REBECCA S. MILTNER | CORI JOHNSON | KATHLEEN E. MILTNER

> **This chapter addresses the following DNP American Association of Colleges of Nursing (AACN) Essentials:**
>
> II. Organizational and Systems Leadership for Quality Improvement and Systems Thinking
> VI. Interprofessional Collaboration for Improving Patient and Population Health Outcomes

INTRODUCTION

Current estimates indicate that healthcare error may be the third most common reason for death in the United States after heart disease and cancer (James, 2013). Despite growing evidence on actions that can improve healthcare systems and processes, failure to implement evidence- based actions that can improve healthcare systems and processes is ongoing (Nembhard, Alexander, Hoff, & Ramanujam, 2012). Nembhard et al. (2012) suggest that there are multiple organizational features that inhibit system changes to improve care. These include the nature of the work (which is high risk and can involve fatalities and requires a high degree of clinical discretion) and a workforce that identifies more with professional boundaries and long-established hierarchies, and less as a member of the organization. Building effective teams can break down these professional boundaries that hinder efforts to improve care.

Quality-improvement methods offer a systematic, data-driven, iterative, problem-solving process that can be adapted to any local context. It is important to note that all quality-improvement works occurs within the context of the team(s). Stated simply, improving healthcare is a team sport. High-quality, safe organizations require reliable, adaptive, and self-correcting teams (Salas, Zajac, & Marlow, 2018). This need is recognized by many healthcare leaders, who seek to build a culture of safety; teamwork improves the safety and quality of care, may improve the coordination of services, increases professional satisfaction, and may maximize resources with more efficient delivery of care (Hughes et al., 2016; Rosen et al., 2018). However, many teams struggle to perform optimally, especially without leadership support or in cultures that do not value teamwork.

What is a team? A simple definition is: a group organized for some kind of work or activity. A common definition used in management is: a small number of people with complementary skills committed to a common purpose and goals who hold each other mutually accountable (Katzenbach & Smith, 1993). The key characteristics of teams include an emphasis on shared goals, group accountability, and mechanisms for mutually respectful communication within the group.

The critical importance of high-functioning teams in healthcare is widely recognized. In 2012, some members of the Institute of Medicine (IOM) Roundtable on Value & Science-Driven Health Care identified core principles of team-based healthcare (Mitchell et al., 2012). These principles include shared goals, clear roles, mutual trust, effective communication, and measurable processes and outcomes (Table 8.1). Conscious use of these principles in teambuilding can enhance the team's ability to accomplish goals, especially in improvement work.

The Science of Teamwork

The science of teamwork has moved beyond early descriptions of team characteristics, such as size, history, classifications by temporal stability,

TABLE 8.1 PRINCIPLES OF TEAM-BASED HEALTHCARE

Principle	Description
Shared goals	The team works to establish shared goals that reflect patient and family priorities and are understood and supported by all team members.
Clear roles	Clear expectations for each team member's responsibilities and accountabilities are defined to optimize team efficiency.
Mutual trust	Team members earn each other's trust.
Effective communication	The team prioritizes and refines its communication skills.
Measurable processes and outcomes	The team agrees on and implements measures that are tracked over time and used to improve performance.

Source: Adapted from Mitchell, P., Wynia, M., Golden, R., McNellis, B., Okun, S., Webb, C. E., . . . Von Kohorn, I. (2012, October). Core principles & values of effectiveteam-based health care. Retrieved from https://nam.edu/wp-content/uploads/2015/06/VSRT-Team-Based-Care-Principles-Values.pdf

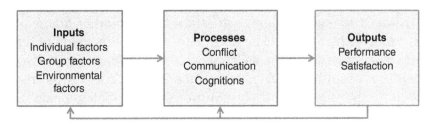

FIGURE 8.1 Conceptual model of teams using the Input—process—outputs model. match text

Source: From Mathieu, J. E., Heffner, T. S., Goodwin, G. F., Salas, E., & Cannon-Bowers, J. A. (2000). The influence of shared mental models on team process and performance. *Journal of Applied Psychology, 85*(2), 273–283. doi:10.1037//0021-9010.85.2.273

authority differentiation, and skill differentiation, and group development frameworks such as the Tuckman (1965) model for team formation (forming, storming, norming, and performing). Currently, the predominant conceptual model for studying team is the input—process—output model (IPO; Figure 8.1).

Team *inputs* are often classified as individual-level factors such as personal traits and experience, group-level factors such as group size and team norms, and environmental factors such as the organizational culture and leadership. Team *processes* can include any behaviors that convert inputs into outputs, but common categories include conflict, communication, and cognitions. Team *outputs* are the results of the work of the team and are generally grouped into either group performance, such as meeting goals or completing a project/product, or team member reactions such as satisfaction and personal development. The main criticism of this IPO model is its linear nature, which does not fully help explain the complexity of teams working with and across other teams (Salas, Reyes, & McDaniel, 2018). Some key concepts within the input and process components of the model that are critical to good teamwork are discussed in the following text.

Team Inputs

Teams in healthcare can be project teams, such as quality-improvement teams, management teams, or work teams, that provide direct functions within the organization, including patient care, administrative processes, and so on (Rosen et al., 2018). Team composition is important to the work and subsequent outcomes of the team. Interprofessional teams in healthcare can lead to better patient outcomes as team members learn to appreciate the expertise of different disciplines, especially if there are clear role boundaries (Salas, Reyes, et al., 2018).

Healthcare teams must function within the context of other teams, and the context is an important structural component of the team. Researchers have primarily focused on small teams, but there is a growing appreciation for the need to examine teams in relationship to other teams when faced with a multiteam system. The multiteam system is a "team of teams which have collective goals" (Salas, Reyes, et al., 2018, p. 598). High- quality patient care requires collaboration across multiple teams in acute care as well as ambulatory and community settings (Salas, Zajac, et al., 2018; Shuffler & Carter, 2018). These multiple teams must solve complex and time-sensitive problems that are individualized to a single patient. It is not clear that the same competencies that help a work team achieve success are the same as those that help teams collaborate with other teams (Salas, Zajac, et al., 2018). Even with shared goals, the contextual features of the individual teams may create problems when collaborating with other required teams. For example, a surgical team may be very confident in its postoperative care of patients, but that confidence may be an impediment to care coordination if the patient has a serious complication and needs intensive care overseen by intensivists. These types of team conflicts play out daily across healthcare organizations among all kinds of teams. More research is needed to advance the science around these multiteam systems (Salas, Reyes, et al., 2018).

Organizational culture is an important input for teamwork. One critical aspect of this culture is psychological safety. Psychological safety is the shared belief that team members can take risks without fear of reprisal or other negative consequences (Edmondson, 1999; Edmondson & Lei, 2014). It is an essential component that allows a team to build mutual trust and respect. Many team members frequently do not speak up because they fear embarrassment or criticism. If psychological safety is practiced, this fear is reduced, and team members are more likely to open up and express different points of view (Edmondson & Lei, 2014).

The concept of psychological safety is defined by its presence within a group; in other words, it is about how members of the team are viewed by other members of the team. This is different from the concept of trust, which is how one individual views another. This difference in these concepts is important. A team member may have a trusting relationship with another member of the team, but if the group as a whole lacks the psychological safety to express different ideas, there is a large risk for personal harm as well as a barrier to team growth. Psychological safety leads to improved team outcomes through team learning and knowledge sharing (Edmondson & Lei, 2014).

Finally, leadership is a critical input to teamwork. Leadership support is critical to creating and sustaining high- functioning teams. Senior leaders primarily impact improvement in two ways. First they provide direction for the organization, align resources to support changes, and hold other leaders accountable for the efforts. The second way they impact improvement is through role modeling commitment to quality that can inspire others within the organization (VanDeusen Lukas et al., 2007).

Senior leaders cannot inspire and lead improvement efforts without the commitment of middle managers and clinical leaders. Healthcare is just beginning to understand the vital role of these local leaders who facilitate change by diffusing information about change efforts, synthesizing information, mediating between strategy and day-to-day activities, and selling the innovation (Birken, Lee, & Weiner, 2012; Engle et al., 2017). To improve quality, advanced practice nurses can frequently serve as the liaison within interprofessional teams (Donahue et al., 2013).

Team Processes

There are several key concepts related to team processes, including conflict, communication, and cognitions. *Conflict* is an inherent part of teamwork and is conceptualized in three ways. *Group conflict* related to the *tasks* of the group involves disagreement about the goals and objectives of the group work. *Relationship conflict* is related to disagreements among members of the group, and can negatively affect team functioning. *Process conflict* focuses on disagreements about how to accomplish the tasks and assigning roles and responsibilities (de Wit, Greer, & Jehn, 2012). *Task conflict*, disagreement about the specifics of the team's work, may be necessary in order to move past the status quo to accomplish team goals (de Wit et al., 2012).

Communication is a process of exchanging information through some system of symbols, signs, or behaviors. Communication includes the ability to ask questions, seek clarification, and acknowledge the message was received and understood. Effective communication is an essential element of teamwork in healthcare in order to deliver safe, high-quality care to patients. Ineffective communication has consistently remained one of the top three root causes for patient sentinel events over the years. Furthermore, researchers estimate that communication inefficiencies result in U.S. hospitals wasting more than $12 billion annually (Agarwal, Sands, & Schneider, 2010).

Many regulatory and advocacy groups have focused on implementing standardized communication tools to reduce errors that could result in patient harm (Leonard, Graham, & Bonacum, 2004). There are four key characteristics of effective communication. The first standard is that communication must be complete in order to be effective. For instance, a team member must include all information that is relevant, while also avoiding unnecessary details that could lead to misunderstanding. Second, the communication must be clear, meaning information must be delivered in language and terminology that is understood by all members of the team. Next, effective communication is brief, concise, and free of all elaborate and unnecessary detail. Last, effective communication must be timely. Team members must all be dependable at information sharing and avoid delays in relaying important information that could impact patient outcomes.

Verifying information by ensuring that what was heard was the intended message of the sender, along with appropriate documentation and frequent updates, are important elements of effective communication (King et al., 2015).

Several tools are used by interprofessional clinical teams to improve communication. One tool that is effective in bridging communication styles among multidisciplinary team members is situation–bBackground–assessment–recommendation (SBAR). SBAR is effective because it structures conversation in a predictable and consistent way, which also facilitates organizing and prioritizing information. Evidence suggests SBAR helps create common expectations and dialog, which minimizes the differences that are caused by different training and experience, which occurs in interprofessional teams (Haig, Sutton, & Whittington, 2006; Manning, 2006).

Another technique used to facilitae effective communication is the call-out technique, in which critical information is yelled out during an emergent event. This ensures all team members are given information simultaneously during an acute event, which helps the team anticipate and prepare for the next steps to be taken. One crucial part of this style of communication is being able to direct specific information to a specific team member when needed (King et al., 2015).

Check-back is another technique useful for effective communication. It uses closed-loop communication to verify and confirm the information exchanged. In this strategy the sender initiates the message, then the receiver taking the message confirms what was communicated, and the sender verifies that the message received was correct. Check-back is an effective tool for all members of a team, even patients and families, because it confirms that the message given was fully understood as meant (King et al., 2015).

Effective communication among all team members is an essential part of healthcare and the ability to achieve good patient outcomes. These communication tools can enhance teamwork by facilitating effective and efficient communication and builds mutual trust among team members.

Cognitions in teamwork theory are the mental processes that occur at the group level. The two most widely studied cognitions are shared mental models and transactive memory systems. *Shared mental model* is a term used to describe the common understanding of how a process functions. In complex environments like healthcare, shared mental models allow team members to act cohesively based on their shared understanding of the tasks that need to be completed by each member and the outcomes expected (Mathieu, Heffner, Goodwin, Salas, & Cannon-Bowers, 2000). For example, in the operating room, an orthopedic surgical team focused on knee replacements has a clear picture of who does what task and the order in which they are completed. But if a couple of team members are on vacation and are replaced with staff from the gynecological service, this shared mental model breaks down and can contribute to delays, misunderstand-ings, and poorer performance.

Transactive memory systems is a concept that is less familiar to nurses, but is defined as a mechanism of group thinking in which the team encodes, stores and retrieves complex bodies of knowledge (Peltokorpi, 2008). Each member of the team has their own expertise, but other members of the group learn who has the expertise needed at the moment and communi-cates to gain access to this knowledge. This transactive memory system (TMS) is ideally developed over time as group members work together. The characteristics of a TMS are specialization or deep knowledge held by members of the group, coordination among members to quickly access the knowledge held by each other, and credibility in that team members believe the others' knowledge is accurate.

Training to Improve Teamwork

Teamwork is important to improving the quality of healthcare, but it is obvious there are many challenges to building high-functioning teams. Fortunately team development interventions can be effective in devel-oping teamwork competencies that improve team functioning (Hughes et al, 2016; Lacerenza, Marlow, Tannenbaum, & Salas, 2018). There are four types of team development interventions. The first is team training, which target team competencies and is represented by programs such as TeamSTEPPS (Strategies and Tools to Enhance Performance and Patient Safety) from the Agency for Healthcare Research and Quality (2015). This program focuses on team leadership, communication skills, situation monitoring, and mutual support of team members and has been imple-mented in a variety of settings across the continuum of care (Lacerenza et al., 2018).

The second type of team development intervention is leadership train-ing, which is targeted at improving leadership knowledge, skills, and abili-ties (KSAs) for people in formal leadership roles. This training can impact leadership functioning, which improves team performance and orga-nizational outcomes (Lacerenza, Reyes, Marlow, Joseph, & Salas, 2017). Optimally, both team and leadership training include elements of provid-ing information, demonstrating skills through videos or other mechanisms, practicing the content such as in role play, and providing effective feedback (Lacerenza et al., 2018).

Two other team development interventions can improve teamwork: team building and team debriefing. Team building can improve the team's ability to solve problems. Many organizations use social events and other casual exercises as their primary team building efforts. But evidence-based team building should include some combination of goal setting, relation-ship management, role clarification, and problem-solving methods and skills (Lacerenza et al., 2018). Goal setting and role clarification especially assist in building the shared mental models needed for teamwork. Relationship management and problem-solving skills can help teams manage the inevitable conflicts that arise in group work.

Finally, team debriefing is an important mechanism for improving team processes. Team debriefs can occur at any point in a project and allow time and space for the team to reflect on what is going right and what requires improvement. Psychological safety is important to the debriefing process. All members of the team need to feel they can speak up without negative consequences.

Evidence-based team development interventions are worth the required investment in time and resources. Team members enjoy and learn from these team development interventions; that knowledge is also transferred to individual and team performance, which leads to improvement in organizational and patient outcomes (Hughes et al., 2016).

Practical Actions to Enhance Improvement Teams

As mentioned earlier, there is poor implementation of evidence-based actions to improve quality. Organizations that have created sustainable transformation of patient care have been characterized by the urgent need to change, leadership commitment to quality, integration across departments and other organizational components, alignment of resources to meet goals, and improvement initiatives to drive the change (VanDeusen Lukas et al., 2007).

Leadership support and psychological safety are critical to building and sustaining high-performing teams that can successfully improve unit, departmental, and organizational level outcomes. Although this chapter has focused on the science of teamwork, there are also practical actions that team leaders can take to facilitate team success in improvement work (Table 8.2).

The first step is clearly defining the goals and objectives for the team. Communicating the expected outcomes of the team's work will help members buy into the work that must be done to improve.

The second step is to select team members for their needed skills and for team competencies. Every team member should know her or his role on the team and actively participate in team activities. Deliberate team-building activities help team members get to know each other and begin to develop mutual respect and trust.

Finally, good team and meeting management can facilitate team functioning. This begins with establishing ground rules for team meetings. It is ideal if at the first meeting, all members of the team establish ground rules that address the following questions:

TABLE 8.2 ACTIONS TO FACILITATE TEAMWORK IN IMPROVEMENT WORK

Actions	Description
Clearly define the purpose of the team	Defined goals and objectives help keep the team on task and limit going beyond the scope of the team's intended work.
Identify team roles and responsibilities	Clear expectations for each team member's responsibilities ensure that each member contributes to the team's work and decreases the risk of relational conflict within the group.
Establish written ground rules for the team	Establishing expectations for attendance, participation, timeliness, and conflict decreases the risk of unnecessary conflict within the group. Writing these rules down codifies the expectations for team members.
Send a timed agenda before the meeting	Use of a detailed agenda with time allocated for each agenda item helps the team stay focused on the required work of the team.
Create and distribute minutes of the meeting soon after the meeting	Meeting minutes are an invaluable tool to keep team members informed and to remind the team of past decision points. Rotating the recorder and/or blocking 30 minutes immediately after a meeting to do this work can reduce the burden of writing minutes.

1. *Attendance:* What are the attendance requirements for team members (e.g., If team member misses more than three meetings in a year, the member will be replaced.)?

2. *Participation:* What are the team member expectations for participation (e.g., All team members are expected to fully participate and contribute.)?

3. *Interruptions:* How will interruptions during the team meetings be handled (e.g., One voice at a time)?

4. *Preparation:* What level of preparation is expected for team meetings (e.g., Be honest about what you can get done before the next meeting.)?

5. *Timeliness:* What are the expectations for meeting start times, what type of preparation is expected (e.g., Everyone's time is valuable, so meetings will start on time.)?

6. *Conflict:* How will conflict between team members be resolved (e.g., Call a stop to the dialogue to stop the escalation.)?

Explicitly addressing each of these potential areas for conflict in the group saves time and trouble down the road. When the inevitable conflicts do occur, the team members can refer back to the ground rules to help resolve the issue and move forward.

In addition to establishing ground rules, the team should use a timed agenda and keep minutes of their team meetings. The timed agenda helps ensure that the team meeting is focused on the goals and objectives the team is trying to accomplish. Meeting minutes remind members of the previous work done, where the work was interrupted, discussion points, and what decisions have been made. The job of taking minutes can rotate among team members as one of the team roles. One tip is to block off 30 minutes after the meeting to ensure minutes are completed and sent out promptly.

Case Study: Improving Care Planning on a Surgical ICU

On a surgical ICU in a large academic medical center, the care team for an individual patient includes the RN assigned to the patient, an advanced practice provider (APP; either a certified registered nurse practitioner or physician assistant), the intensivist attending physician (MD), a pharmacist (PharmD), a physical therapist (PT) or occupational therapist (OT), a social worker/case manager (SW/CM), and others as needed. This ICU has a long history of interprofessional collaborative practice. There is ongoing professional development, including weekly educational lectures, monthly journal article review, high-fidelity simulation for highrisk scenarios. All members of the care team are encouraged to reach the full scope of practice, and each discipline's input into the plan of care is welcomed and valued.

The patient care team conducts interprofessional rounds daily, and patient and family members are encouraged to attend and participate. Rounds begin with the bedside nurse giving a brief presentation of the patient. The APP provides a systems-based presentation with a summary assessment and plan of care. After rounds, the APP is responsible for facilitating changes in the plan of care and adjusts as needed for changing patient conditions.

When two new physicians were hired from outside the organization for this unit, this process began to break down. The new attending physicians had not worked with the APP model on their previous teams, so they routinely made changes in the plan of care through the bedside RN. The APP would find out about the plan-of-care changes only after the RN would request orders supporting those changes in the electronic health record. Incidents of patient harm, organizational waste, and many near misses increased. In one instance, the lack of communication led to a patient receiving unnecessary imaging studies. In another incident, a medication change resulted in a drug being discarded that cost the hospital over $10,000. Team morale broke down as changes in plans of care were made unilaterally.

The ICU coleaders, including the lead APP, the unit medical director, and the nurse manager, realized the new team members were not oriented appropriately to the unit and the teamwork expectations within this ICU. There was no clear resolution to the issue, so a team meeting was called to discuss the issue and seek resolution. The APP's expressed concern that they were being left out of decision-making, undervalued for their input into patient care, and felt like their role had been diminished to being a scribe who put in orders. The attending physicians were surprised by the comments, and many stated their intent was to relieve some of the workload of the APPs. Other physicians did not understand the APP's concerns. RNs expressed concern that they

(continued)

Case Study: Improving Care Planning on a Surgical ICU (*continued*)

were "in the middle" of disagreements between attendings and APPs, which increased stress on the unit. They also described several incidents that caused harm to patients because of the lack of communication from provider to provider.

During the final PDSA (plan–do–study–act) cycle, a process was agreed upon. The process is as follows: If the attending physician wants to change the plan of care, first he or she contacts the APP responsible for the patient to discuss the change. The two providers will then come to an agreement on the change and will determine who will notify the rest of the care team of the change.

QUESTIONS

1. List ideas to address this issue within the team.
2. What type of communication strategy could be used during the conversation between the APP and attending physician to ensure clear, effective communication?
3. Describe an example of psychological safety seen within the case study and how this impacted the team.
4. Discuss traits a team leader must possess in order to self-correct as the team did in this case study.

CONCLUSIONS

As the overview of the science of teamwork show, teams differ in terms of their purpose, size, membership and experience, level of authority, history and chemistry. Teams do not necessarily need to have a long history of working together, or have members who even like each other. It is more important that team members have teamwork competencies such as team orientation, mutual performance monitoring, backup behavior, adaptability, and leadership (Salas, Rosen, Burke, & Goodwin, 2009). More importantly those teamwork competencies can be effectively taught and positively impact team performance as well as organizational outcomes (Hughes et al., 2016). Using the evidence from the science of teamwork can facilitate improvement activities within interprofessional teams.

REFERENCES

Agarwal, R., Sands, D. Z., & Schneider, J. D. (2010). Quantifying the economic impact of communication inefficiencies in U.S. hospitals. *Journal of Healthcare Management, 55*(4), 265–282. doi:10.1097/00115514-201007000-00007

Birken, S. A., Lee, S. D., & Weiner, B. J. (2012). Uncovering middle managers' role in healthcare innovation implementation. *Implementation Science, 7,* 28. Retrieved from http://www.implementationscience.com/content/7/1/28

de Wit, F. R. C., Greer, L. L., & Jehn, K. A. (2012). The paradox of intragroup conflict: A meta-analysis. *Journal of Applied Psychology, 97*(2), 360–390. doi:10.1037/a0024844

Donahue, K. E., Halladay, J. R., Wise, A., Reiter, K., Lee, S. D., Ward, K., . . . Qaqish, B. (2013). Facilitators of transforming primary care: A look under the hood at practice leadership. *Annals of Family Medicine, 11*(Suppl. 1), S27–S33. doi:10.1370/afm.1492

Edmondson, A. C. (1999). Psychological safety and learning behavior in work teams. *Administrative Science Quarterly, 44,* 350–383. doi:10.2307/2666999

Edmondson, A. C., & Lei, Z. (2014). Psychological safety: The history, renaissance, and future of an interpersonal construct. *Annual Review of Organizational Psychology and Organizational Behavior, 1,* 23–43. doi:10.1146/annurev-orgpsych-031413-091305

Engle, R. L., Lopez, E. R., Gormley, K. E., Chan, J. A., Charns, M. P., & Lukas, C. V. (2017). What roles do middle managers play in implementation of innovative practices? *Health Care Management Review, 42*(1), 14–27. doi:10.1097/HMR.0000000000000090

Haig, K., Sutton, S., & Whittington, J. (2006). SBAR: A shared mental model for improving communication between clinicians. *Journal on Quality and Patient Safety, 32,* 167–175. doi:10.1016/S1553-7250(06)32022-3

Hughes, A. M., Gregory, M. E., Joseph, D. L., Sonesh, S. C., Marlow, S. L., Lacerenza, C. N., . . . Salas, E. (2016). Saving lives: A metaanalysis of team training in healthcare. *Journal of Applied Psychology, 101,* 1266–1304. doi:10.1037/apl0000120

James, J. (2013). A new, evidence-based estimate of patient harms associated with hospital care. *Journal of Patient Safety, 9*(3), 122–128. doi:10.1097/PTS.0b013e3182948a69

Katzenbach, J. R., & Smith, D. K. (1993). The discipline of teams. *Harvard Business Review, 71*(2), 111–120.

King, H. B., Battles, J., Baker, D. P., Alonso, A., Salas, E., Webster, J., . . . Salisbury, M. (2015). *TeamSTEPPS: Team strategies and tools to enhance performance and patient safety.* Rockville, MD: Agency for Healthcare Research and Quality. Retrieved from http://www.ahrq.gov/teamstepps/instructor/fundamentals/index.html

Lacerenza, C. N., Marlow, S. L., Tannenbaum, S. I., & Salas, E. (2018). Team development interventions: Evidence-based approaches to improving teamwork. *American Psychologist, 73,* 517–531. doi:10.1037/amp0000295

Lacerenza, C. N., Reyes, D. L., Marlow, S. L., Joseph, D. L., & Salas, E. (2017). Leadership training design, delivery, and implementation: A meta-analysis. *Journal of Applied Psychology, 102,* 1686–1718. doi:10.1037/apl0000241

Leonard, M., Graham, S., & Bonacum, D. (2004). The human factor: The critical importance of effective teamwork and communication in providing safe care. *Quality & Safety in Health Care, 13*(Suppl. 1), i85–i90. doi:10.1136/qshc.2004.010033

Manning, M. (2006). Improving clinical communication through structured conversation. *Nursing Economic$, 24*(5), 268–271.

Mathieu, J. E., Heffner, T. S., Goodwin, G. F., Salas, E., & Cannon-Bowers, J. A. (2000). The influence of shared mental models on team process and performance. *Journal of Applied Psychology, 85*(2), 273–283. doi:10.1037/0021-9010.85.2.273

Mitchell, P., Wynia, M., Golden, R., McNellis, B., Okun, S., Webb, C. E., . . . Von Kohorn, I. (2012). Core principles & values of effective team-based health care. From the Best Practices Innovation Collaborative of the IOM Roundtable on Value & Science-Driven Health Care. Retrieved from https://nam.edu/wp-content/uploads/2015/06/VSRT-Team-Based-Care-Principles-Values.pdf

Nembhard, I., Alexander, J., Hoff, T., & Ramanujam, R. (2012). Why does the quality of health care continue to lag? Insights from management research. *Academy of Management Perspective, 23*(1), 24–42. doi:10.5465/AMP.2009.37008001

Peltokorpi, V. (2008). Transactive memory systems. *Review of General Psychology, 12*(4), 378–394. doi:10.1037/1089-2680.12.4.378

Rosen, M. A., DiazGranados, D., Dietz, A. S., Benishek, L. E., Thompson, D., Pronovost, P. J., & Weaver, S. J. (2018). Teamwork in health care: Key discoveries enabling safer, high quality care. *American Psychologist, 73,* 433–450. doi:10.1037/amp0000298

Salas, E., Reyes, D. L., & McDaniel, S. H. (2018). The science of teamwork: Progress, reflections, and the road ahead. *American Psychologist, 73,* 593–600. doi:10.1037/amp0000334

Salas, E., Rosen, M. A., Burke, C. S., & Goodwin, G. F. (2009). The wisdom of collectives in organizations: An update of the teamwork competencies. In E. Salas, G. F. Goodwin, & C. S. Burke (Eds.), *Team effectiveness in complex organizations* (pp. 39–82). New York, NY: Routledge.

Salas, E., Zajac, S., & Marlow, S. L. (2018). Transforming health care one team at a time: Ten observations and the trail ahead. *Group and Organization Management, 43*(3), 357–381. doi:10.1177/1059601118756554

Shuffler, M. L., & Carter, D. R. (2018). Teamwork situated in multiteam systems: Key lessons learned and future opportunities. *American Psychologist, 73,* 390–406. doi:10.1037/amp0000322

Tuckman, B. (1965). Developmental sequence in small groups. *Psychological Bulletin, 63*(6), 384–399. doi:10.1037/h0022100

VanDeusen Lukas, C., Holmes, S., Cohen, A., Restuccia, J., Cramer, I., Shwartz, M., & Charns, M. (2007). Transformational change in health care systems: An organizational model. *Health Care Management Review, 32*(4), 309–320. doi:10.1097/01.HMR.0000296785.29718.5d

9

LEADING PROGRAM EVALUATION

SHARON SABLES-BAUS

This chapter addresses the following DNP American Association of Colleges of Nursing (AACN) Essentials:

I   Scientific Underpinnings for Practice
III Clinical Scholarship and Analytic Methods for Evidence-Based Practice
IV Information Systems/Technology and Patient Care Technology for the Improvement and Transformation of Healthcare
VI Interprofessional Collaboration for Improving Patient and Population Health Outcomes
VII Clinical Prevention and Population Health for Improving the Nation's Health

INTRODUCTION

Choosing program development, implementation, and evaluation methodologies for the DNP scholarly project depends on many factors, including the school's expectations and timeline for completion. At many schools, even in the event of a tight deadline, evaluation of an existing program, or specific processes within a program, can meet expectations for a strong evidence-based translational project. The word *evaluation* has been defined as a critical appraisal or assessment; a judgment of the worth or effectiveness of something; a measurement of progress. In healthcare, there are three common definitions of *evaluation*: the first is the process of determining the merit, worth, or value of something (Scriven, 1980); the second is the use of systematic, data-based inquiries about whatever is being evaluated (American Evaluation Association, 2018); and the third is the process undertaken for purposes of improvement, decision-making, enlighten-ment, and/or persuasion (Shadish, Cook, & Leviton, 1991).

For the purposes of the DNP scholarly project, program evaluation includes evaluation of the implementation process for a new program and assessment of (a) how well the processes within the program are working and (b) whether or not the program is meeting the needs of its specific con-stituents, such as chief operating officer, unit manager, or the target popu-lation. Evaluation projects can also include systematic methods to judge the effectiveness of specific practices, technology, or policies (Newcomer, Hatry, & Wholey, 2015). A structured evaluative process is a translational methodology that can be utilized by a DNP student to meet five of the AACN DNP Essentials (see previous listing; Graham et al., 2006).

WHAT IS A PROGRAM?

Typically, organizations identify several overall goals that must be reached to accomplish their mission. A nonprofit organization works from its overall mission/purpose to identify service goals and typi-cally organizes these goals into specific programs. Programs in the non-profit world can be thought of in terms of inputs, process, outputs, and outcomes: *Inputs* are the various resources needed to run the program (e.g., money, facilities, and program staff), *process* is how the program is carried out (e.g., the counseling of clients), *outputs* are the units of service (e.g., the number of clients counseled or impacts on the clients receiving those services), and *outcomes* are the effects anticipated from the program.

A program can also be thought of as a one-time effort to produce a new product or line of products. For a hospital, programs can be defined by a service line, such as women's health, or by use of a certain technology, such as a gait-and-motion program for children with special healthcare needs. Specifically, a program can be defined as "a set of resources and activi-ties directed toward one or more common goals, typically under the direc-tion of a single manager or management team" (Newcomer et al., 2015, p. 7). A program can be held in an acute care setting (e.g., a fall-prevention program) for a certain population (e.g., patients with similar health prob-lems). A program can also be thought of at the community level (e.g., a local health department or educational system). The focus of programs in a community may be on preventing disease and injury, improving health, and enhancing quality of life. An example of a community-based educa-tion program is The American Academy of Family Physicians' Tar Wars Program, which targets fourth- and fifth-grade students to educate them about the consequences of tobacco use (The American Academy of Family Physicians, 2018).

A DNP project could be focused on implementing a Tar Wars Program in a school that does not have one or on the evaluation of the outcomes of a newly implemented program at one or more schools (Cain, Dickinson, Fernald, Bublitz, Dickinson, & West, 2006). The project could involve identifying a gap (e.g., a school that does not have this program), implementing the program to address the need, and evaluating the outcome of the implementation process and/or the outcomes of the program from the perspective of one or more constituents.

PROGRAM PERFORMANCE

Organizations must be concerned with how they are performing, and one way to measure performance is through metrics and key performance indicators (KPIs). The term *performance management* captures the use of performance measurement information to allocate and prioritize resources, to confirm or change current policy, or to report on success of meeting performance goals (Berenson, Pronovost, & Krumholz, 2013; DeGroff & Cargo, 2009; Loeb, 2004). A KPI (kpi.org) is a measurable value that can span departments and demonstrate how effectively a company is achieving key business objectives (see Table 9.1 for examples of KPIs in hospitals and

TABLE 9.1 EXAMPLES OF KEY PERFORMANCE INDICATORS IN HOSPITALS

Inpatient Flow	Outpatient Flow	Medication Management
Inpatient raw mortality rate	CMS outpatient measures	Adverse drug events per 1,000 patient days
CMS core measures	Compliance with care coordination pathways	Medication errors per 1,000 patient days
Harm events per 1,000 patient days	Cost per outpatient episode	High-risk adverse drug events per 1,000 doses
Bed turnover	No-show rate	Percentage of unreconciled medications
30-day readmission rate	Patient satisfaction	Number of self-reported medication errors
Patient satisfaction		Compliance with drug monitoring protocols
Average length of stay		
Average cost per discharge		

CMS, Centers for Medicare & Medicaid Services.

Source: From Martinez, D. A., Kane, E. M., Jalalpour, M., Scheulen, J., Rupani, H., Toteja, R., . . . Levin, S. R. (2018). An electronic dashboard to monitor patient flow at the Johns Hopkins Hospital: Communication of key performance indicators using the Donabedian Model. *Journal of Medical Systems, 42*(8), 133. doi:10.1007/s10916-018-0988-4

TABLE 9.2 EXAMPLES OF KEY PERFORMANCE INDICATORS IN PUBLIC HEALTH

Illustrative Program	Input	Process	Output	Outcome	Efficiency
Childhood immunization	Number of measles vaccination doses purchased	Percentage of children (ages X and Y) who receive measles vaccination	Measles deaths per child receiving measles vaccination	Measles deaths per 1,000 population	Measles vaccinations administered per employee-day
HIV/AIDS treatment	Number of ARV drug-treatment centers established	Number of HIV-infected patients receiving sustained ARV drug treatment	Opportunistic infection per 100 patients receiving ARV treatment	Rate of deaths due to HIV infection	Cost per unit of ARV drug treatment

ARV, antiretroviral.

Source: From Rozner, S. (2013). *Developing and using key performance indicators: A toolkit for health sector managers.* Bethesda, MD: Abt Associates.

Table 9.2 for examples of KPIs in public health). KPIs are often the building blocks of DNP program evaluations.

KPIs can be financial; customer, client, or patient related; or process related. In the public sector, sectors or organizations use KPIs to define success and track progress in meeting strategic goals. Well-designed KPIs should help health sector decision makers to do a number of things, including the following:

• Establish baseline information (i.e., the current state of performance).
• Set performance standards and targets to motivate continuous improvement.
• Measure and report improvements over time.
• Compare performance across geographical locations.
• Benchmark performance against regional and international peers or norms.
• Allow stakeholders to independently judge health sector performance.

Metrics, on the other hand, are quantifiable measures used to track and assess the status of a specific process. Metrics illuminate process effectiveness within a program or organization. They are collected at regular intervals to try to determine the progress of a particular intervention or service against a set of targets or objectives. Project management metrics are vital to implementing practical and sustainable project management practices and processes in any organization. The key is to keep the metrics simple, practical, and relevant to the organization. Whether measuring outcomes, patient experiences, and/or costs, metrics are critical to the effectiveness of the program or organization and should be the basis for the DNP project.

Measuring the performance of a healthcare organization or program can be difficult due to the various perspectives of success among the key stakeholders, such as the professionals in the healthcare organization, patients or clients receiving services, and regulatory agencies (Barry et al., 2018; Berenson et al., 2013; Mant, 2001). Donabedian (1966) was a germinal figure in developing measures of healthcare quality/performance, proposing a three-element model (structure, process, and outcome). Donabedian's linear evaluation model purposely does not account for patient, economic, or social factors outside of the care delivery system. His framework posits that improvements in structure of care should lead to improvements in clinical processes, which should in turn improve patient outcomes. He emphasized the importance of metrics. These concepts of structure, process, and outcome remain the foundation of quality assessment today, and his model may be useful for evaluating quality of care in an organization or a program (Ayanian & Markel, 2016; Moore, Lavoie, Bourgeois, & Lapointe, 2015).

Since Donabedian's time, many agencies have developed quality and patient safety indicators, the first being the National Quality Forum (NQF). NQF was created in 1999 "to promote and ensure patient protections and healthcare quality through measurement and public reporting" (The National Quality Forum, 2018). Specific to nursing is the National Database of Nursing Quality Indicators (NDNQI), which lists nursing-sensitive structure, process, and outcomes measures that monitor relationships between quality indicators and outcomes (National Database of Nursing Quality Indicators, 2018). It is often helpful for the student or project lead to obtain such reliable performance measures and build them into the program evaluation.

WHAT IS PROGRAM EVALUATION?

Programs must be evaluated to decide whether they are indeed useful to constituents. Evaluation can involve ongoing monitoring or a one-time study of program outcomes, processes, or impact. Program evaluation entails carefully collecting information about a program or some aspect of a program in order to make necessary program-related decisions. It is concerned with developing understanding and supporting strategic decision-making, such as whether/how an intervention should continue and whether the program itself should continue to be funded. The purposes of program evaluation include establishing who needs the evaluation and why, what stakeholders want to know, and who is going to use the evaluation results. The design of the evaluation extends from the primary purpose of the evaluation and the key questions that need to be answered (Newcomer et al., 2015; Shadish et al., 1991).

The primary purpose of a program evaluation can be to provide useful information to those who hold a stake in whatever is being evaluated. The key stakeholder can be those involved in the operations of a certain program, such as the program manager, the employees in the program, or a funding agency. Stakeholders can be those who are served by the program, such as clients or patients. Program evaluation can be defined as a systematic, standards-guided assessment of the processes and/or outcomes of a program, conducted in order to make judgments regarding the program, improve its effectiveness, and guide further development (Centers for Disease Control and Prevention [CDC], 1999). If it is important to establish causality with considerable confidence, a research methodology should be used; a primary goal of most research is to demonstrate that a particular independent variable (the cause) has an effect on the dependent variable of interest (Hirschhorn et al., 2018).

Program evaluation investigates the value, importance, or significance of something. It measures program merit and effectiveness (Mant, 2001). Program evaluation has been used routinely in public health but is becoming more common in clinical practice as hospital leaders consult stakeholders, set program goals, develop program evaluation plans, collect/analyze/interpret data, and share lessons learned. Often, program evaluation is used to examine the outcomes of an evidence-based program and may be paired with process evaluation, which measures within-program efficiencies of component interventions. The object of evaluation engenders the choice of evaluation method, which can include cost/benefit analysis (i.e., comparative assessment of all benefits anticipated from a project and all costs associated with introducing, performing, and supporting the changes resulting from a project). A program may seek evaluation to attract more funding or expand community partnerships. The type of evaluation depends on what the evaluator wants to learn about the program. For quality evaluation, methodological rigor and collection of reliable/valid data are critical.

Evaluation methodology entails following certain steps and fully incorporating ethical standards. Although program evaluation is a scientific process, it is not research. Program evaluation is typically concerned with making judgments about the effectiveness, efficiency, and sustainability of a program; it is a management tool for providing feedback so that future work can be improved or altered. Different from research methodology—where the research leads to conclusions, adds knowledge to a field, or contributes to expansion of a theory—a program evaluation, again, leads to judgments. *Research* makes statements about relationships among two or more variables, and its purpose is to explore and establish causal relationships using a hypothesis that is chosen by investigator. In contrast, *evaluation* seeks to examine and describe a particular entity and consider its value. Research is generalizable, whereas evaluation is context specific (Hirschhorn et al., 2018).

Furthermore, although traditional research is concerned with (a) internal validity, (b) success at establishing causality, (c) external validity, and (d) generalizability, program evaluations are judged by accuracy, utility, feasibility, and propriety (Figure 9.1):

- Accuracy—The extent to which the information obtained is an accurate reflection of how the program is really working
- Utility—The extent to which the results serve the practical information needs of intended users
- Feasibility—The extent to which the evaluation is realistic, practical, and economical
- Propriety—The extent to which the evaluation is done legally and ethically, protecting the rights of those involved (Yarbrough, Shulha, Hopson, & Caruthers, 2011).

TYPES OF PROGRAM EVALUATION

The different purposes of and motivations for conducting evaluations determine the evaluation type. Program evaluators can then determine whether, for example, a lack of expected results was due to poor implementation practices or flaws in the program activities themselves.

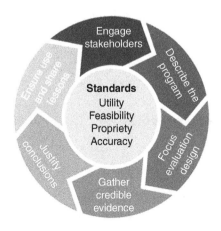

FIGURE 9.1 Framework for public health program evaluation: Steps and standards.

Source: From Centers for Disease Control and Prevention. (1999). Framework for program evaluation in public health. Retrieved from http://www.cdc.gov/eval/framework.html

Formative Evaluations

Generally speaking, if the identified need is to improve the way a program is delivered, then a formative evaluation would be the approach to use. *Formative* means the evaluation is looking at program activities or processes that are *forming* or in progress. A formative evaluation may also be called an internal evaluation and should provide information for program improvement. A formative evaluation ensures that the program is feasible, appropriate, and acceptable, and it generally is performed when a new program is being developed or when a currently functioning program is being considered for/requies modification for a new setting (Issel, 2014).

Summative Evaluations

Summative evaluation, or outcome evaluation, captures the overall quality and outcomes of a program (i.e., presents a "summing up"). This type of evaluation provides information about the program's adoption, continuation, or expansion with an audience of potential customers, funding sources, or officials. It can be used to (a) support long-term organizational learning and continuous improvement or (b) help organizations consider future directions, changes, or adaptions. Summative evaluation is most often associated with objective, quantitative methods of data collection and will detect whether the program is working (i.e., meeting intended outcomes relative to cost). This type of evaluation looks at the accountability of the program and lends itself to finding out what works, what does not work, and why certain program elements do or do not work. The evaluator can use the knowledge gained from the summative evaluation to improve future project design/implementation. Summative evaluations seek to determine whether the program should be continued, replicated, or curtailed; in contrast, formative evaluations are intended to help program designers, managers, and implementers address challenges to program effectiveness.

In short, summative evaluations assist in answering questions such as the following:

- Should the program be continued?
- If so, should it be continued in its entirety?
- Is it possible to implement the program in other settings?
- How sustainable is the program?
- What elements could have helped or hindered the program?
- What recommendations have evolved out of the program?

Process Evaluations

Evaluation of within-program processes is an important step that occurs typically during the program's early and midcycle phases of implementation and is often a part of a formative evaluation. The word *process*, as defined in business literature, refers to a series of logically related activities or tasks (e.g., a service or product) that, when performed together, produce a defined set of results. In other words, a process is an organized group of related activities that creates a result valuable to customers. Besides differing in importance, processes can be either simple or complicated, involving many people or many steps. Processes are what create the results that a company, program, or hospital delivers to its clients, patients, or populations. A process evaluation can help determine whether the program activities or processes have been implemented as intended, or it can be used to collect and analyze data to see how a program outcome or impact was achieved. Information from process evaluations is useful for program replication (Bilimoria, 2015; Saunders, Evans, & Joshi, 2005). This type of evaluation attempts to determine how successfully the project followed the strategy laid out in the planning stages.

Process goals are very different from outcome goals. When we engage in true process improvement, we seek to learn what causes things to happen in a process and use this knowledge to reduce variation, remove activities that contribute no value to the product or service produced, and improve customer satisfaction. When evaluation is focused on the outcome, workers will attach worth to the outcome and resist trying new things or putting forth their best effort. When the evaluation is focused on processes, a worker's sense of worth is attached to the effort, and she or he will put forth her or his very best. Thus, the process itself becomes exciting and rewarding, regardless of the outcome.

Specific processes within a program can be measured as specific, observable, and measurable indicators. An indicator will detect genuine differences in quality. Process measures are more sensitive than outcome measures to differences in the quality of care as long as a link has been demonstrated between a given process and outcome (Kirwin et al., 2012; Mant, 2001). Similar to process indicators, process measures are the specific steps in a process that lead to a particular outcome metric. In healthcare, process measures are the evidence-based best practices that represent the health system's improvement efforts. For example, all infants on a neonatal iIntensive care unit should be assessed for the risk of skin breakdown. The infants at risk should receive care based on an evidence-based care protocol. A process map could be used to examine the steps needed to identify high-risk infants and the application of the protocol for those identified as being in need. By tracking this process, if there is a skin breakdown, then the root cause of the system's failure can be identified. The goal of process measurement is to reduce process variation. When process metrics are established at potential points of variation in a care process, the inappropriate variation can be monitored and reduced.

Process evaluation will help answer program-specific questions, such as the following:

- Has the project reached the target group?
- Are all project activities reaching all parts of the target group?
- Are participants and other key stakeholders satisfied with all aspects of the project?
- Are all activities being implemented as intended? If not, why?
- What, if any, changes have been made to intended activities?
- Are all materials, information, and presentations suitable for the target audience?

Impact or Outcome Evaluations

An impact evaluation is aligned with objectives and is used to measure the immediate effect of the program, project, or policy on its participants, clients, or patients. The following are examples of the types of interventions in which impact evaluation would be useful:

- Innovative schemes
- Pilot programs that are due to be scaled up substantially
- Interventions for which there is scant solid evidence of impact in the given context, and
- A selection of other interventions across an agency's portfolio on an occasional basis

Impact evaluation can also help the evaluator decide whether or not the design was appropriate, providing policy-relevant information for redesign and/or the design of future programs. It is a contextual evaluation and should reveal both intended and unintended consequences for up to 6 months after completion. It should not be confused with the need to find causality. Impact evaluation will help answer questions such as the following:

- How well has the project achieved its objectives (and subobjectives)?
- How well have the desired short-term outcomes been achieved?

An outcome evaluation is concerned with long-term effects and is generally used to measure the outcome of the program, project, or policy 6 months or more after implementation. Outcome evaluation will help answer questions such as the following:

- Has the overall program goal or outcome been achieved?
- What, if any, factors outside the program have contributed to or hindered the desired change?
- What, if any, unintended change has occurred as a result of the program?

GUIDING THE PROGRAM EVALUATION

Program Theory

A theory is a description of how something works. It is an educated guess, a hypothesis, about what will happen, and it contains statements about relationships among the variables. We use theories in everyday life: In theory, if I touch a hot stove, I assume that it will cause me to burn my finger. We also use theories based on science, such as Nightingale's Environment Theory, which posits that environmental conditions assist or inhibit patient recovery. In program evaluation, after deciding on the health problem, the next step is to articulate an explanation of what caused the problem: This is the program theory. Program theories are often used in public health and are a necessary component of program evaluations.

Similarly, a program theory is the assumption that a program's design, processes, and execution will lead to the achievement of the intended outcomes for a specified population. A program theory explains how and why a program is supposed to work. It provides a logical and reasonable description of why the program activities and processes should lead to the intended results or benefits. It should be based on credible evidence for assuming that the specific processes will actually lead to the intended results. A program theory must contain relevant variables or factors and indicate the direction of the interactions among those variables related to the health problem.

A program theory consists of a set of statements that (a) describe a particular program; (b) explain why, how, and under what conditions the program effects occur; (c) predict the outcomes of the program; and (d) specify the requirements necessary to bring about the desired program effects. Program theories can often be captured in a series of "if/then" statements— if something is done with or for the program participants, then something should change. Examination of the evidence for each process and outcome is important to ensure that the program theory is correct and the evaluation accurate.

There are two parts of program theory: normative theory and causative theory. Normative theory offers a hypothesis about what is right/ wrong or desirable/undesirable, and when used in evaluating programs, its meaning suggests a description of the program as it should be, its goals and outcomes, its attendant interventions, and the rationale for these from the perspectives of various stakeholders. On the other hand, causative theory uses existing research to describe the potential outcomes of the program based on characteristics of the program itself and those of the clients, populations, or patients. Use of both normative and causative theories is necessary to develop a complete logic model (Fitzpatrick, Sanders, & Worthen, 2011).

A program theory should be developed prior to the beginning of the program. Effective planning results in a program design that is evidence based and well organized and identifies which intervention or group of interventions will be most effective in addressing the health problem. Program theory modeling (i.e., logic modeling) uses three components to describe the program: (a) the program activities or inputs, (b) the intended outcomes or outputs, and (c) the mechanisms through which the intended outcomes are achieved. A logic model is more diagrammatic, working forward from the actions that need to take place to drive the change that is likely to result in the desired improvement. Both Theory of Change (ToC; Weiss, 1995) and logic model approaches are based on structured thinking processes used to understand how and why a desired change is expected to result from an intervention. Once a program theory has been established, the process of conducting a theory-based evaluation can begin.

Logic Models

Program theory explains why a program is expected to work, and a logic model illustrates a program theory. A program theory needs to lay out the evidence for claiming that one thing will lead to the next; as its name suggests, a logic model is a commonly used tool for depicting an underlying program theory, the underlying logic of a planned initiative. A logic model helps communicate to stakeholders/target populations the relationships between program elements. It shows the relationships between resources (inputs), planned activities (outputs), and expected results (outcomes). The following components are usually included in a logic model:

- Inputs—Any resources or materials used by the program to provide its activities (e.g., money, staff, volunteers, facilities, equipment, supplies)

- Activities—Any services or treatments provided by the program

- Outputs—Amount of activity provided, described in quantifiable terms (e.g., number of classes taught, people served, educational materials distributed, hours of service delivered)

- Outcomes—Any characteristics of the participants that, according to the program theory, are expected to change as a result of the participant's receiving services (Wilder Research, 2009).

Logic models should also identify (a) key factors that are outside the control of program staff but are likely to affect the achievement of desired outcomes; and (b) mediating factors such as changes in staff, new polices, or competing programs. One benefit of a logic model is that it guides the choice of program evaluation design and methodology.

A logic model that is constructed in these five stages guides an evaluation plan:

1. Collect the relevant information.
2. Clearly define the problem that the program will address or solve and describe the context.
3. Define the elements of the program in a table.
4. Draw the model to reveal the program's ToC.
5. Verify the program logic with stakeholders (Newcomer et al., 2015).

Process Theory

A process theory predicts that all of the steps in a process will lead to a certain outcome. Development of the theory must include evidence to support not only the steps of the process but also the ways that people can be motivated or educated to follow each step. Process variation leads to outcome variation. If a company or a program wants to reproduce a certain outcome, it will duplicate the process used to reach the objective. A process theory should incorporate input about resources and actions from clients, best practices, guidelines, and change ideas or concepts.

Process theory design may be completed using business process re-engineering (i.e., conceptualizing the organization as a process). In manufacturing, the basic principles of process flow analysis—using Little's Law—are often used to seek information on throughput time and flow rate (i.e., organizational capacity; Gustafson, 2011). In healthcare, Little's Law is applied in Lean Six Sigma. Lean Six Sigma is a combination of two process-improvement methods: Lean and Six Sigma. This team-focused managerial approach seeks to improve program performance by eliminating waste of physical resources, time, effort, and talent while ensuring quality in production and organizational processes. Simply put, under the tenets of Lean Six Sigma, any use of resources that does not create value for the end customer is considered waste and should be eliminated. Persons using Lean Six Sigma are required to complete training. The organization where the DNP leader is working may use Lean Six Sigma and may employ trained professionals who can help with the process design of the scholarly project (goleansixsigma.com/what-is-lean-six-sigma).

Process Mapping

Healthcare agencies may use something similar to process flow analysis: process mapping. A process map is a tool that depicts workflow and is used to improve efficiency. Process mapping uses flowcharts that focus on work performed rather than job titles, hierarchies, specific units, or locations. A process map can reveal unexpected complexity or redundancy. Such maps are intended to (a) represent a process in such a way that all steps are included, even if those steps cross departments or professional duties and (b) show inputs, outputs, and tasks that are linked (Figure 9.2).

EFFECT THEORY

Effect theory can describe the relationship between interventions and desired outcomes. The theory must be based on evidence-based interventions and the effect these interventions have shown on certain outcomes. Examples of interventions that have an effect on program participants and can be used in a DNP scholarly project include coaching, counseling, educating, assessing, coordinating, or treating. Interventions should be evidence based, tailored to the population, and conducive to health gains. They should also be technologically, logistically, and politically feasible as well as cost-effective. Data can be sought from program budgets and data information systems. Effect theory can also show the effect of interventions on programmatic outcomes, thereby giving the evaluator information about the design of the program.

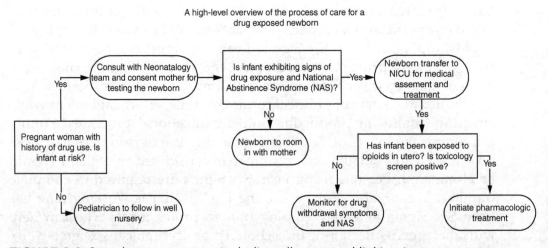

A high-level overview of the process of care for a drug exposed newborn

FIGURE 9.2 Sample process map, including all steps and linking inputs, outputs, and tasks.

A MODEL FOR PROGRAM EVALUATION

One of the best-known approaches to planning, implementing, and evaluating health programs is the PRECEDE–PROCEED Model of health program planning and evaluation (Green & Kreuter, 2005). It is a health-promotion model informed by epidemiology, social/behavioral/educational sciences, and health administration, and it emphasizes two fundamental propositions: (a) health and health risks are multifactorial and (b) because health and health risks are multifactorial, behavioral, environmental, and social change must be affected by multidimensional/multisector, participatory programs (Green & Kreuter, 2005).

PRECEDE–PROCEED is an acronym for predisposing, reinforcing, and enabling constructs in educational diagnosis and evssaluation (PRECEDE); and policy, rRegulatory, and organizational constructs in educational and environmental development (PROCEED). The model offers a detailed process for program planning and evaluation that considers the impact of organizational and environmental systems on the selected intervention. It has been applied in various situations, including cross-cultural programs to change health behavior. The model is most useful when planning an intervention and including the evaluative components up front while providing analysis at every step in the process. The eight phases (some versions have six phases) walk the evaluator through situational analysis, development, and evaluation of the intervention (Glanz, Rimer, & Viswanath, 2008; Porter, 2015).

The PRECEDE part of the model (phases 1 – 4) focuses on program planning, and the PROCEED part (phases 5–8) focuses on implementation and evaluation (Table 9.3). The PRECEDE phases move logically backward from a desired result to where and how an intervention is warranted, and then to administrative and policy issues that need to be addressed in order to have a successful intervention. PROCEED covers intervention implementation and evaluation, working forward to the original starting point.

BEGINNING STEPS OF THE EVALUATION

Step 1: Choose a Project Setting.

Examples of viable project settings are as follows:

- Work environment
- School connections
- Community
- Big data
- Policy at local, state or federal level—outcomes that are linked to policy goals are measured at the level of large groups of people

TABLE 9.3 PHASES OF THE PRECEDE–PROCEED MODEL OF HEALTH PROGRAM PLANNING AND EVALUATION

PRECEDE	1	Social assessment	Health, social problems, cultural needs, quality of life
	2	Epidemiological assessment	Determinants of health
	3	Educational and ecological assessment	Analyze the determinants of health for behavioral and environmental determinants
	4	Administrative and policy assessment and intervention alignment	Individual determinants of health; choice
PROCEED	5	Implementation	Interventions
	6	Process evaluation—identifies operational challenges; output measures, stakeholder observation	Puts into effect the interventions in phase 5
	7	Impact evaluation	Process evaluation of the implemented interventions
	8	Outcome evaluation	Impact produced by the interventions

Furthermore, the person conducting the DNP project should choose a particular area of interest in a particular setting. This is called an *opportunity assessment*—and refers to what can be evaluated in the period of time allotted with the resources available to conduct such an evaluation. The following are examples of within-setting areas of interest:

- Exploring symptoms of a dysfunctional process in a work setting
- Asking people in control/management or coworkers on the front line what the opportunities for evaluation and improvement are
- Collecting data or using data that have already been collected (surveys, analyses of administrative data, key informant interviews, observations, focus groups)
- Asking customers of the service or program what they would like to see evaluated or improved
- Examining health information systems (HIS)

Step 2: Define the Actual Problem.

The following are ways of defining the problem:

- Do a gap analysis.—Examine the way things should be and the way things are, and then decide how to reconcile the gap between these two.

- Conduct this exercise.—If the activity is provided, then what, realistically, should be the result for participants?
- Reflect on why you, the client, or the customer believes the process or the program will lead to this result.
- Ask what evidence you have that the process or the program will lead to this result.
- Find processes and procedures impacted by budget shortfalls, staffing, information technology infusion, and external pressures for greater accountability and responsiveness.
- Reflect on organization, market, and customer requirements, seeking to understand how things are currently done and determine strengths and weaknesses of the organization or program compared to the competition.

Step 3: Choose the Program Outcome and/or Process Measure to Be Evaluated.

First, choose the outcome you or the organization would like to see evaluated and then work backward to learn about all of the processes that take place in order to get to the outcome.

- Understand the feasibility of doing the project. Determine the organizational commitment for such an evaluation. Ensure the project fits with the organization's mission and vision.
- Seek to develop a solid understanding of the organizational culture and its dynamics and politics before the evaluation begins. Determine whether the evaluation is a priority for the organization.
- Think about the project costs—not just monetary costs, but also the time costs for the people who are involved in the program.
- If evaluating the outcome of a program, a decision to evaluate one or more processes in the program may be made, along with measuring the outcomes of the program. Due to time constraints of the DNP scholarly project, it is helpful to choose someone to spearhead each process evaluation.
- Understand and document the workflow for the process.—Use tools to illustrate this.
- Review relevant documentation and any available data from the process or the program.
- Include people on your team who are invested in the processes you want to measure.

- Be sure to include the customer/client/patient perspective on the process and the program outcome.

- Determine whether the data needed for the evaluation are easily obtainable in that organization.

Step 4: Choose a Change Model

There are many change models that can be used in the DNP scholarly project. Two of the more common change models used in program evaluation are the ToC and Kurt Lewin's Change Model.

A ToC is built on a causal framework, a process wherein program stakeholders identify goals and determine ways that those goals can be reached (Clark & Taplin, 2012). A ToC accounts for how interventions yield a result chain that leads to the final intended outcome. It can be developed for any level of intervention (e.g., a specific process within a program or an entire program within one organization). A ToC can also be developed for a specific policy. The DNP-prepared clinician can use this ToC framework not only to explain how interventions lead to an outcome but also to serve as a working model against which to test the program theory. It is important to note that every outcome in the theory must be explicitly defined. All outcomes should be given at least one indicator of success. The project lead will collect and analyze data on key indicators to monitor progress on the project ToC.

Kurt Lewin's Change Model (1951) focuses on the perception that a change is needed, moves toward the desired behavior, and solidifies that new behavior as the norm. The Change Model includes three steps: unfreezing, changing, and refreezing. *Unfreezing* creates awareness that the way things are being done is negatively affecting the program outcomes. This part of the model can be the most difficult to achieve because people typically do not like change. The DNP-prepared nurse must showcase leadership and communication skill to get people on board with the need for change. The next step in the model, *changing*, is the transitioning step during which change is implemented. The last step is called *refreezing*, which reinforces or stabilizes the new postchange state (Figure 9.3).

There are many ways of implementing change. However, planned change (i.e., a purposeful, calculated, and collaborative effort to bring about improvements) requires the leadership of a change agent, such as a DNP-prepared nurse. A DNP-prepared nurse leading a project must provide a change framework by identifying an appropriate change theory or model.

CONCLUSIONS

All nurses are knowledgeable about the nursing process as a scientific method for ensuring the quality of patient care. The process is broken down

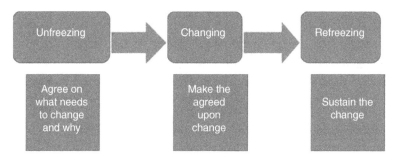

FIGURE 9.3 Lewin's (1951) Three-Stage Change Model: Unfreezing, changing, and refreezing.
Source: Adapted from Mitchell, G. (2013). Selecting the best theory to implement planned change. *Nursing Management, 20*(1), 32–37. Retrieved from http://www.ncbi.nlm.nih.gov/pubmed/23705547

into five separate steps: assessment, diagnosis, planning, implementation, and evaluation.

Nurses use evaluation in the final step of the nursing process. Evaluation is crucial to determining whether, after application of all of the steps of the nursing process, the client's condition or well-being has improved due to the nursing care provided. The nurse conducts evaluation measures to determine whether expected (i.e., evidence-based) outcomes have been met. In short, during the evaluative step, the nurse compares client behavioral responses with predetermined client goals and outcome criteria.

Program evaluation is a macro version of micro-scale, client-specific nursing evaluation. The DNP nurse can apply program evaluation to evaluate whether all processes in a program are effectively being implemented to ensure broader programmatic outcomes. Program evaluation can be defined as the judgment of effectiveness of the processes within a program to meet client goals.

Case Study

Illicit drug use among pregnant women is on the rise. Intrauterine opioid exposure can result in neonatal abstinence syndrome (NAS). Newborns exposed to addictive substances during the mother's pregnancy begin withdrawal as soon as the umbilical cord is cut. Most infants born to drug-dependent mothers will undergo NAS (between 55% and 94%). The severity of presentation is based on the infant's level of exposure in utero. Of exposed infants, 60% to 80% will have moderate to severe symptoms requiring medical intervention. Infants with NAS may exhibit a constellation of central nervous system, gastrointestinal, autonomic nervous system, and respiratory symptoms (Finnegan & MacNew, 1974; Hudak, Tan, Committee on Drugs, Committee on Fetus

(continued)

Case Study (*continued*)

and Newborn, & American Academy of Pediatrics, 2012). According to the severity of the withdrawal, the duration of symptoms is anywhere from 6 days to 8 weeks (Finnegan & MacNew, 1974; Patrick et al., 2012). Studies of inpatient populations of infants with NAS report a wide range of length of stay (LOS), from 1 to 122 days; (Burns & Mattick, 2007; Johnson, Greenough, & Gerada, 2003; Seligman et al., 2008).

Clinical practice guidelines for NAS provide evidence-informed recommendations that address the needs of substance-using pregnant women and newborns at risk of NAS. Reducing the incidence and impact of NAS requires immediate action in order to improve the care of affected women and infants. This includes optimizing and standardizing treatment strategies, assessing and managing social risk, monitoring of prescribing practices, and facilitating the implementation of better treatment and prevention strategies as they become available. These clinical practice guidelines provide the framework to inform and support the development of a coordinated strategy to address this important issue and to promote safe, effective care.

Toward this end, an evaluation of inpatient services, both maternal and infant, was designed with the objective to improve NAS inpatient outcomes. An interdisciplinary team was put together to optimize care strategies for substance-using pregnant women and their infants.

QUESTIONS

1. What type of program evaluation can be conducted to address the goal of improving NAS inpatient outcomes?
2. What is the project setting?
3. How would the actual problem be defined?
4. Working backward from the identified outcome, what are all of the processes that take place in order to get to the outcome?
5. What is the best change model for this evaluation?

ADDITIONAL RESOURCES

- Getting To Outcomes 2004. Promoting accountability through methods and tools for planning, implementation, and evaluation: www.rand.org
- Introduction to Program Evaluation for Public Health Programs: a Self-Study Guide: https://www.cdc.gov/eval/ www.cdc.gov
- W.K. Kellogg Foundation - Logic Model Development Guide: https://www.wkkf.org/resource-directory#pp=10&p=1&q=logic%20model%20development%20guide
- Human Services Research Institute- Selecting process measure for quality improvement in mental healthcare: http://hsri.org
- Wisconsin's University Extension: https://fyi.uwex.edu/programdevelopment/logic-models/
- University of Minnesota: https://cyfar.org/learning-mods-home)

- University of Kansas, Community Tool Box: https://ctb.ku.edu/en/table-of-contents/overview/models-for-community-health-and-development/logic-model-development/main
- Program Evaluation and Performance Measurement at the EPA: https://www.epa.gov/evaluate/program-evaluation-and-performance-measurement-epa
- Developing Key Performance Indicators: A Toolkit for Health Sector Managers (2013). https://www.hfgproject.org/wp-content/uploads/2014/10/03-Developing-Key-Performance-Indicators.pdf
- Evaluation Toolbox: http://evaluationtoolbox.net.au/

REFERENCES

The American Academy of Family Physicians. (2018). Tar Wars program. Retrieved from https://www.aafp.org/about/initiatives/tar-wars.html

American Evaluation Association. (2018). Application and exploration of program evaluation. Retrieved from www.eval.org

Antonacci, G., Reed, J. E., Lennox, L., & Barlow, J. (2018). The use of process mapping in healthcare quality improvement projects. *Health Services Management Research, 31*(2), 74–84. doi:10.1177/0951484818770411

Ayanian, J. Z., & Markel, H. (2016). Donabedian's lasting framework for health care quality. *New England Journal of Medicine, 375*(3), 205–207. doi:10.1056/NEJMp1605101

Barry, D., Kimble, L. E., Nambiar, B., Parry, G., Jha, A., Chattu, V. K., . . . Goldmann, D. (2018). A framework for learning about improvement: Embedded implementation and evaluation design to optimize learning. *International Journal for Quality in Health Care, 30*(Suppl. 1), 10–14. doi:10.1093/intqhc/mzy008

Berenson, R., Pronovost, P., & Krumholz, H. (2013). Achieving the potential of health care performance measures: Timely analysis of immediate health policy issues. Robert Wood Johnson Foundation. Retrieved from https://www.rwjf.org/en/library/research/2013/05/achieving-the-potential-of-health-care-performance-measures.html

Bilimoria, K. Y. (2015). Facilitating quality improvement: Pushing the pendulum back toward process measures. *Journal of the American Medical Associasion, 314*(13), 1333–1334. doi:10.1001/jama.2015.12470

Burns, L., & Mattick, R. P. (2007). Using population data to examine the prevalence and correlates of neonatal abstinence syndrome. *Drug and Alcohol Review, 26*(5), 487–492. doi:10.1080/09595230701494416

Cain, J. J., Dickinson, W. P., Fernald, D., Bublitz, C., Dickinson, L. M., & West, D. (2006). Family physicians and youth tobacco-free education: outcomes of the Colorado Tar Wars program. *Journal of the American Board of Family Medicine, 19*(6), 579–589.

Centers for Disease Control and Prevention. (1999). Framework for program evaluation in public health. Retrieved from https://www.cdc.gov/eval/framework/index.htm

Clark, H., & Taplin, D. (2012). *Theory of change basics: A primer on the Theory of Change.* New York, NY: Actknowledge.

DeGroff, A. C., & Cargo, M. (2009). Policy implementation: Implications for evaluation. *New Directions for Evaluation, 2009*(124), 47–60. doi:10.1002/ev.313

Donabedian, A. (1966). Evaluating the quality of medical care. *Milbank Memorial Fund Quarterly, 44*(3), 166–206. doi:10.2307/3348969

Finnegan, L. P., & MacNew, B. A. (1974). Care of the Addicted Infant. *American Journal of Nursing, 74*(4), 685–693. doi:10.1097/00000446-197404000-00051

Fitzpatrick, J. L., Sanders, J. R., & Worthen, B. R. (2011). *Program evaluation: Alternative approaches and practical guidelines* (3rd ed.). New York, NY: Pearson.

Glanz, K., Rimer, B. K., & Viswanath, K. (2008). *Health behavior and health education: Theory, research, and practice* (4th ed.). San Francisco, CA: John Wiley & Sons.

Graham, I. D., Logan, J., Harrison, M. B., Straus, S. E., Tetroe, J., Caswell, W., & Robinson, N. (2006). *Journal of Continuing Education in the Health Professions, 26*(1), 13–24. doi:10.1002/chp.47

Green, L. W., & Kreuter, M. W. (2005). *Health program planning: An educational and ecological approach* (4th ed.). New York, NY: McGraw-Hill Higher Education.

Gustafson, J. L. (2011). Little's Law. In D. Padua (Ed.). *Encyclopedia of parallel computing* (pp. 1038–1041). Boston, MA: Springer.

Hirschhorn, L., Ramaswamy, R., Devnani, M., Wandersman, A., Simpson, L.A., & Garcia-Elorrio, E. (2018). Research versus practice in quality improvement? Understanding how we can bridge the gap. *International Journal for Quality in Health Care, 30*(1), 24–28. doi:10.1093/intqhc/mzy018

Hudak, M. L., Tan, R. C., Committee on Drugs, Committee on Fetus and Newborn, & American Academy of Pediatrics. (2012). Neonatal drug withdrawal. *Pediatrics, 129*(2), e540–e560. doi:10.1542/peds.2011-3212

Institute for Healthcare improvement. (2018). 5 steps for creating value through process mapping and observation. Retrieved from http://www.ihi.org/communities/blogs/5-steps-for-creating-value-through-process-mapping-and-observation

Issel, L. M. (2014). *Health program planning and evaluation: A practical, systematic approach for community health.* Burlington, MA: Jones & Bartlett Learning.

Johnson, K., Greenough, A., & Gerada, C. (2003). Maternal drug use and length of neonatal unit stay. *Addiction, 98*(6), 785–789. doi:10.1046/j.1360-0443.2003.00391.x

Kirwin, J., Canales, A. E., Bentley, M. L., Bungay, K., Chan, T., Dobson, E., . . . Spinler, S. A. (2012). Process indicators of quality clinical pharmacy services during transitions of care. *Pharmacotherapy: The Journal of Human Pharmacology and Drug Therapy, 32*(11), e338–e347. doi:10.1002/phar.1214

Lewin, K. (1951). *Field theory in social science: Selected theoretical papers.* New York, NY: Harper & Row.

Loeb, J. M. (2004). The current state of performance measurement in health care. *International Journal for Quality in Health Care, 16*(Suppl. 1), i5–i9. doi:10.1093/intqhc/mzh007

Mant, J. (2001). Process versus outcome indicators in the assessment of quality of health care. *International Journal for Quality in Health Care, 13*(6), 475–480. doi:10.1093/intqhc/13.6.475

Martinez, D. A., Kane, E. M., Jalalpour, M., Scheulen, J., Rupani, H., Toteja, R., . . . Levin, S. R. (2018). An electronic dashboard to monitor patient flow at the Johns Hopkins Hospital: Communication of key performance indicators using the Donabedian Model. *Journal of Medical Systems, 42*(8), 133. doi:10.1007/s10916-018-0988-4

Moore, L., Lavoie, A., Bourgeois, G., & Lapointe, J. (2015). Donabedian's structure-process-outcome quality of care model: Validation in an integrated trauma system. *Journal of Trauma and Acute Care Surgery, 78*(6), 1168–1175. doi:10.1097/TA.0000000000000663

National Database of Nursing Quality Indicators. (2018). Retrieved from https://nursingandndnqi.weebly.com/ndnqi-indicators.html

National Quality Forum. (2018). NQF's history. Retrieved from www.qualityforum.org/about_nqf/history

Newcomer, K. E., Hatry, H. P., & Wholey, J. S. (2015). *Handbook of practical program evaluation* (4th ed.). Hoboken, NJ: John Wiley & Sons.

Patrick, S. W., Schumacher, R. E., Benneyworth, B. D., Krans, E. E., McAllister, J. M., & Davis, M. M. (2012). Neonatal abstinence syndrome and associated health care expenditures: United States, 2000–2009. *Journal of the American Medica Association, 307*(18), 1934–1940. doi:10.1001/jama.2012.3951

Porter, C. M. (2015). Revisiting PRECEDE-PROCEED: A leading model for ecological and ethical health promotion. *Health Education Journal, 75*(6), 753–764. doi:10.1177/0017896915619645

Rozner, S. (2013). *Developing and using key performance indicators: A toolkit for health sector managers.* Bethesda, MD: Abt Associates.

Saunders, R. P., Evans, M. H., & Joshi, P. (2005). Developing a process-evaluation plan for assessing health promotion program implementation: A how-to guide. *Health Promotion Practice, 6*(2), 134–147. doi:10.1177/1524839904273387

Scriven, M. (1980). *Evaluation thesaurus* (2nd ed.). Inverness, CA: Edgepress.

Seligman, N. S., Salva, N., Hayes, E. J., Dysart, K. C., Pequignot, E. C., & Baxter, J. K. (2008). Predicting length of treatment for neonatal abstinence syndrome in methadone-exposed neonates. *American Journal of Obstetrics and Gynecology, 199*(4), 396.e1–396.e7. doi:10.1016/j.ajog.2008.06.088

Shadish, W. R., Cook, T. D., & Leviton, L. C. (1991). *Foundations of program evaluation: Theories of practice.* Thousand Oaks, CA: Sage.

Weiss, C. (1995). Nothing as practical as good theory: Exploring theory-based evaluation for comprehensive community initiatives for children and families. In J. Connell, A. Kubish, L. Schorr & C. Weiss (Eds.), *New approaches to evaluating community initiatives.* Washington, DC: Aspen Institute.

Wilder Research. (2009). Program theory and logic models. Evaluation resources from Wilder Research. Retrieved from http://www.evaluatod.org/assets/resources/evaluation-guides/logicmodel-8-09.pdf

Yarbrough, D. B., Shulha, L. M., Hopson, R. K., & Caruthers, F. A. (2011). *The program evaluation standards: A guide for evaluators and evaluation users* (3rd ed.). Thousand Oaks, CA: Sage.

IMPROVEMENT AND BIG DATA

JOHN M. WELTON | SHARON SABLES-BAUS |
CATHERINE KLEINER

This chapter addresses the following American Association of Colleges of Nursing (AACN) DNP Essentials:

I.   Organizational and Systems Leadership for Quality Improvement and System Thinking
III. Clinical Scholarship and Analytical Methods for Evidence-Based Practice
IV. Technology and Information for the Improvement and Transformation of Patient-Centered Healthcare
VII. Clinical Prevention and Population Health for Improving the Nation's Health

INTRODUCTION

Quantities of data are growing every day, everywhere, and the advent of the electronic health record (EHR) has expanded the number of large, complex, information-enriched datasets in the healthcare industry. In turn, developing the abilities to (a) extract useful knowledge hidden in these large numbers of data and (b) act on that extracted knowledge is becoming increasingly important. The term *data mining* (often termed *knowledge discovery*) is frequently used when referring to the method of analyzing data from different perspectives and distilling it into valuable information. The DNP scholar can examine correlations or patterns among dozens of fields in large relational databases to problem solve such healthcare issues as readmissions, triage, and decompensation, thereby reducing preventable harm, as well as delivery of evidenced-based information to increase efficiencies.

In this chapter, techniques for extracting, setting up, and cleaning data from existing clinical and operational datasets are examined. Considerations for analyzing various large datasets and disseminating the results of those analyses are also discussed.

WORKING WITH BIG DATA

Big data refers to a form of data that is of high volume, velocity, and variety (Krumholz, 2014; Roski, Bo-Linn, & Andrews, 2014). From a clinical standpoint, many, if not most, patient care data are now entered into the EHR. These data are contained within core EHR components such as provider order entry, pharmacy systems, lab order, and results reporting, and clinical documentation modules.

One such dataset captured in hospital EHRs is obtained from bar coding of medication administration (BCMA). This bar code system was specifically designed to prevent medication errors in healthcare settings. Medications can be barcode-scanned to populate relevant data into the BCMA system. The BCMA system captures key information: to whom, what, when, and how much medication is to be administered. With the data captured, it can be shared with pharmacists to process medication orders and with nurses to properly administer medication. It might also be used to ensure the correct medication was ordered, that it was administered, that the proper dose was used, and more. These data provide a steady high-volume, high-velocity stream of clinically relevant information about the care a patient receives in a certain setting. A DNP scholarly project focused on analysis of these data to find the types and causes of delays in administering antibiotics (e.g., differences in practice patterns among nurses in administering pro re nata [PRN] analgesics) would both fall within the core competencies of a DNP-educated professional and benefit the institution. Analysis of these data and feedback of the results to clinicians and administrators can lead to a decrease in medication errors and prevention of serious or fatal consequences (Seibert, Maddox, Flynn, & Williams, 2014). Another way that BCMA data analysis may be useful is in preventing overdose of medications, including opioids, within a clinical setting.

ROLE OF THE DNP-PREPARED NURSE IN USING BIG DATA

The inherent value of a DNP-prepared nurse is his or her proximity to practice. This clinical expertise and experience within a care setting or patient population provides valuable insights. There are many potential roles and relationships with data.

Role as Clinical Expert

A DNP-prepared nurse can identify key data used in the clinical setting and assist with preparation of data for analysis. For example, a DNP-prepared nurse leading a quality-improvement project on improvement of pain management for neonates can identify (a) differences in pain assessment methods and use of pain scores by nurses and (b) the practice patterns of providers ordering pain medication by pulling data from the EHR and BCMA.

Role as Data Expert

A DNP-prepared nurse skilled in descriptive and inferential statistics and analysis can summarize data in a meaningful way. As a result, patterns can emerge from the data and generalizations can be made about the populations from which the samples were drawn. Inferential tests require the user to make educated, theory-based guesses.

Role in Supporting Research Teams by Providing Clinical Guidance and Relevance

A DNP-prepared nurse can identify ways data are collected in the clinical setting and potential causes for missing or aberrant data. The DNP-prepared nurse can conduct or assist with data-extraction techniques for clinical or administrative use.

Role as Expert in Applying Existing Research to Practice

A DNP-prepared nurse is knowledgeable about literature-search strategies. As such, she or he can identify key studies and other relevant literature that can be translated and applied in the clinical domain for specific issues and problems encountered in a particular clinical setting. This can be beneficial in relating the findings from a formal study to a clinical context.

Role in Assisting Research Teams to Interpret Analysis Findings and Put Into Clinical/Operational Context

The DNP-prepared nurse can interpret unexpected results of a project or study based on clinical knowledge of the patient population and setting or context of care.

Specialist DNP Roles in Leadership and Informatics

Some DNP-prepared nurses have specialty roles in clinical practice. For example, a nurse informaticist has expert knowledge of data systems and information technology (IT) used in the clinical environment; the nurse informaticist can thus act as liaison between the clinical/research teams and the programmers who will extract data from the EHR. A DNP-prepared nurse leader can guide the formulation of clinical questions, identify problems that are a priority for analysis, and shepherd dissemination of findings from projects and studies within the organization.

Ultimately, any results from data analysis have the potential to provide actionable interventions or strategies, leading to overall improvement of patient care. Use of big data across multiple settings and populations can support and maintain quality of care and patient safety.

USE OF DATA IN DNP PRACTICE

First and foremost, how will DNP-prepared nurses identify and use data to improve practice and care outcomes across a broad range of settings, including school-based clinics, public health organizations, home care, primary care, as well as acute care hospitals and clinics? What is the overall intended use of these data, and how can these be used for quality analysis, to identify differences in practice and association with outcomes of care in a particular care setting?

Clinical data captured in a typical care setting include the following:

- Patient demographic data such as age, gender, race, ethnicity, income, education, and employment
- Patient-generated health data, including, but not limited to, health history, diagnosis, treatment history, biometric data, symptoms, lifestyle choices, vital signs, lab values, physical/mental assessments, and test results
- Data related to treatments (e.g., medications administered, surgeries/other procedures) or use of devices (e.g., assisted ventilation, surgical drains, or intravenous catheters)
- Provider-specific information (e.g., the name of the person directly responsible for care and what care was given), provider-specific characteristics (e.g., experience level and credentials) and provider–patient relationship (e.g., a day shift assignment of nurses to patients on an inpatient unit)
- Organizational data such as the location care was received (e.g., hospital) and costs charges related to care

Measures, such as the ones described in Table 10.1, provide a rich environment for a DNP scholarly project on evaluating the quality, cost, effectiveness, and outcomes of care offered by different providers in a particular setting during a specific time frame. The data can also be aggregated to identify differences in groups of patients, populations, providers, and

TABLE 10.1 TYPES OF NURSE–PATIENT MEASURES FOR DNP PROJECTS

One Nurse to One Patient (Nurse–Patient Measures)	Many Nurses to One Patient (Patient Level Measures)	Many Nurses to Many Patients (Unit/Organization Measures)
Direct-care hours (intensity) and cost per unit of service (e.g., home visit, patient day, clinic appointment, etc.)	Sum of direct-care time and costs by case, diagnosis, DRG, procedure, etc.	Aggregate intensity and cost per unit of outcome (e.g., intensity and cost per case, per DRG, episode of care, per number of client, etc.)
Units of service, interventions, procedures, surveillance, assessments	Demand for nursing care (hours needed) compared to hours and services delivered	Intensity/cost variability, trends, and differences by age, diagnosis, nursing case mix, day of stay or day of service, etc.
Acuity, complexity of care	Aggregate acuity and intensity of care, complexity of case, interventions, etc.	Nursing costs/intensity vs. reimbursement
Nurse experience, wage, education, competencies, certifications	Environmental scanning (number and time of admissions, transfers and discharges, clinic appointment volume, home visits, etc.)	Benchmark nursing time and costs/case across settings (e.g., hospitals, clinics, home health care, etc.)
Performance measures such as giving medications on time, effective pain management, etc.	Outcomes of care, quality indicators such as infections, pressure ulcers, injuries, etc.	Sum of indirect (nonpatient) time, such as vacation or sick time, costs by unit of time, and nursing intensity/costs by level of acuity or severity of illness (productivity)

Efficiency and effectiveness; quality and outcomes |

DRG, diagnosis-related group.

Source: Reprinted with permission from Welton, J. M., & Harper, E. M. (2015). Nursing care value-based financial models. *Nursing Economics, 33*(1), 1–25.

settings. For example, a project could be developed examining the effects of follow-up care in a primary care clinic for diabetic patients to assess how such care is helping this population maintain healthy glycemic control by analyzing hemoglobin A1c (HbA1c) levels over time. This could be done in a single primary care setting or across many different locations.

Working with large sets of clinical and administrative data has both advantages and disadvantages. Extracting data from a healthcare system that encompasses many hospitals and clinics can give insight into variation of outcomes between certain hospitals or clinics, or even variation of types of patients accessing a certain hospital or clinic within one system.

The comparison of care across many settings can result in sharing results that can improve practice and provide data indicating meaningful differences in care (e.g., information about one or two locations producing superior results could be disseminated across the system). A DNP professional could utilize a large-system dataset to examine delays in antibiotic administration and the subsequent effects on care outcomes such as development of sepsis.

But the complexity of both extraction and analysis of these data can be daunting. The challenge for the DNP-prepared nurse will be to prompt the interdisciplinary team of healthcare professionals to identify, utilize, and analyze large datasets to effect improvement in care or to implement evidence-based clinical care guidelines. This can be done in a leadership role to identify and interpret continuous streams or groups of data, thereby identifying changes in care, outliers, patterns of practice, or significant trends.

PREPARING DATA FOR ANALYSIS

It is imperative that the DNP professional be familiar with the Health Insurance Portability and Accountability Act (HIPAA) Privacy Rule when accessing healthcare data. Protected health information (PHI) can be stripped of identifying features and added anonymously to large databases of patient information. Such de-identified data can contribute to population health management efforts and value-based care programs. There are no restrictions on the use or disclosure of de-identified health information captured in a database, which is an organized collection of data, stored and accessed electronically. A relational database (Codd, 1970) is a tabular database in which data are defined so that they can be reorganized and accessed in a number of different ways. Relational databases are made up sets of tables with data that fit into predefined categories. Each table has at least one data category in a column, and each row has a certain data instance for the categories defined in the columns. The power of relational databases comes from the fact that tables can be linked, enabling users to gain access to data across tables.

Two tables are linked when they have a matching field (i.e., a field in each table containing similar data). For example, suppose you want to link a "patients with a hip replacement" table with another table called "hip replacement product." Both tables must have at least one field in common. If you insert the primary key field of the patient-centered table (e.g., PtID) into the product-centered table (e.g., ProdID), the two tables will have a matching field: PtID. The tables are now linked, and you can access their data together. In the case of the patient identifier, one central table can house all unique information about a patient (e.g., age, gender, and race), and these data can then be linked to other tables that contain clinical or operational data. This linkage allows information about a patient, such as age, to be "pulled" at the time the nurse enters assessment data. Figure 10.1 links nurses as providers

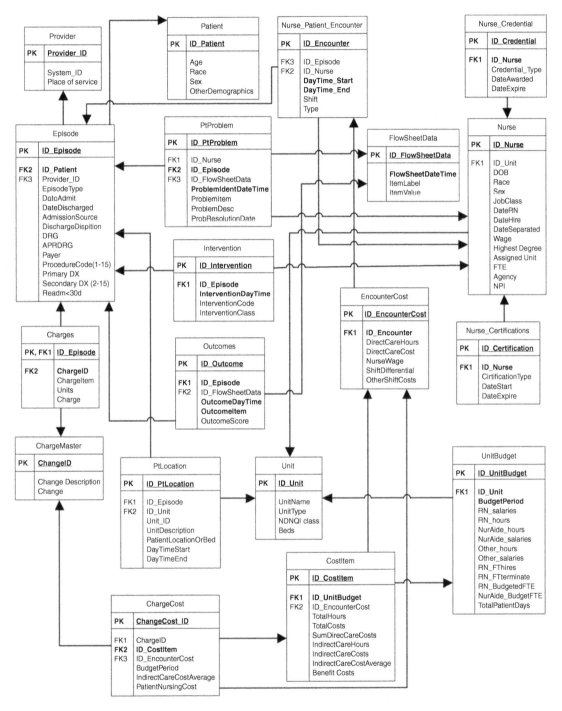

FIGURE 10.1 Nursing Value Data Model.

DOB, date of birth; DRG, diagnosis-related group; FTE, full-time equivalent; NDNQI, National Database of Nursing Quality Indicators; NPI, national provider identifier; Pt, patient.

Source: From Welton, J. M., & Harper, E. M. (2015). Nursing care value-based financial models. *Nursing Economics, 33*(1), 14–19, 25; Welton, J. M., & Harper, E. M. (2016). Measuring nursing care value. *Nursing Economics, 34*(1), 7–14.

TABLE 10.2 DATA FILE EXAMPLE: ID_PATIENT AND ID_NURSE EXTRACTED DATA

ID_Patient	ID_Nurse	Age	Location	Pain Score	Medication	Dose	Route	Date Time
12345678	ABCD	69	SICU	7	Morphine	2 mg	IV	8/1/2018 12:00
12345678	ABCD	69	SICU	4				8/1/2018 12:23
12345678	ABCD	69	SICU	8	Morphine	4 mg	IV	8/1/2018 18:50
12345678	ABCD	69	SICU	7				8/1/2018 19:07

SICU, surgical intensive care unit.

of care directly to a patient (Welton & Harper, 2016). In this data model, nursing care can be examined at the individual nurse–patient relationship level. For example, a patient is admitted to a hospital and a nurse provides specific interventions such as pain assessment and PRN opioid administration. The primary keys that link the tables (i.e., ID_Patient and ID_Nurse) would result in the extracted data seen in Table 10.2.

This example would be derived from a large and complex EHR that could provide additional data such as patient age, gender, and diagnosis. Also, the nurse is directly identified, and additional data about the nurse could be included (e.g., length of experience, whether the nurse is floating from another unit or is a contract or travel nurse). Based on this relatively simple example, a DNP professional working in an acute care setting could include several analyses to answer the questions on the amount of PRN opioid versus nonopioid PRN medications being given, differences in PRN medication administered by different nurses, or the amount and prevalence of PRN opioids administered over change of shift. A DNP student could examine practice patterns of nurses and other providers in administrating pharmacologic and nonpharmacologic treatments for pain to identify best practices across multiple settings by linking individual nurses to each patient.

Figure 10.1 shows a more complex data model from elements of the EHR that can be used to extract clinical and operational data across patients and settings. This is relevant to identify and link nurses directly to patient care and include pertinent information about the clinical care the patients have received and the clinicians administering that care.

COLLECTING AD CONFIGURING DATA FOR ANALYSIS

This conceptual data model leads to specification of all the variables and the relationship of these variables (see Figure 10.1). From this data model, a data dictionary is produced. A data dictionary provides information about each attribute, also referred to as *fields*, of a data model. An attribute is a place in the database that holds information. It is typically organized in a spreadsheet format. Each attribute is listed as a row in the spreadsheet, and each column labels an element of information that is useful to know about the attribute. The most common elements included in a data dictionary are as follows:

- Attribute name—A unique identifier, typically expressed in business language, that labels each attribute
- Optional/required—Indicates whether information is required in an attribute before a record can be saved
- Attribute type—Defines what types of data are allowable in a field (e.g., text, numeric, date/time, enumerated list, look-ups, booleans, and unique identifiers)

Data dictionaries do not contain any actual data from the database; instead they are used by IT professionals to extract the requested data from the EHR or a data warehouse in a suitable format that can be used in traditional statistical analysis software. Table 10.3 is an example of a data dictionary based on the data in Table 10.2.

WORKING WITH DATA

Because quality-improvement activities are data-driven and involve human participants, it is vital that they be executed in a manner that is ethical and respects the rights and welfare of the human participants.

First, if the project requires patient- or provider-level data, an institutional review board (IRB) should be engaged, and a protocol for use of the data must be approved before data extraction can begin. Protected health identifiers will need to be removed or anonymized to hide the identity of each patient or provider in the study. Typically, QI projects used for internal purposes within the healthcare institution do not need IRB approval. However, it is imperative that the person leading the project knows the agency and school requirements for review.

Extraction of data from data warehouses or EHRs typically requires working with key information technology (IT) programmers to identify which data are needed, where they are to be extracted from, and what format the data need to be in in order to conduct an analysis. Unfortunately, this can take time as programmers have a primary responsibility for overseeing the clinical application of the various IT systems. Students requesting data for a project must (a) build in plenty of lead time to obtain the data and (b) anticipate spending time in setting up and cleaning the data prior to analysis.

TABLE 10.3 DATA FILE EXAMPLE: ID_PATIENT AND ID_NURSE EXTRACTED DATA

Field Name	Label	Data Type	Format	Value Set	Description
ID_Patient	Patient ID	Char (8)	xxxxxxx		Unique to each patient and admission, actual value will be anonymized prior to analysis
ID_Nurse	Nurse ID	Char (5)	xxxxx		Unique to each nurse, linked to nurse table in database
Age	Patient Age	Num	xx.x		Age greater than 90 will be converted to 90 to meet IRB approved protocol
Loc	Unit Location	Char (5)	xxxxx	CCU; ICU; 2E 2W 3E; 3W	At time of assessment or intervention
PainScor	Pain Score	Int	x	Scale 0–10	Patient verbal score of pain based on nurse assessment
Med	Medication	Char (15)			Linked for hospital formulary data
Dose	Dose	Num	xx.x		In milligrams
Route	Route	Char (10)		IV; Oral; SubQ; IM; Other	
DateTime	Date Time	Date	Mm/dd/yy HH:MM		Time assessment completed or medication was administered based on 24-hour clock

CCU, coronoary care unit; IM, intramuscular; SubQ, subcutaneous.

Nomenclature:

Char, Character or text, can be mix of letters and numbers, length of field in parenthesis; Date, numeric representation of date and time; Int, Numeric data stored as an integer (no decimal place); Num, Numeric data.

Data cleaning, also called *data cleansing* or *data scrubbing*, deals with detecting and removing errors and inconsistencies from the data in order to improve the data quality. Data-quality problems are present in single data collections, such as files and databases, for example, due to misspellings during data entry, missing information, or other invalid data. When multiple data sources need to be integrated (e.g., in data warehouses, federated database systems, or global web-based information systems), the need for data cleaning increases significantly. This is because the sources often contain redundant data in different representations. To provide access to accurate and consistent data, consolidation of different data representations and elimination of duplicate information become necessary. The first step is to identify each continuous numerical variable and produce preliminary statistics such as mean, median, maximum, minimum, and standard deviation values. A histogram can be used to depict distribution of the data for each variable and identify outliers or oddly shaped curves that may indicate problems with the underlying variable. Likewise, for categorical data, frequency tables and percentage distribution are created to identify the distribution and missing variables.

Prior to any data analysis, there needs to be a discussion and decision about how to handle aberrant or missing data. For example, using age as a variable, a value of 200 would be impossible and likely a data-entry error. There needs to be a decision about how to trap such errors (e.g., write code that changes any age greater than 100 to a null value). If the value were changed to 0 (zero), that data point would be included in descriptive analysis and potentially bias the results by pulling down the mean age.

For categorical data, one of the primary issues is how to deal with missing data. For example, in the medication administration example discussed previously (see Table 10.2), many pain scores could be missing. That may bias results from the analysis. There are no easy answers for how best to deal with missing data. The best practice for addressing aberrant, skewed, or missing data should be determined prior to data extraction/setup and corrected, if possible, before data are extracted.

TRANSFORMATIONS AND NEW VARIABLES

Additional variables (e.g., time-referenced data) can be calculated based on data obtained from data- collection instruments other than what is pulled from a table. In the medication administration example, one key issue may be late-scheduled doses. One way to calculate late doses is to look at the scheduled administration time provided by the pharmacy and the actual administration time provided by the BCMA data. A simple date–time calculation can provide the number of minutes a dose was early or late. If an antibiotic was due at 12:00 (noon), and the BCMA was time-stamped at 12:50, the medication administration is 50 minutes past the actual scheduled time. If the hospital policy is to give all antibiotics within a ±30-minute window, a second variable could be calculated that would indicate "1" if outside the 30-minute window or "0" if not.

Time-referenced data can be used in other interesting ways. Trends and patterns could be identified from existing data, such as the number of late medications by shift (day or night), by weekend or holiday, by staffing patterns, or in larger time groups such as months, quarters, or years.

These are helpful in identifying short-term issues that may be isolated to individual units or clinicians or could identify subtle long-term changes (e.g., increase/decrease in the number of late doses with changes in staffing patterns or patient case mix and severity of illness). One benefit of having access to very large datasets is the ability to identify small changes over time that otherwise would be difficult or impossible to capture.

DATA-ANALYSIS PLAN

A data-analysis plan is a road map for organizing and analyzing the data. The data-analysis project plan illustrates many basic requirements of the project. The plan outlines the structure of the data, declares the objectives of the project, describes the data sources, and identifies the procedures used to carry out the project. The plan document becomes a vital part of the project because it shows the methods and purpose of the project to supervisors, administrators, the QI team, and/or the school. The data-analysis plan is produced prior to the start of data collection (Simpson, 2015).

DATA ANALYSIS

After data are extracted, organized, cleaned, and validated, overall data analysis can begin. Typically, an overall descriptive analysis of the sample, key variables, and summary data by unit of analysis is completed first. Describing the population under study provides a number of important indicators. The analysis shows whether there are any differences, outliers, or identifiable characteristics in the populations. This initial analysis also depicts the project population in relationship to the project aims or objectives. One or several tables and graphs can be constructed. If the purpose is an internal review or QI project, the various graphics and tables can be copied and pasted into a report for distribution. If these are to be used for presentation or publication, care should be used to identify the needs of the journal or conference for table formatting and size.

Tables are very effective in condensing large amounts of data and organizing columns and rows to provide clarity and information. Review the different ways that the data can be organized. For example, for categorical data; the total number, row, or column percentage; and total table percentage can include subtotals with different percentages. When examining a continuous variable with categorical data, consider ways to make the table user-friendly and convey the most information without becoming too cluttered. Sometimes, it is easier to separate data into two tables rather than force too much information into a single table.

There are several tips for improving the overall "product" of the analysis. Avoid complex tables and graphs that are hard to read. If submitting for publication, it is worthwhile to do all initial analysis in black and white to avoid issues in ultimate production (i.e., needing to change graphics submitted in color to black and white for the final proof for publication). For presentation graphics, use limited color for maximum utility (e.g., use green to indicate positive results or red to show negative results). Generally, avoid three-dimensional graphs as they can be difficult to read and interpret in a presentation setting. Last, remember that simpler is better: This approach will enhance clarity and readability of the output of your study or project. When attempting to show changes in a patient or among a group of patients over time, a basic line or bar graph with time on the x (bottom) axis can show differences clearly, and a pie graph can effectively show proportions within a population under study.

The DNP-prepared nurse can be instrumental in identifying the best way to disseminate key findings and relevance to practice. Different stakeholders (e.g., bedside clinicians, nurse managers, or "C-suite" executives) will need different information, and therefore, the presentation and written materials produced should be adapted to meet the needs of the intended audience.

DISSEMINATION PLAN

Developing a dissemination plan is also good practice, and this can be included in the analysis plan or generated as a stand-alone document. Dissemination-plan development is a key part of the collaborative planning process. Although the decision-makers and QI leaders working together will not know the results of the project until it is completed, working through a dissemination plan early in the project can help the team focus the project and identify key audiences. The plan should include activities and tools (e.g., printed materials, posters, and presentations) and face-to-face meetings that will inform the target audience. Each member of the project team should be responsible for carrying out at least one dissemination activity.

For small internal projects, the dissemination plan may specify reporting responsibilities and internal meetings to discuss results. If the project will be disseminated outside of the institution, a list of conferences/due dates for abstracts and potential journals for submission should be drafted, with responsibility for completing action items clearly identified.

ISSUES WITH BIG DATA

One of the vexing problems in using big data for a DNP scholarly project is that there is potential for overwhelming desktop computers with large data files. These large files may need to be broken into many smaller files to be able to extract, load, and analyze the data. Therefore, prior to conducting analyses of large datasets, the computational power of available computers should be considered, including processor speed, amount of random access memory (RAM), and storage space on a hard drive or other permanent medium. Long-term storage needs to be considered in that these large files may take up valuable space or require an upgrade of local computer resources. The computation power of the computers used for analysis could provide a challenge.

Moving data, especially very large datasets, from multiple sites to a central location for analysis can also provide challenges. First, data must be protected by anonymizing protected health identifiers, such as names, addresses, and other patient identifiers (Yaraghi & Gopal, 2018). Then, the data need to be transferred securely. Last, the central data repository needs to be protected and HIPAA compliant to prevent unauthorized access.

Transfer of large data from outside sites to a central site can produce unique challenges and barriers (e.g., not having the necessary internet bandwidth could significantly prolong data transfer). Any patient-level data will require a secure file transfer over a network that can handle the large dataset. Second, the storage medium and processing power at the next site used for analysis needs to be considered. Corruption of data either during the initial data extraction from the EHR or during file transfer is possible. Finally,, opening very large files using typical software on a desktop or laptop can be problematic and may inadvertently alter the data if opened then saved. For example, there is a limit to the number of rows of data that the commonly used Microsoft Excel spreadsheet program can handle. If a data extraction from the EHR exceeds this limit, data will be truncated. File size can also present issues with regard to how much RAM a computer has or the amount of available permanent storage available. The size of the file can also affect how fast large amounts of data can be processed and analyzed.

CONCLUSIONS

This chapter reviews the potential for a DNP-prepared nurse to conduct a project using large clinical and operational datasets. The skillset inculcated in and provided by DNP-prepared nurses supports the overall effort to extract EHR-based data; select appropriate variables; develop and execute a data- analysis plan; interpret results; and disseminate the findings to the bedside, classroom, or boardroom.

There is a move toward making more data-informed decisions in caring for patients instead of just making experienced-informed decisions.

The creation of sophisticated predictive analytic-driven solutions based on big data are needed to improve health outcomes. With this changing environment, there is a growing need for DNP-prepared nurses who can work with these data and help craft actionable interventions that improve care, decrease overall costs, and ultimately, add value to the healthcare system.

Case Study

Medication administration is a primary responsibility of nurses. A safety net hospital in the Rocky Mountain region partnered with a local college of nursing to evaluate the practice patterns of nurses when administering medications. Data entered in the EHR for day-to-day patient care allow for the evaluation of processes to improve nurse-centered workflow and quality of care. The case study accessed data from several systems that were merged to supply additional information, allowing for a more complete picture of medication administration practices. Approximately 700 nurses administered over 3,000,000 medication doses to 50,000 patients over a 3-year period. Data for this evaluation came from the EHR, the pharmacy database, BCMA, and human resources systems data.

Obtaining data from multiple software systems was the first challenge to overcome. Data from most of the systems were stored in a unified data warehouse, making retrieval somewhat easier. In order to retrieve the data, a programmer with the proper training and credentials was needed to access the information in the warehouse (i.e., the available data that identified medication administration patterns and the tables that contained those data). Most organizations limit access to the data warehouse, making it difficult to obtain data if no one in the department is trained/cleared and sometimes requiring a long wait time if there is a queue of multiple requests to obtain data.

For the nurse medication administration project, the primary objective was to describe overall practice patterns in administering both scheduled and PRN (as needed) drugs. A key focus was the difference between scheduled times and administered times to allow calculation of time differences and estimate overall early or late doses (as well as delayed doses for high-alert medications such as antibiotics). When a nurse administers medications at the bedside, she or he uses a badge to access the system, which enters the unique identifier of the nurse. The BCMA scans the patient's bracelet, entering the unique patient identifier. These two identifiers create a direct link between a nurse and patient.

Data used in this project included administrative data (demographic and encounter-level), medication orders, medication administration, Pyxis cabinet administration data, and staff-focused data (e.g., licensure and clocking data). Although the EHR is one system, it has many parts, and data can be retrieved from multiple areas. The case study pulled data from two areas of the EHR: provider order entry of medication (order entry) and the BCMA system. Physicians' orders were used to identify the drug, drug class, dose, route, and scheduled versus PRN medication. Data were also pulled from the human resources system to identify the nurses' education/certification levels and years of experience.

(continued)

Case Study (*continued*)

Matching data to the same patient and nurse from disparate systems was a time-consuming undertaking. Having one unique identifier for a nurse would prevent some of the issues encountered when trying to match nurses from several of these systems. Different data sources had different unique identifiers, and many links had to be created manually. For example, one of the objectives was to calculate the time from when a nurse pulled a drug from the dispensing cart on the unit (Pyxis) to when it was bar coded at the bedside to detect whether there were patterns of delays. Unfortunately, the lack of common nurse identifiers made this very problematic, and it was ultimately abandoned in the final analysis.

Missing data are an issue that must be dealt with when undertaking a project. The project lead or statistical specialist needs to determine whether there is a way to retrieve the data from another source or in another way. Time and attention needs to be given to obtaining the most complete dataset possible. Do not just remove observations simply because obtaining missing data is inconvenient or time-consuming. For example, the data from the human resources system linked to each nurse had intermittent and sometimes sparse data for credentials, certifications, and academic preparation. These data often were not updated as each nurse or nurse manager had to manually enter them. There are some of the realities in working with existing clinical and operational data.

Time-stamped data can provide information on the amount of time required to perform tasks, such as medication administration, because multiple time stamps are documented. These include the time the medication was pulled from the dispensing cart, the time the medication was due (scheduled), and the time it was administered using BCMA. The sequence of time stamps can provide a picture of how long it takes to administer medications to patients. These time stamps also allow a determination of whether medications were given on time over a patient encounter or by the mix of different nurses.

When joining data from multiple systems, it is best to consult with someone who has expertise in this area. Data can be dropped or not joined correctly for a variety of reasons, and if this is not evaluated and errors corrected, the results of any analysis will be invalid. The outliers in a dataset must also be evaluated to determine whether they should be included in the analysis. Making a determination about outliers is usually done by the team working on the project because statistical knowledge and clinical knowledge are needed to make these decisions. Any decisions on inclusion/exclusion criteria or protocols for manipulation/transformation of data should be clearly identified in the analysis plan.

QUESTIONS

1. Can EHR data alone answer the question of practice patterns of nurses when administering medications?
2. Why is data cleaning so difficult in this case?
3. Who needs to be involved in the collection, cleaning, and analysis of these data?

REFERENCES

Codd, E. F. (1970). A relational model of data for large shared data banks. *Communications of the ACM, 13*(6), 377–387. doi:10.1145/362384.362685

Krumholz, H. M. (2014). Big data and new knowledge in medicine: The thinking, training, and tools needed for a learning health system. *Health Affairs, 33*(7), 1163–1170. doi:10.1377/hlthaff.2014.0053

Roski, J., Bo-Linn, G. W., & Andrews, T. A. (2014). Creating value in health care through big data: opportunities and policy implications. *Health Affairs, 33*(7), 1115–1122. doi:10.1377/hlthaff.2014.0147

Seibert, H. H., Maddox, R. R., Flynn, E. A., & Williams, C. K. (2014). Effect of barcode technology with electronic medication administration record on medication accuracy rates. *American Journal of Health-System Pharmacy, 71*(3), 209–218. doi:10.2146/ajhp130332

Simpson, S. H. (2015). Creating a data analysis plan: What to consider when choosing statistics for a study. *Canadian Journal of Hospital Pharmacy, 68*(4), 311–317. doi:10.4212/cjhp.v68i4.1471

Welton, J. M., & Harper, E. M. (2015). Nursing care value-based financial models. *Nursing Economic$, 33*(1), 14–19, 25.

Welton, J. M., & Harper, E. M. (2016). Measuring nursing care value. *Nursing Economic$, 34*(1), 7–14.

Yaraghi, N., & Gopal, R. D. (2018). The role of HIPAA omnibus rules in reducing the frequency of medical data breaches: Insights from an empirical study. *Milbank Quarterly, 96*(1), 144–166. doi:10.1111/1468-0009.12314

VALUE-BASED PAYMENT MODELS IN HEALTHCARE

BARBARA J. MARTIN

This chapter addresses the following DNP American Association of Colleges of Nursing (AACN) Essentials:

II. Organizational and Systems Leadership for Quality Improvement and Systems Thinking
V. Healthcare Policy for Advocacy in Healthcare
VI. Interprofessional Collaboration for Improving Patient and Population Health Outcomes
VII. Clinical Prevention and Population Health for Improving the Nation's Health

INTRODUCTION

DNP-prepared advanced practice registered nurses (APRNs) work across the healthcare continuum, often serving populations most in need of care in underserved or rural areas of the country. These patient populations are often covered by public health insurance, such as Medicare and Medicaid. Increasingly, APRNs are reimbursed directly by commercial health insurance plans. Healthcare delivery is influenced by many complex systems inputs, most important of which is financing. It is imperative for APRNs to understand the history of healthcare financing and policy, and how this affects their ability to deliver high-quality, cost-effective care. It is also helpful to have context for the ways in which healthcare has evolved so that APRNs can play a pivotal role in shaping the future of healthcare delivery (DesRoches et al., 2013; Everett et al., 2013).

Although the U.S. healthcare system is based on a market economy, there are basic economic principles that are unmet, creating a system that is, at times, unchecked. There are traditionally two main actors within an economic transaction: the buyer and the seller. Historically in healthcare this is represented by the patient and the provider. The market-based principles require that the buyer have information about price and quality when making the decision to buy goods or services (Buchanan, Dranove, & White, 1988). In the U.S. healthcare system, information about price and quality is not typically available to the patient in a form that he or she can utilize. A third party, the insurer or payer, has emerged during the last 50-plus years in the healthcare market, which adds complexity and influences the basic tenets of supply and demand, and the role of buyer and seller in healthcare. Because the nursing profession holds health as a universal right, the transactional and financial aspects of healthcare delivery and payment are not well researched in nursing literature. Yet that disconnect can limit the ability to influence future healthcare delivery designs that ensure better patient health outcomes and the avoidance of unnecessary costs. An exploration of the history and evolution of the complex healthcare delivery system reveals the influence all three of these actors have on healthcare financing and policy. As the U.S. healthcare system has evolved, reactions to the financial impact, public voice, and market forces have all influenced the delivery of care. Healthcare financing invariably impacts healthcare delivery design. APRNs are at the center of these complex systems, often in leadership positions, which is why they can influence effective delivery design and maintain a focus on evidence-based treatment and patient-centered outcomes. Understanding the history and current status of financing and payment reform, as summarized in the text that follows, is core to a DNP leader's role.

This chapter provides a summary of the history of healthcare financing, including the role of healthcare insurance and its subsequent impact on healthcare quality, cost, and health outcomes. The history of healthcare can be broken into three time periods: The Industrial Era and the advent of modern medicine: (1900–1950), public and private insurance expansion and the escalation of health-care costs: 1950–2001, and the era of healthcare delivery and payment reform: 2001–present.

The concept of value-based payment (VBP), which was catalyzed by the 2001 Institute of Medicaid report: *Crossing the Quality Chasm*, is also explored. This chapter concludes with the practical implications for the DNP leader, exploring a case study on bundled or episode of care payments for maternity care. Taking a systems approach is necessary to understand healthcare financing, the evolution of healthcare reform, and the emergence of VBP as a paradigm shift. Emerging VBP models are, in many ways, meant to fix problems that have been present since the beginning of the country's healthcare system.

HISTORY OF HEALTHCARE FINANCING AND EVOLUTION OF HEALTHCARE INSURANCE

1900–1950: The Industrial Era and Advent of Modern Medicine

The healthcare system in the United States is primarily based on a health insurance model that has evolved over the last two centuries. Along with economic and medical advances, the social structure and household economy in the United States has changed and created a need for insurance against financial costs related to medical care and lost wages. In the beginning of the 20th century, the concern focused on an individual's medical costs and lost wages if the individual was the family's primary breadwinner (Berkowitz, 2005). The medical costs had less of an impact than the social costs of foregone wages (Martin & Weaver, 2005; Starr, 1982). Because of this, health insurance began as social insurance. As early as 1883 Germany created a program to protect against the financial cost of sickness with a focus on lost wages for specific workers. As this practice spread across Europe, periodic attempts to introduce social insurance policies were not successful in the United States (Berkowitz, 2005; Starr, 1982). Key opponents included physician groups, which maintained that medical care should be a transaction between a patient and provider without third party interference (Berkowitz, 2005).

During this time, medical education and training were maturing, yet the doctor maintained a direct relationship with the patient, often providing care based on ability to pay (Starr, 1982). The first part of the 20th century saw a shift—medical costs escalated beyond the social cost of forgone wages, a changing paradigm influenced by improvements in medical care and increased access to hospitals (Berkowitz, 2005). A committee, formed in the 1920s to evaluate the costs of medical care, called for some type of social system to ensure a sufficient supply of medical care and mechanisms to pay for it. The 1930s and the Great Depression diverted attention from the cost of medical care as societal concerns again focused on income security.

The passage of the 1935 Social Security Act, one of the most sweeping welfare reform acts of the 20th century, did not tackle sickness or health insurance. The Act did, however, provide for unemployment insurance, old-age insurance, and means-tested welfare programs (Martin & Weaver, 2005). Perhaps most important, it laid the groundwork for the role of the federal government in providing a safety net for its citizens, an important foundation for future healthcare legislation. With the advent of World War II, advocates for health insurance continued to develop policy solutions, and during the postwar period proposals for national health insurance were proposed in 1943, 1945, and 1947. This is an important context because often effective policy is achieved only after sufficient policy softening lays the groundwork for acceptability within government or policy networks, or larger constituent groups.

Although the debate about a public health insurance solution continued during the 1940s, private health insurance became increasingly available across the country. The Stabilization Act of 1942 imposed controls over wages and prices during World War II and the aftermath to avoid inflation and stabilize prices in the county. However, it did not apply to fringe benefits. Because of this, employer-sponsored insurance was a tool that employers used to attract employees (Buchmueller & Monheit, 2009). Largely due to this, there was an expansion of private, often employer-based health insurance in the 1940s. By 1951 more than half of hospitalized patients had some type of insurance (Berkowitz, 2005).

Legislation passed in the 1940s had a significant impact on the healthcare system. The Hospital Survey and Construction Act, more commonly known as the *Hill–Burton Act of 1946*, which was signed into law by President Truman, provided federal dollars to subsidize the construction of new healthcare facilities. The purpose of the Act was to infuse dollars into community hospitals, clinics, or similar care settings, to provide access to care for all people in the community (Dowell, 1987). The Hill–Burton Act required provision of free or reduced cost services for facilities that received funding, and stipulated that facilities could not discriminate. In many ways, this legislation—which was meant to increase equitable access to needed care—ultimately led to construction of facilities in areas where the demand was not in line with the supply. During the next 40 years, the federal government pumped significant dollars into construction of healthcare facilities (states were required to match federal dollars) for 6,800 facilities in 4,000 communities. Although the Act was intended to target rural areas, construction was much more expansive and although it was meant to increase access, especially for poor Americans, it ultimately resulted in excess capacity within the system. In many ways, this supply-side economic policy created the paradigm of filling hospital beds that would drive a volume-based system in the ensuing decades (Dowell, 1987; Mantone, 2005).

1950–2001: Public and Private Insurance Eexpansion and the Escalation of Healthcare Costs

An important development in physician and provider reimbursement dates to the early 1950s. The California Medical Association, which was concerned that variable pricing set by physicians for services would lead third-party insurers to set prices, set service codes with associated relative value units (RVUs) for each service provided across primary and specialty care (Sandy, Bodenheimer, Pawlson, & Starfield, 2009). This process was expanded into a national model of fee-setting and has become entrenched in the payment system and fee schedules for providers. The Relative Value Scale Update Committee (RUC), a body of the American

Medical Association (AMA), maintains and updates the RVU system. This system has been blamed for perpetuating the imbalance in reimbursement for primary care versus specialty care. The RVU is a factor of physician (or provider as this applies to APRNs) work, practice expense, and malpractice costs. This historical price-setting process remains a core component of the healthcare fee-for-service (FFS) reimbursement models of today.

The idea of focusing a national health insurance solution on the elderly gained traction during the 1950s and 1960s. Because of the increase in employer-sponsored health insurance for working-age Americans, the focus turned toward a solution for seniors, a population typically not eligible for employer-sponsored insurance. In the early 1960s, elderly individuals with insurance were 25% more likely to be admitted to a hospital than those without insurance. This was thought to indicate that a lack of insurance was a barrier to accessing care for the elderly (Lave & Silverman, 1983). During this time, the elderly comprised a vulnerable population with nearly one in four living in poverty. By 2000 that number was one in 10 and by 2015 the percentage of seniors, who were older than 65 and at the poverty level had decreased to 8.8% (Centers for Disease Control, n.d.; Lave, & Silverman, 1983).

The concept of using Medicare to cover the elderly was introduced in 1961, and the bill went through various iterations until it was passed in 1965 as Titles XVIII and XIX of the Social Security Act, which forever changed the healthcare dynamics in this county and is known as the *Medicare and Medicaid Act*. Medicare Part A, which covers hospitalizations, was the core component of the bill until the eleventh hour when Medicare Part B, which covers physician services and Medicaid, was added. This addition is attributed in large part to Wilbur Mills, the head of the Ways and Means Committee at the time, who proposed combining the hospital insurance proposal (Part A) with the physician services proposal (Part B) and expanding the existing Kerr–Mills program (Medicaid), and ensured that all three components made it into law (Berkowitz, 2005).

Medicaid, the medical program to cover the poor (those eligible for cash assistance under the Social Security Act at the time of passage), was not a key component of the health insurance debate. However, advocates for expanding healthcare coverage to the poor were interested in expanding The Kerr–Mills program of 1962, which provided grants to states to cover care for medically indigent elderly. Proponents at the time were interested in expanding coverage to other populations on welfare, especially children. A supplemental program that expanded the Kerr–Mills eligible population was included in the 1965 amendment to the Social Security Act, and it was renamed *Medicaid* (Berkowitz, 2005).

Much of the current policy considerations in healthcare are a result of the provisions of the 1965 bill. If Medicare Part B were not added, or the Kerr–Mills program were not expanded, the healthcare ecosystem would look much different today. Effects of the sweeping legislation led to unanticipated growth in healthcare spending. At the time the bill passed in 1965, healthcare accounted for approximately 6% of the gross domestic product (GDP), 80% of which was out of pocket or paid for by private insurance companies. The federal portion was 8% and the state portion was 12%. The dramatic shift that occurred after passage of the Medicare and Medicaid Act has both a direct and indirect impact on society and influenced policy in later decades (Feldstein, 2011).

In the first half of the 20th century medical care was based on an FFS model. The passage of the Medicare and Medicaid Act of 1965 did not change this—it did not alter how healthcare was purchased, it just expanded coverage so that more individuals could purchase healthcare. This provided financial security to physicians in a way that was not possible with the direct-pay (often using a sliding scale) model used early in the century (Berkowitz, 2005; Starr, 1982). For the first time there was a guaranteed source of payment for physicians. The FFS model meant that the more services delivered, the more a provider or hospital would be paid. Combined with the expansion of hospitals and health facilities, which was spurred by the Hill–Burton Act, the amount spent on healthcare quickly escalated. By the early 1970s, the percentage of GDP spent on healthcare prompted the passage of legislation that tried to alter how care was paid for with the introduction of health maintenance organizations (HMOs). Prior to this time, policy was aimed directly at ensuring access to care. With the escalating costs, policy became focused on how care was delivered and financed (Table 11.1).

By the early 1970s, the impact of the increased supply prompted by the Hill–Burton Act, the increased demand through employer-sponsored insurance, and the passage of the Medicaid and Medicare Bill, led to an alarming increase in healthcare expenditure. By 1974, nearly 8% of the GDP was spent on healthcare, and the healthcare system employed twice the number of employees it had 25 years earlier (Health Planning and Resources Development Act of 1974, 1975). The duality of the problem began to emerge at this time: The healthcare system as a whole became responsible for uncontrolled healthcare expenditures and it became an increasingly important employer. Legislation emerged in the early 1970s to address the growing issue of healthcare costs.

The Health Planning and Resource Development Act of 1974 created an organized structure for the prioritization of health facilities and introduced the concept of Certificate of Need (CON) to establish criteria for the construction of new health facilities. This has been an important policy lever for states to limit new facilities (Havighurst, 1973; Health Planning and Resources Development Act of 1974, 1975). The Act required states to develop a process for obtaining approval for major capital projects such as building expenses or high-tech devices. In addition, states had to identify

TABLE 11.1 SUMMARY OF MEDICARE AND MEDICAID: ROLES, SERVICES, AND POPULATIONS COVERED

Title	Authority	Federal and State Role	Services and Population Covered	Beneficiary Role	Services Not Covered
Medicare Part A	Social Security Title XVIII (Medicare and Medicaid Bill) 1965	Federally funded and administered	Individuals over 65, ESRD, SSI Inpatient hospital, limited skilled nursing postacute Hospice and home health services	Automatically enrolled Deductible 1,184/ benefit period Copay/coinsurance if in hospital >60 days or skilled nursing >20 days	Dental, vision, hearing aids, long-term services
Medicare Part B	Social Security Title XVIII (Medicare and Medicaid Bill) 1965	Federally funded and administered	Individuals over 65, ESRD, SSI Doctor and clinical lab services Outpatient and preventive care Home healthcare Screenings, surgical fees and supplies Physical and occupational therapy	Need to opt-in Cost-sharing Deductible $147/year Premium: $104.90–$335.70/month depending on income Co-pays: 20%	Outpatient services—consumer choice drafted as part of last-minute negotiations includes components that are funded in part by the beneficiaries
Medicare Part C (also called Medicare Advantage)	TEFRA 1982	Federally funded Administered through private health plans in risk-based contracts	Medicare Advantage covers part A and B services in one plan. Can also include part D.	Opt into a Medicare Advantage plan	Plan may choose to cover more comprehensive benefits

TABLE 11.1 SUMMARY OF MEDICARE AND MEDICAID: ROLES, SERVICES, AND POPULATIONS COVERED *(continued)*

Title	Authority	Federal and State Role	Services and Population Covered	Beneficiary Role	Services Not Covered
Medicare Part D	Medicare Prescription Drug Improvement and Modernization Act 2003	Federally funded through private health plans Stand alone or part of Part C	Helps cover the cost of prescription drugs May help lower prescription drug costs and protect against higher costs in the future Copays and deductibles varies with plan	Choose plan Cost-sharing	Subsidizes cost of prescription drugs Does not cover total cost History of the "donut hole," which put seniors at risk for out-of-pocket expenses
Medicaid	Social Security Title XVIX (Medicare and Medicaid Bill) 1965	Federally funded with state matching State administered	Began as coverage for poor on cash assistance Coverage has expanded to pregnant women and children under a certain percentage of FPL ACA authorized states to expand to individuals under 65 with income below 133 FPL	Must enroll—some states have 12 months continuous eligibility others monthly Meet income criteria	Basic coverage requirements, state flexibility

(continued)

TABLE 11.1 SUMMARY OF MEDICARE AND MEDICAID: ROLES, SERVICES, AND POPULATIONS COVERED (continued)

Title	Authority	Federal and State Role	Services and Population Covered	Beneficiary Role	Services Not Covered
Medicare Supplemental		Private insurance	Covers co-payments and co-insurance and deductibles not covered by Medicare Supplements original Medicare benefits—does not cover new benefits	Voluntary Choose plan and pay premiums	Cost may exceed actual out of pocket for many seniors
The CHIP	The BBA of 1997	Federally funded with state matching State Administered	Children and pregnant women up to a certain percentage of FPL (may vary by state)	Must enroll Covers basic Medicaid package of services plus dental	

BBA, Balanced Budget Act; CHIP, Children's Health Insurance Program; ESRD, end-stage renal disease; FPL, federal poverty level; SSI, supplemental security income; TEFRA, Tax Equity and Fiscal Responsibility Act.

Source: From De Lew, N. (2000). Medicare: 35 years of service. *Health Care Financial Review, 22*(1), 75–103; Havighurst, C. C. (1973). Regulation of health facilities and services by "Certificate of Need." *Virginia Law Review, 59*(7), 1143–1232. doi:10.2307/1072049; McGuire, T. G., Newhouse, J. P., & Sinaiko, A. D. (2011). An economic history of Medicare part C. *Milbank Quarterly, 89*(2), 289–332. doi:10.1111/j.1468-0009.2011.00629.x; Oliver, T. R., Lee, P. R., & Lipton, H. L. (2004). A political history of medicare and prescription drug coverage. *Milbank Quarterly, 82*(2), 283–354. doi:10.1111/j.0887-378x.2004.00311.x

an entity responsible at the state level for approving such proposals. Partly in response to the expansion of building facilities spurred by the Hill–Burton Act, CON was a regulatory mechanism states could use to control the escalation of healthcare spending to meet the needs of the community (Havighurst, 1973).

The HMO Act of 1973 was unlike any previous piece of legislation. Its goal was not financing healthcare services or regulating facilities but changing the way healthcare was delivered (Dorsey, 1975). This Act was the culmination of several reports issued during the late 1960s and early 1970s on the increasing cost of healthcare. The concept of HMOs emerged in the early 1970s as an alternative to the FFS model that was codified by the passage of the Medicare and Medicaid Act of 1965. The basic premise of the HMO was a fixed periodic payment for services and an organized delivery system of providers, who were contractually responsible to provide services under the periodic payment model. The bill identified basic services that should be covered under a federally qualified HMO plan. In addition, several key concepts were introduced in this law. For example, annual open-enrollment periods were required, quality standards were set, and employers were required to offer both an HMO and indemnity option for employer-sponsored coverage. Although it is said that the Act had a limited impact, it was foundational to the acceptance of managed care, a concept that was embraced by employers in the late 1970s and 1980s and led to the emergence of the managed care boom in the 1980s (Mitka, 1998). Before the advent of managed care, indemnity plans were considered the classic model of healthcare insurance, and scope of coverage and payment was based on services delivered. These traditional health insurance models often included the following three dimensions: a premium, a set of covered benefits (such as inpatient hospitalization), and a set of cost-sharing provisions that apply to those benefits (possibly including an out-of-pocket payment limit and limits on annual or lifetime payments). In traditional indemnity insurance plans, medical services are unbundled and reimbursed on an FFS basis. Profits are linked to volume, which provides a perverse incentive to prescribe unnecessary or marginally beneficial treatments (Dugan, 2014).

By 1980, the percentage of GDP tied to medical care was more than 8.8%. In addition to the emergence of managed care as a way to manage the delivery and financing of healthcare delivery, a new model, the prospective payment system (PPS) for hospital services, which was based on diagnosis-related groups (DRGs) was introduced in 1984 (Chen & Ackerly, 2014). The hospital PPS was a departure from Medicare's per diem cost-based system, which reimbursed based on the number of days a patient stayed in the hospital and the cost of each day of care. In the PPS program, payment would be based on the diagnosis and average cost of resources used based on the national average cost to treat patients with similar diagnoses

(Altman, 2012). The prospective payment amount would be set by the government every year. DRGs were developed to categorize illnesses and associated resource usage. Of note, physicians remained on an FFS reimbursement model even within the hospital setting, where the facility was paid within the PPS.

Managed care models emerged in the late 1970s and 1980s, and by 1985, 20% of the insured population was in some type of managed care plan. By 1993, more than 70% of Americans were enrolled in a managed care plan (Glied, 2000). By 1996, 12% of Medicare beneficiaries and 39% of Medicaid beneficiaries were in some type of managed care plan. Managed care is a broad concept that has evolved and seeks to bring together the financing and delivery of healthcare. There are generally three components: selection and organization of providers, choice of payment methods (including capitation, FFS, or salary payment if a physician is employed) and assessment of utilization of care. Within this broad context, models emerged in which insurance and service delivery are fully integrated, such as staff and group model HMOs; arrangements in which insured people are restricted to a defined set of providers, such as an independent practice association (IPA); and arrangements in which the choice of providers is unrestricted but insurers provide incentives to use selected providers and monitor the care provided, such as preferred provider organizations (PPOs) that conduct utilization management reviews of costly services. HMOs are the strongest form of managed care arrangement. The selection and organization of participating providers is an instrument to incent the right type of care at a lower cost. A notable gap in managed care models is the absence of quality and patient experience metrics (Glied, 2000; Gold, Hurley, Lake, Ensor, & Berenson, 1995).

Capitation arrangements within managed care can require physicians face the full financial cost of their patients' services use, which gives the physician an incentive to reduce utilization. This model may also incentivize appropriate preventive care, as providers seek to minimize future service utilization. The scope of services covered may vary. Under broad arrangements, the provider may be responsible for services regardless of whether he or she provided the service, such as those received through referral or hospitalizations. This was a new role for physicians—to share in the financial risk of illness—and one that many were not fully prepared to handle. Many think of gatekeeper arrangements when thinking of managed care. In some managed care arrangements, an individual requires a referral from a primary care provider or other designee before he or she can see a specialist.

The rise and fall of managed care during the 1980s and 1990s, which is outlined in the following text, exemplifies the key voice of the patient and provider in driving healthcare policy and influencing the market. There is some evidence that managed care lowered overall healthcare costs.

However, patient and provider objections to the reimbursement and management mechanisms—namely, too much risk for the provider and the potential for denial of service—led to consumer backlash and the decline of managed care models. This culminated in federal legislation limiting *drive-by deliveries*, a term coined to describe the short period of time new mothers were allowed to stay in the hospital after delivery (Konetzka, Zhu, Sochalski, & Volpp, 2008). Rapid disenrollment was observed between 1998 and 2003 as HMO models gave way to PPOs and other forms of managed care that were less restrictive from a patient perspective but had fewer incentives for providers to manage cost and utilization (Barnes, Unruh, Chukmaitov, & van Ginneken, 2014; Dugan, 2014).

During this tumultuous phase of managed care, legislation was once again passed to curtail escalating healthcare costs within the Medicare program, specifically, physician services. The Resource-Based Relative Value Scale (RBRVS) system was created in 1989 in an attempt to recalibrate the RVUs based on input costs rather than historical data. This was combined with a geographic cost index (GPCI) and monetary conversion factor to determine the Medicare Physician Payment Schedule. The RVU/RBRVS and physician fee schedule continued to be the basis for reimbursement for Medicare Part B services. Section 1848(f) of the 1997 Balanced Budget Act of 1997 amended the Social Security Act to introduce the sustainable growth rate (SGR) provision, which was meant to control the growth in expenditures for physician part-B services by setting yearly SGR targets for physician services under Medicare. One component required an estimated 10-year average tied to the annual change in real GDP per capita. This would ultimately lead to legislative and programmatic challenges until its final repeal in 2015 (Center for Medicare & Medicaid Services [CMS,] 2015).

2001–Present: The Era of Healthcare Delivery and Payment Reform

The turn of the century marked an era of increasing healthcare complexity as medical and technological advancements continued and health information technology (HIT) and electronic medical records appeared. The burden on providers to retain an increasingly untenable amount of information hit a tipping point. In 2001, the Institute of Medicine (IOM) published its seminal publication, *Crossing the Quality Chasm*. The report not only called for large-scale system and payment redesign to meet the evolving needs and challenges of the healthcare system, but also defined a key role the federal government could play in support of this transformation (IOM, 2001). The report called on coordinated payment reform and delivery-system redesign, the double-edged sword that historically had not been managed effectively through policy and program implementation. A key concept that emerged from the publication is the concept of VBP. This concept, bolstered by the work of defining the Triple Aim, has emerged as a core goal of the CMS in assuming its role as a public payer and influencer of healthcare policy (Berwick, Nolan, & Whittington, 2008). The Triple Aim, which refers to the achievement of improvements in patient experience, population health, and cost of care through efficient delivery and coordination of healthcare, has become a rallying cry of health policy experts working to define the new policy era of delivery-system redesign nestled within VBP models.

The concept of VBP is a complex compilation of incentives and delivery-system redesign meant to drive providers and care strategies toward value-based outcomes. *Value* is hard to define in healthcare because of the complexities of the market-based system (Porter, 2008). There are several characteristics and core elements of VBP models that will be explored: the base payment method, the mechanism for incentivizing value, the expected delivery redesign, and the anticipated outcome. The anticipated outcome is key to achieving value in healthcare delivery—most policy makers have agreed that the Triple Aim, now evolved into the Quadruple Aim, represents the core principles of value-based delivery-model design: improved patient experience; improved population health outcomes; reduced cost of care; and more recent, provider and care team well-being.

DNP leaders can play a unique role in the era of healthcare delivery and payment reform. APRNs are providers who often bill directly for services, and certainly are at the forefront of impacting care delivery and improving care outcomes. Although the role of the APRN within the specific payment model may vary depending on his/her practice setting and employment structure, all APRNs can play a role in navigating their organization through the care delivery redesign necessary to be successful in VBP models.

Healthcare Legislation in the 21st Century

The passage of the Patient Protection and Affordable Care Act (ACA) of 2010 was the most sweeping healthcare reform legislation since the amendment to the Social Security Act produced the Medicare and Medicaid bill in 1965. The ACA gave states the ability to expand Medicaid to previously ineligible populations, mandated healthcare for individuals, and created health insurance exchanges for the individual market to expand access to coverage. It also contained several reform provisions that can be traced back to the IOM report of 2001. These provisions continued to drive VBP models in Medicare (Patient Protection and Affordable Care Act, 42 U.S.C. § 18001 et seq, 2010). The ACA created the Center for Medicare and Medicaid Innovation (CMMI), and authorized Health and Human Services (HHS) to oversee the development and testing of new healthcare delivery and payment models to catalyze cost-effective care (Kocher, Emanuel, & DeParle, 2010). After passage of the ACA, the VBP models that emerged in the early

2000s continued to expand: pay-for-performance (P4P) models continued to proliferate, the Accountable Care Organization (ACO) model was further developed, bundled payments and exploration of global budget models also emerged as important considerations within VBP.

The passage of the Medicare Access and CHIP Reauthorization Act (MACRA) of 2015 marked another pivotal transition in the healthcare landscape. This Act, which abolished the SGR, reconfirmed the federal government's commitment to moving toward value in the healthcare delivery system. Several CMS programs set to sunset in 2019 have been rolled up into the MACRA Quality Payment Program (QPP), including the Meaningful Use (MU) program, the Physician Quality Reporting System (PQRS), and the Value-Based Modifier System (VBMS). The shift in provider reimbursement builds on the P4P, patient-centered medical home (PCMH), and ACO models in the two tracks of provider reimbursement with the QPP. MACRA changes the way Medicare rewards clinicians to incentivize value over volume, streamlines programs, and offers bonus payments for participation in eligible alternative payment models (APMs; Tsai, Joynt, Wild, Orav, & Jha, 2015).

The two tracks of the QPP include merit-based incentive payments (MIPS) and APMs. MIPS encompasses the sunset MU, PQRS, and VBPMS, and is based in a P4P-incentive structure. All eligible professionals who bill Medicare Part B are subject to QPP, and this includes APRNs. Advanced APMs are the second track of the QPP. Eligible clinicians in an advanced APM may earn a 5% incentive for reaching a threshold level of patients in an APM and meeting its reporting and quality requirements. This alleviates the additional burden of separate reporting for providers enrolled in an approved advanced APM (Miller & Mosley, 2016).

The language used to discuss VBP has shifted somewhat since the passage of MACRA and the introduction of the QPP. APMs are increasingly referred to in the health policy literature and can be confusing because advanced APMs in the QPP denote a specific model that meets specific criteria for track two of the QPP. According to the CMS, in general an APM is a "payment approach that gives added incentive payments to provide high-quality and cost-efficient care. APMs can apply to a specific clinical condition, a care episode, or a population" (Center for Medicare & Medicaid Services, n.d.). For the advanced APM model, providers must bear more than nominal financial risk for losses. There are specific models that qualify as advanced APMs such as the Medicare Shared Savings Program (MSSP) track 2 and 3 and the oncology care model (two-sided risk; (Miller & Mosley, 2016).

MACRA remains popular among legislators, providers, and health system advocates because it repealed the SGR and laid a path for sustainable provider reimbursement. There have been calls to further evaluate MIPS track one of the QPP due to the mixed results from the PQRS/VBMS program as well as other P4P models. However, both QPP tracks remain intact (Frakt & Jha, 2018; Roberts, Zaslavsky, & McWilliams, 2018). A review of the major legislation enacted thus far in the 21st century illustrates the background legislation and role the federal government has taken to advance emerging models that fall under the VBP umbrella. The DNP can advance the role of APRNs in influencing the financing and policy of healthcare, and impact system redesign to improve health outcomes and quality of care.

The Rise of VBP Models in the 21st Century

At the time the IOM released its publication in 2001, healthcare as a percentage of the GDP had risen to 13.8%. After relative stable growth in the 1990s, due in large part to managed care efforts, the percentage began to increase again in the early 2000s. FFS reimbursement remained the predominant payment model in healthcare, despite evidence that FFS incentivizes volume of care delivery without ensuring appropriateness or quality of care delivery (Reinhardt, Hussey, & Anderson, 2004).

During the early 2000s, the increasing role that medical technology and HIT played added further complexity to the healthcare system. HIT has become an essential component of evolving care delivery and payment models. The collection, sharing, and use of data have propelled population health management as a core construct of comprehensive care, which requires providers and practice teams to learn new skills and redesign their workflows.

VBP is inclusive of performance-based strategies that link financial incentives to providers' performance on the set of defined measures to achieve better value by driving improvements in quality and slowing the growth in health spending (Damberg et al., 2014). Several evolving payment models fall under the umbrella of VBP and are meant to move the delivery system away from FFS payment toward payment that incentivizes quality (Damberg et al., 2014; Dudley et al., 2000; Dudley, Miller, Korenbrot, & Luft, 1998; Ryan & Damberg, 2013). Alleviating the pressure to drive volume of care to maintain a revenue allows providers and care teams the ability to appropriately manage a patient population. Using modalities, such as telehealth and asynchronous communication, maximizing care coordination and chronic disease management, and using data for quality improvement are all activities that are traditionally not reimbursed in an FFS model. By changing how care is paid for, VBP models can provide flexibility for the provider and care team to focus on what is best for the patient. In reality, current VBP models, most notable are those offered by Medicare, are still based on FFS (Ginsburg & Patel, 2017). With the continued base payment in FFS, these models create a conflicting paradigm for providers. Many are still entrenched in productivity targets and RVU generation, even while trying to build a business model to be successful in VBP.

VBP MODELS

Pay-for-Performance

Pay-for-performance (P4P) is defined as "any performance-based provider payment arrangements including those that target performance on cost measure" (Bardach et al., 2013). P4P models are one of the most common VBP models that emerged early in the 2000s, usually offered on top of a base FFS payment (Ginsburg & Patel, 2017). These P4P models have been implemented in different sectors of healthcare, including hospitals, nursing homes, primary care, and specialty practices. Performance metrics are identified at the onset of a P4P program. The program setting (primary care, hospital setting, etc.), the population, and the benchmark, or target performance goal, should be defined over a designated time period. The program may or may not include resources for delivery system redesign. The provider or organization may be eligible for incentive payments or penalties based on performance within the predetermined quality metrics. P4P models are often the first VBP model a provider or organization may engage in because it is added on top of the existing payment structure and most often carries minimal risk. The contractual agreement is negotiable and may include an opportunity for shared savings if benchmark targets are met. These models continue to proliferate, arguably because it is feasible to implement as an add-on to incentivize focused quality outcomes within an FFS environment. In some cases, P4P programs begin with a pay-for-reporting period that gives the provider organization time to develop the tools and resources to effectively report the data.

There are, however, multiple sources of data and types of measures that can be considered in P4P and other VBP models. Data sources include electronic clinical quality measures (eCQMs), claims-based measures, and patient satisfaction surveys. Types of measures include process measures, outcome measures, and cost measures, as well as patient-reported survey data and patient-reported outcome measures. Emerging reports of provider burnout and fatigue have been traced to the rise of performance-based reporting and lack of alignment of metrics used in performance-based contracts across public and private payers (Bodenheimer & Sinsky, 2014).

There is no substantial evidence that P4P payment models positively influence health outcomes (Jha, Joynt, Orav, & Epstein, 2012; Ryan, Burgess, Pesko, Borden, & Dimick, 2015; Ryan & Damberg, 2013; Van Herck et al., 2010). After launching the Premier Hospital Quality Incentive Demonstration (HQID) in 2003, CMS enrolled 216 hospitals across the United States in a performance-based incentive program (Blumenthal & Jena, 2013). Jha and colleagues evaluated the long-term effects of the HQID program and found no evidence that there was a reduction in 30-day mortality for the participating hospitals (Jha et al., 2012). Despite mixed results from the HQID and other P4P programs, CMS launched the Hospital Value-Based Purchasing (HVBP) program in 2012, which required participation for most acute care hospitals (Blumenthal & Jena, 2013). An evaluation of the early implementation of HVBP showed no improvement in clinical process or patient experience during the study period, a result that may have been confounded by existing quality-improvement projects at the time the P4P model was implemented (Ryan et al., 2015; Ryan & Damberg, 2013).

An early study evaluating the impact of a P4P program on quality of care in the outpatient setting found only cervical cancer screening rates improved compared to a provider group that was not subject to a P4P program (Rosenthal, Frank, Li, & Epstein, 2005). A recent publication by Roberts and colleagues assessed the impact of Medicare's Value-Based Modifier Payment program, the precursor to the MACRA QPP, analyzing data from 2014 to 2015. The authors found that "differences in exposure" of physician practices to financial incentives were not associated with meaningful differences in hospitalizations for ambulatory sensitive conditions, readmissions, mortality, or Medicare spending. Authors cite potentially weak incentives, lack of awareness of the program, and the 2-year time period between measure reporting and incentive payment as potential reasons for this. The authors further concluded that the inadequate risk adjustment in the program might contribute to health disparities, a significant unintended consequence (Roberts et al., 2018).

Patient-Centered Medical Home

PCMH has expanded as a primary care model since the joint principles were first published in 2007 (American Academy of Family Physicians, 2008). However, the concept of a medical home first emerged in the 1960s when the American Association of Pediatricians used the term to define primary care. The medical home model is a framework for organizing care delivery. It has also become a mechanism for contracting with payers, most notably for dollars to support care coordination and care management, population health management, and potential opportunities for shared savings based on meeting quality targets. However, it originally was not created as a VBP model, but a model of care redesign. Core components of the PCMH include team-based care that is comprehensive, coordinated and patient centered. In additiony, access to care is a key component and one that supports effective delivery of care at the appropriate setting, with a promise of avoiding costly, unnecessary care. The National Committee for Quality Aassurance (NCQA) is the largest national organization to recognize and certify practices for meeting designated criteria. Quality and safety are core tenets of the NCQA certification and much of the work required includes implementing continuous quality-improvement activities in the clinical setting.

Two strategies that enable effective team-based care and care coordination and management are empanelment and risk stratification. Empanelment of a patient population enables a practice to utilize a defined methodology to determine which patients they are responsible for—often the empaneled list of patients can be compared with a health plan's list of attributed patients to ensure a shared understanding of the patients under the practices care for a defined model. Once the patient population is empaneled patients can be assigned to care teams and risk stratified based on patients' social and medical risk. Risk stratifying patients can ensure effective care coordination and management of high-risk patients. For example, patients who are frequent users of the emergency department may be considered high risk and appropriate for care coordination and care management. These strategies can be deployed as part of population health management in any of the VBP models.

Early evidence on PCMH was mixed, largely due to the wide variation in the definition and implementation. A large-scale evaluation of impact of a PCMH model within the Veterans Health Administration showed reduction in utilization rates as well as staff burnout (Nelson et al., 2014). A systematic review of 19 comparative studies found a small but positive effect on patient and staff experience, preventive service delivery, and emergency room visits (Jackson et al., 2013).

The APRN plays a key role within the PCMH. Core tenets of the PCMH philosophy include team-based care, care coordination, and care management—aspects of comprehensive primary care that APRNs have embraced for years. APRNs can influence the practice's ability to succeed within a PCMH model by understanding the quality or performance targets and taking a leadership role in the quality-improvement process as well as the population health management interventions. Within an evolving team-based care paradigm, APRNs are often the team lead, which enhances the role of the ARPN leader within the PCMH model.

Bundled Payments

Bundled payment models, sometimes referred to as *clinical episode payments (CEP)* or *episode-based payments* date back to the Medicare PPS of the 1980s, which bundled hospital services. Within the Medicare PPS program, reimbursement to the hospital is based on DRGs. However, the physician is still reimbursed on an FFS model, which can create a disincentive to work collaboratively to ensure cost and quality outcomes (Scamperle, 2013). The new iteration of bundling payments is meant to incentivize coordination across individuals or organizations during an episode of illness or surgery. An episode of a bundle may include the hospital, physician and provider, as well as post discharge services for a defined period of time. There is considerable variation in the contractual arrangement within bundled payment models. Payment can be prospective or retrospective, based on a global budget for an episode of care or based on FFS with a retrospective review of costs to target. Bundled payments connect clinical care services and providers across the delivery system that serves patients during an episode of care (Scamperle, 2013). An orthopedic bundle may begin when a patient is admitted for surgery and last 30 or 60 days postdischarge. This requires the surgeon coordinate care with the postacute team to ensure cost-effective care that meets quality and cost targets.

Public and private payers began adopting bundled payment models in the 1990s, with many private insurers covering transplantation as a bundle or episode of care (U.S. Government Accountability Office, 2011). In 2008, the PROMETHEUS payment project was launched. In 2009, CMS launched the Acute Care Episode (ACE) Demonstration Project, focused on global payments for cardiovascular or orthopedic episodes of care. Section 3021 of the ACA granted authority to CMMI to test new payment delivery models to reduce expenditures. A specific requirement mandated implementation of a national bundled payment pilot by 2013. Since its inception, CMMI has launched the Bundled Payments for Care Improvement (BPCi), the Joint Replacement Model (CJR), and the Oncology Care Model (OCM). Although there has been pushback from legislators concerned with implementation of mandatory bundles, they continue to be offered within the Medicare program on a voluntary basis (Press, Rajkumar, & Conway, 2016). Bundled payment models that have emerged since the passage of the ACA typically bundle hospital services, as well as the care given by the providers and any care for a defined 30-, 60- or 90-day period after discharge. This is a dramatic shift in healthcare financing that creates an opportunity for providers across the continuum to coordinate care and collectively account for the management of an episode of care (Altman, 2012). Usually the episode or bundle is triggered by a hospital admission, and with most of the CMS demonstration projects the provider group is able to elect the postacute period (Press et al., 2016). Bundles are meant to incentivize effective care coordination and ensure delivery of the appropriate volume of services and procedures. One attractive feature of bundled payments is that they can be nestled within other VBP models such as ACO arrangements. Historically, bundled payments have focused on surgical or procedure-based episodes. However, the Oncology Care Model covers an episode of care that starts with chemotherapy and lasts for six months.

Commercial health plans are increasingly offering global budgets or bundled payments for maternity care. The Health Care Payment Learning & Action Network (HCP LAN), a public and private organization tasked with advancing VBP models, published a report on CEPs highlighting maternity care in 2016. A key opportunity for providers is the flexibility in design and service delivery in bundled payment models. Effective partnerships and accountability can drive efficiencies in the system. Maternity care and hospital births account for the majority of hospitalizations in the United States. Although there are a variety of mechanisms to pay for maternity services, episode or bundled payments have emerged among both commercial and Medicaid programs as an effective way to incentivize and coordinate value-driven care to avoid unnecessary caesarean sections and elective deliveries. Despite spending significant dollars on maternity care services, the United States has worse maternal and infant mortality, higher caesarian rates, and racial and ethnic disparities in outcomes than many other industrialized nations (Health Care Learning & Action Network, 2016).

Bundled payments for maternity care, like other models, bring together providers in the outpatient and inpatient setting and encourage alignment and cooperation with the hospital or facility, holding each other accountable for cost and quality. Bundled payment models are attractive to physicians and other providers because there is some room for flexibility in negotiating terms of the contract, defining the episode, and in determining necessary services (Nijagal, Shah, & Levin-Scherz, 2018).

Early evidence to support bundled payment models was limited by the variation in implementation. However, AHRQ found that bundled payment programs on average had a spending reduction of less than 10% from baseline and a decline in utilization. Impact on quality was variable (Hussey, Mulcahy, Schnyer, & Schneider, 2012a; Hussey, Mulcahy, Schnyer, & Schneider, 2012b; Hussey, Ridgely, & Rosenthal, 2011). In 2011, three years after the PROMETHIUS bundled payment model project was launched, none of the sites had implemented the model. Authors cited early challenges that have since become important implementation considerations: defining the "bundle," defining the payment model, implementing quality measurement, determining accountability, engaging providers, and, most important, delivery redesign (Hussey et al., 2011).

More recent evidence in support of payment models continues to reflect the need for ongoing evaluation. An evaluation of the Bundled Payments for Care Improvement Initiative (BPCI) quality outcomes for lower extremity joint replacement episodes found that the mean Medicare episode payment declined by $1,166 for BPCI episodes than comparison episodes, with no statistically significant improvement in claims-based quality measures, 30-day unplanned readmissions, 30-day emergency department visits, or 30- and 90-day postdischarge mortality (Dummit et al., 2016). An evaluation of teaching hospital experience implementing one of the four models of BCPI bundled payments found the first-phase participants generated savings in major joint replacement, congestive heart failure, and cardiac valve episodes, and lost money in stroke, percutaneous coronary intervention, and spine surgery. One of the key insights of participation in a bundled payment program was access to the "black box" of postacute cost and utilization data. The authors cite access to this data enabled their cohort of hospitals to develop effective partnerships across the continuum.

The authors did not report on quality or patient experience outcomes (Kivlahan et al., 2016). As with other emerging APMs, more research is necessary to understand the implementation and effects of bundled models.

Accountable Care Organizations

The core concepts of ACO models often have features of both managed care and P4P and include PCMH principles. These models developed from Medicare's Physician Group Practice (PGP) demonstration project, which was implemented from 2005 to 2010. After the limitations identified with the managed care concept of the 1990s, PGP signaled a return to the realm of risk-based contracting with physician groups. With the payment system still firmly entrenched in FFS, the demonstration project provided incentives to coordinate care for Medicare beneficiaries. In aAddition, there were 32 cost and quality performance metrics. Bonuses were given to practices that achieved quality targets. The term *ACO* was coined in 2006 by Fisher and colleagues, who recognized that fragmentation of the system and lack of coordination could be remedied by creating organizations that were accountable for the management of a population across a continuum of care (Fisher, Staiger, Bynum, & Gottlieb, 2007).

The ACA established ACOs as a payment model under Medicare and encouraged alignment with private payers and Medicaid. Private payers have initiated their own ACO models, which have proliferated following the passage of the ACA. ACO models generally consist of providers, including provider organizations, hospitals, or health systems, and can include insurance companies, all of which are jointly held accountable for improvements in quality and reductions in the cost of care (Fisher & Shortell, 2010). The goal of ACOs is to improve quality and lower costs employing many of the concepts of PCMHs, such as disease management programs, care coordination, and data-driven population health and performance improvements. Medicare defines *ACOs* as "groups of doctors, hospitals and other healthcare providers, who come together voluntarily to give coordinated, high quality care to the Medicare patients they serve" (Centers for Medicare & Medicaid Services, 2015, p. 32695). All providers assume financial responsibility and clinical accountability for the care provided to a defined population regardless of whether they are directly responsible for the patient. This encourages effective care management and care coordination (Barnes et al., 2014; Colla & Fisher, 2017). Most ACO arrangements are based on an FFS model with opportunity for shared savings and potentially shared risk. Less often, ACO models can be based on a global budget or population-based payments. A comprehensive set of clinical and cost performance measures are identified at the onset of the model.

Medicare has experimented with different ACO models. Provider or hospital organizations are eligible to enter into a phased implementation strategy, beginning with a focus on shared savings with an eventual requirement that the organization move into a risk-bearing arrangement after a prescribed period in the program. Less often organizations have entered into two-sided risk-sharing ACO models. There is an exception ACO model for rural areas that enables them to participate in shared saving opportunities within an ACO model without requiring full transition to downside risk. However, most begin with a shared savings component with a transition to the acceptance of downside risk. Entry requirements into a Medicare ACO include at least 5,000 beneficiaries, a 3-year commitment, acceptance that primary care determines retrospective attribution, and responsibility for total cost of care. Both care coordination and HIT have become increasingly important in ACO models that rely on coordinating care across systems and providers. Implementing successful ACO models requires key components that are necessary for success: governance and partnerships, linking and coordinating care across a continuum, HIT to facilitate effective care coordination and disease management, and structures to negotiate aligned contracts with commercial payers (Barnes et al., 2014). The payment methods, contractual arrangements, and participating organizations vary across public and private payers, which leaves significant room for variation across ACOs.

Early evaluation of the MSSP compared changes in spending per beneficiary and quality of care by cohort the year an organization joined the MSSP. A variation in savings between the 2012 and 2013 cohort revealed a savings of 1.4% in the 2012 cohort compared with no statistically significant change in cost for the 2013 cohort. Quality metrics, including 30-day readmissions, preventive service delivery, and diabetes management, did not show any statistically significant change during the 18-month evaluation period (McWilliams, Hatfield, Chernew, Landon, & Schwartz, 2016). An evaluation of 114 ACOs in the 2012 cohort found a 9% reduction in post-acute spending, which was related to a reduced number of beneficiaries, who were admitted to skilled nursing facilities as well as reduced length of stay. There was no significant positive or negative impact on quality outcomes as measured by 30-day readmission or outcomes (McWilliams et al., 2017). Evidence is still emerging about how ACOs influence quality and outcomes. A study evaluating the impact of ACOs on preventive screening found a 2.4% increase in colorectal screening relative to baseline, a 1.8% reduction in breast cancer screening, and a 3.4% reduction in prostate cancer screening. Age was strongly associated with changes in breast cancer screening, with women older than 75 years of age having a 6.2% reduction. This suggests age-appropriate screening and appropriate screening of those in the highest risk category. There was also a 0.36% increase in screening for colorectal cancer among beneficiaries who were younger than 75 years old, which suggests positive screening and avoidance of overscreening. Prostate cancer screening rates were lower across the age continuum for both ACO and non-ACO beneficiaries (Resnick et al., 2018). A study examining preventive services, patient experience, and healthcare expenditures for patients 18 to 64 years of age found no difference in preventive screening rates for ACO and non-ACO patients, nor was there a difference in interaction quality with providers or overall satisfaction. IN addition, no statistically significant difference in cost of care, emergency department utilization or hospitalization was found with between ACO-patients and non-ACO patients (Hong, Sonawane, Larson, Mainous, & Marlow, 2018).

A systematic review of commercial and public payer ACO models evaluated 42 research articles spanning Medicare, Medicaid, and commercial ACOs. Reduced inpatient use, emergency department visits, improved preventive care and chronic disease management were seen most consistently across the studies. Although there was no evidence of worse patient outcomes or experience of care, further research is warranted to investigate the impacts on cost and quality (Kaufman, Spivack, Stearns, Song, & O'Brien, 2017).

Shared savings is a key concept that can be considered a model in its own right, but is often a component of a larger model. As opposed to P4P models that seek to incentivize behavior by identifying key performance or outcome metrics, shared savings offers an opportunity to spread the net savings generated in care delivery and financing due to the implementation of a model. ACO models often have a shared savings component, as do PCMH and bundled or episode care models. There are usually predetermined quality metrics that must be met, and the savings can be achieved at the provider, practice, region, or plan level, which creates different levels of buy-in from provider groups. Providers might not believe they can effectively influence the performance metrics of a region, and many become frustrated that they might not share in savings despite achieving the quality metrics if their neighbors in the model do not.

CONCLUSIONS

There are many iterations of the models presented in this chapter, and given the evidence compiled thus far on emerging models, there is work to be done to continue to evaluate and implement models that improve outcomes, experience, and cost of care. APRNs with a DNP education play a crucial role in the evolving healthcare landscape. Not only do they provide care in a variety of care settings, they provide practice and systems leadership. A foundational knowledge of VBP models in practice and policy will enable DNP leaders to shape the healthcare of tomorrow. Nurse-led clinics are some of the innovators in advancing the scope of performance metrics, thereby improving the financial reimbursement in VBP models. Nurse system leaders and APRNs are well poised to make important contributions to emerging value-based models.

Case Study

ABC Birth and Women's Health Center located in the Southwest United States, is a freestanding birth center staffed entirely by certified nurse midwives (CNMs). Housed within a larger community federally qualified health center (FQHC), the CNM-led birthing center offers women an option of delivery in the freestanding birthing center or the hospital. The CNMs have an agreement with a materna–fetal medicine (MFM) group of physicians at the hospital if higher risk patients need to be comanaged during labor and delivery or postpartum period. The FQHC and ABC Birth and Women's Health Center is deemed a Federal Tort Claims Act facility. The Federal Tort Claims Act enables Health Resources and Servies Administration-supported health centers to receive medical malpractice liability protection with the federal government as the primary insurer. This collaboration is a core reason why ABC Birth and Women's Health Center has been able to support a freestanding birthing center.

The CNM-led birth center provides core services to women in the community. In the Tucson community, The Center is known for high patient engagement, patient-centered care models, and strong CNM-patient rapport. All CNM providers at the center enjoy full patient panels. The philosophy at the birth center is that quality care focuses on helping patients thrive, not just avoiding harm. Patients and families who receive care are so satisfied with the model of care at the ABC Women's Birth and Health Center, the practice manager and CNMs are exploring expanding the practice to include women's health nurse practitioners (WHNP) to provide primary care for women of all ages.

The clinic has contracts with private insurance companies and Medicaid. The practice manger negotiates these contracts and has entered into several bundled payment or episodes-of-care model contracts with health plans and participates in the Medicaid bundled payment program for maternity services. Table 11.2 outlines elements of the CEP model relevant to this nurse-run clinic.

TABLE 11.2 HCP LAN SUMMARY OF MATERNITY CARE EPISODE RECOMMENDATIONS

Episode definition	The episode is defined to include the large majority of births, including the newborn care that is lower-risk. Although not necessarily lower risk, episode payment might also be considered appropriate for women who may be at elevated risk due to conditions that have defined and predictable care trajectories, such as gestational diabetes. As the CEP model matures, some groups with significant high-risk pregnancy experience and capacity may seek to manage the entire continuum of risk.
Episode timing	The episode should begin 40 weeks before the birth and end 60 days postpartum for the woman, and 30 days after the birth of the baby.
Patient opulation	The episode should primarily include the large majority of births, including newborn care that is lower-risk. The work group also supports CEP for women who may be at elevated risk because of predictable risk factors that have defined care trajectories, such as gestational diabetes.

(continued)

Case Study (*continued*)

TABLE 11.2 HCP LAN SUMMARY OF MATERNITY CARE EPISODE RECOMMENDATIONS (*continued*)

Patient engagement	Engaging women and their families is critical in all three phases of the episode—prenatal, labor and birth, and postpartum/newborn—to contribute to the foundation for healthy women and babies.
Accountability	The accountable entity should be chosen based on readiness to re-engineer change in the way care is delivered to the patient and to accept risk. In this model, the accountable entity will likely require a degree of shared accountability, given the number of clinicians working to care for a patient.
Payment flow	The unique circumstances of the episode initiative will determine the payment flow. The two primary options are: (a) a prospectively established price that is paid as one payment to the accountable entity or (b) upfront FFS payment to individual providers within the episode with retrospective reconciliation and a potential for shared savings/losses.
Episode price	The episode price should strike a balance between provider-specific and multiprovider/regional utilization history. The price should: (a) acknowledge achievable efficiencies already gained by previous initiatives, (b) reflect a level that potential provider participants see as feasible to attain, and (c) include the cost of services that help achieve the goals of episode payment.
Type and level of risk	The goal should be to utilize both upside reward and downside risk. Transition periods and risk mitigation strategies should be used to encourage broad provider participation and support inclusion of as broad a patient population as possible.
Quality metrics	Prioritize use of metrics that capture the goals of the episode, including outcome metrics, particularly patient-reported outcome and functional status measures; use quality scorecards to track performance on quality and inform decisions related to payment; and use quality information and other supports to communicate with and engage patients and other stakeholders.

CEP, clinical episode payments; FFS, fee for service; HCP LAN, Health Care Payment Learning & Action Network.

Source: From Health Care Learning & Action Network. (2016). Accelerating and aligning clinical episode payment models. Retrieved from https://hcp-lan.org/workproducts/cep-whitepaper-final.pdf

Quality and performance metrics are included as core components of the bundled contracts for this clinic, but are limited in scope. Clinicians at the birthing center track outcomes related to labor and delivery but are also actively seeking outcome measures that represent the integrated comprehensive care they provide to their clients. Historically, maternity care VBP models were based in P4P with a focus on incentivizing process and outcome measures such as screening rates for Group B *Streptococcus* or avoiding early deliveries.

(continued)

Case Study (*continued*)

From the CNM perspective, bundled payments for maternity care offer benefits and risks. Often it starts with the terms and conditions that are negotiated in the contract. Most OB GYN providers and CNMs would argue that patients presenting with an upper respiratory infection or other diagnosis not related to the pregnancy should not be included in the bundle. For this clinic, CNMs are encouraged to code any visit not related to the pregnancy as a problem visit. If this is not negotiated within the contract, the providers may be at risk for nonpregnancy- related illnesses. A practice manager or APRN leader adept at negotiating contracts is essential.

One of the challenges with a global or episode-of-care payment for maternity care and delivery is the reimbursement. Some contractual arrangements cover the comprehensive 10 months of care: prenatal care plus labor and delivery and postpartum care.

The ABC clinic is an example of a nurse-led clinic that has embraced VBP, yet still seeks to improve the model development. Improving performance metrics and ultimately improving the financial reimbursement are two key considerations moving forward.

QUESTIONS

1. What are the positive aspects of the bundled payment model for CNMs at ABC Clinic?
2. What are the challenging aspects or limits of the bundled payment model for CNMs at ABC Clinic?
3. Based on the CNMs' desire to expand their practice to include WHNPs, what negotiations would the practice manager want to have with the payer?
4. If ABC Clinic is able to expand to include WHNP, how might the quality metrics of the CEP model shift?

REFERENCES

Altman, S. H. (2012). The lessons of Medicare's prospective payment system show that the bundled payment program faces challenges. *Health Affairs, 31*(9), 1923–1930. doi:10.1377/hlthaff.2012.0323

American Academy of Family Physicians. (2008). Joint principles of the patient-centered medical home. *Delaware Medical Journal, 80*(1), 21.

Bardach, N. S., Wang, J. J., DeLeon, S. F., Shih, S. C., Boscardin, W. J., Goldman, L. E., & Dudley, R. A. (2013). Effect of pay-for-performance incentives on quality of care in small practices with electronic health records: a randomized trial. *Journal of the American Medical Association, 310*(10), 1051–1059.

Barnes, A. J., Unruh, L., Chukmaitov, A., & van Ginneken, E. (2014). Accountable care organizations in the USA: Types, developments and challenges. *Health Policy, 118*, 1–7. doi:10.1016/j.healthpol.2014.07.019

Berkowitz, E. (2005). Medicare and Medicaid: The past as prologue. *Health Care Financial Review, 27*(2), 11–23.

Berwick, D. M., Nolan, T. W., & Whittington, J. (2008). The Triple Aim: Care, health, and cost. *Health Affairs (Millwood), 27*(3), 759–769. doi:10.1377/hlthaff.27.3.759

Blumenthal, D., & Jena, A. B. (2013). Hospital value-based purchasing. *Journal of Hospital Medicine, 8*(5), 271–277. doi:10.1002/jhm.2045

Bodenheimer, T., & Sinsky, C. (2014). From Triple to Quadruple Aim: Care of the patient requires care of the provider. *Annals of Family Medicine, 12*(6), 573–576. doi:10.1370/afm.1713

Buchanan, A., Dranove, D., & White, W. D. (1988). Principal/agent theory and decision making in health care Agency and the organization of health care delivery. *Bioethics, 2*(4), 317–333. doi:10.1111/j.1467-8519.1988.tb00057.x

Buchmueller, T. C., & Monheit, A. C. (2009). Employer-sponsored health insurance and the promise of health insurance reform. *Journal of Health Care Organization, Provision, and Financing, 46*(2), 187–202. doi:10.5034/inquiryjrnl_46.02.187

Centers for Disease Control. (n.d.). Historical poverty tables: People and families– 1959–2017. Retrieved from https://www.census.gov/data/tables/time-series/demo/income-poverty/historical-poverty-people.html

Centers for Medicare & Medicaid Services. (2015). Medicare program; Medicare shared savings program: Accountable care organizations. Final rule. *Federal Register, 80*(110), 32691–32845.

Centers for Medicare & Medicaid Services. (n.d.). Alternative payment model overview. Retrieved from https://qpp.cms.gov/apms/overview

Chen, C., & Ackerly, D. C. (2014). Beyond ACOs and bundled payments: Medicare's shift toward accountability in fee-for-service. *Journal of the American Medical Association, 311*(7), 673–674. doi:10.1001/jama.2014.11

Colla, C. H., & Fisher, E. S. (2017). Moving forward with accountable care organizations: Some answers, more questions. *JAMA Internal Medicine, 177*(4), 527–528. doi:10.1001/jamainternmed.2016.9122

Damberg, C. L., Sorbero, M. E., Lovejoy, S. L., Martsolf, G. R., Raaen, L., & Mandel, D. (2014). *Measuring success in health care value-based purchasing programs*: Santa Monica, CA: Rand Corporation.

DesRoches, C. M., Gaudet, J., Perloff, J., Donelan, K., Iezzoni, L. I., & Buerhaus, P. (2013). Using Medicare data to assess nurse practitioner–provided care. *Nursing Outlook, 61*(6), 400–407. doi:10.1016/j.outlook.2013.05.005

Dorsey, J. L. (1975). The Health Maintenance Organization Act of 1973 (P.L. 93-222) and Prepaid Group Practice Plans. *Medical Care, 13*(1), 1–9. doi:10.1097/00005650-197501000-00001

Dowell, M. A. (1987). Hill–Burton: The unfulfilled promise. *Journal of Health Politics Policy and Law, 12*(1), 153–175. doi:10.1215/03616878-12-1-153

Dudley, R. A., Landon, B. E., Rubin, H. R., Keating, N. L., Medlin, C. A., & Luft, H. S. (2000). Assessing the relationship between quality of care and the characteristics of health care organizations. *Medical Care Research and Review, 57*(Suppl 2), 116–135. doi:10.1177/1077558700057002s07

Dudley, R. A., Miller, R. H., Korenbrot, T. Y., & Luft, H. S. (1998). The impact of financial incentives on quality of health care. *Milbank Quarterly, 76*(4), 649–686. doi:10.1111/1468-0009.00109

Dugan, J. (2014). Trends in managed care cost containment: An analysis of the managed care backlash. *Health Economic&, 24*, 1604–1618. doi:10.1002/hec.3115

Dummit, L. A., Kahvecioglu, D., Marrufo, G., Rajkumar, R., Marshall, J., Tan, E., . . . Gu, Q. (2016). Association between hospital participation in a Medicare bundled payment initiative and payments and quality outcomes for lower extremity joint replacement episodes. *Journal of the American Medical Association, 316*(12), 1267–1278. doi:10.1001/jama.2016.12717

Everett, C., Thorpe, C., Palta, M., Carayon, P., Bartels, C., & Smith, M. A. (2013). Physician assistants and nurse practitioners perform effective roles on teams caring for Medicare patients with diabetes. *Health Affairs, 32*(11), 1942–1948. doi:10.1377/hlthaff.2013.0506

Feldstein, P. J. (2011). *Health policy issues: An economic perspective* (5th ed.). Chicago, IL: Health Administration Press.

Fisher, E. S., & Shortell, S. M. (2010). Accountable care organizations: Accountable for what, to whom, and how. *Journal of the American Medical Association, 304*(15), 1715–1716. doi:10.1001/jama.2010.1513

Fisher, E. S., Staiger, D. O., Bynum, J. P., & Gottlieb, D. J. (2007). Creating accountable care organizations: The extended hospital medical staff. *Health Affairs, 26*(1), 44–57. doi:10.1377/hlthaff.26.1.w44

Frakt, A. B., & Jha, A. K. (2018). Face the facts: We need to change the way we do pay for perfor-mance. *Annals of Internal Medicine, 168*(4), 291–292. doi:10.7326/M17-3005

Ginsburg, P. B., & Patel, K. K. (2017). Physician payment reform—Progress to date. *New England Journal of Medicine, 377*(3), 285–292. doi:10.1056/NEJMhpr1606353

Glied, S. (2000). Managed care. In A. J. Culyer & J. P. Newhouse (Eds.), *Handbook of health econom-ics* (Vol. 1, pp. 707–753). Philadelphia, PA: Elsevier.

Gold, M. R., Hurley, R., Lake, T., Ensor, T., & Berenson, R. (1995). A national survey of the arrangements managed-care plans make with physicians. *New England Journal of Medicine, 333*, 1678–1683. doi:10.1056/NEJM199512213332505

Havighurst, C. C. (1973). Regulation of health facilities and services by "certificate of need." *Virginia Law Review, 59*(7), 1143–1232. doi:10.2307/1072049

Health Care Learning & Action Network. (2016). Accelerating and aligning clinical episode pay-ment models. Retrieved from https://hcp-lan.org/workproducts/cep-whitepaper-final.pdf

Health Planning and Resources Development Act of 1974. (1975). *Journal of the National Medical Association, 67*(6), 489–494.

Hong, Y. R., Sonawane, K., Larson, S., Mainous, A. G., III, & Marlow, N. M. (2018). Impact of pro-vider participation in ACO programs on preventive care services, patient experiences, and health care expenditures in US adults aged 18–64. *Medical Care, 56*, 711–718. doi:10.1097/MLR.0000000000000935

Hussey, P. S., Mulcahy, A. W., Schnyer, C., & Schneider, E. C. (2012a). *Bundled payments: Effects on health care spending and quality. Closing the quality gap: Revisiting the State of the Science.* Rockville, MD: Agency for Healthcare Research and Quality.

Hussey, P. S., Mulcahy, A. W., Schnyer, C., & Schneider, E. C. (2012b). *Closing the quality gap: Revisiting the state of the science: Vol. 1.Bundled payment: Effects on health care spending and qual-ity* (pp. 1–155). Rockville, MD: Agency for Healthcare Research and Quality.

Hussey, P. S., Ridgely, M. S., & Rosenthal, M. B. (2011). The PROMETHEUS bundled payment experiment: Slow start shows problems in implementing new payment models. *Health Affairs, 30*(11), 2116–2124. doi:10.1377/hlthaff.2011.0784

Institute of Medicine. (2001). *Crossing the quality chasm: A new health system for the 21st century.* Washington, DC: National Academies Press.

Jackson, G. L., Powers, B. J., Chatterjee, R., Bettger, J. P., Kemper, A. R., Hasselblad, V., . . . Kendrick, A. S. (2013). The patient-centered medical home: a systematic review. *Annals of Internal Medicine, 158*(3), 169–178. doi:10.7326/0003-4819-158-3-201302050-00579

Jha, A. K., Joynt, K. E., Orav, E. J., & Epstein, A. M. (2012). The long-term effect of premier pay for performance on patient outcomes. *New England Journal of Medicine, 366*(17), 1606–1615. doi:10.1056/NEJMsa1112351

Kaufman, B. G., Spivack, B. S., Stearns, S. C., Song, P. H., & O'Brien, E. C. (2017). Impact of accountable care organizations on utilization, care, and outcomes: A systematic review. *Medical Care Research and Review, 76*(3), 255–290.

Kivlahan, C., Orlowski, J. M., Pearce, J., Walradt, J., Baker, M., & Kirch, D. G. (2016). Taking risk: Early results from teaching hospitals' participation in the Center for Medicare and Medicaid Innovation Bundled Payments for Care Improvement Initiative. *Academic Medicine, 91*(7), 936–942. doi:10.1097/ACM.0000000000001121

Kocher, R., Emanuel, E. J., & DeParle, N.-A. M. (2010). The Affordable Care Act and the future of clinical medicine: The opportunities and challenges. *Annals of Internal Medicine, 153*(8), 536–539. doi:10.7326/0003-4819-153-8-201010190-00274

Konetzka, R. T., Zhu, J., Sochalski, J., & Volpp, K. G. (2008). Managed care and hospital cost containment Trends in Managed Care Cost Containment: An analysis of the managed care backlash. *Inquiry, 45*(1), 98–111. doi:10.5034/inquiryjrnl_45.01.98

Lave, J. R., & Silverman, H. A. (1983). Financing the health care of the aged. *Annals of the American Academy of Political and Social Science, 468*, 149–164. doi:10.1177/0002716283468001010

Mantone, J. (2005). The big bang. The Hill–Burton Act put hospitals in thousands of communities and launched today's continuing healthcare building boom. *Modern Healthcare, 35*(33), 6–7.

Martin, P. P., & Weaver, D. A. (2005). Social Security: A program and policy history. *Social Security Bulletin, 66*(1). Retrieved from https://www.ssa.gov/policy/docs/ssb/v66n1/v66n1p1.html

McWilliams, J. M., Gilstrap, L. G., Stevenson, D. G., Chernew, M. E., Huskamp, H. A., & Grabowski, D. C. (2017). Changes in postacute care in the medicare shared savings program. *Journal of the American Medical Association, 177*(4), 518–526. doi:10.1001/jamainternmed. 2016.9115

McWilliams, J. M., Hatfield, L. A., Chernew, M. E., Landon, B. E., & Schwartz, A. L. (2016). Early performance of accountable care organizations in medicare. *New England Journal of Medicine, 374*(24), 2357–2366. doi:10.1056/NEJMsa1600142

Miller, P., & Mosley, K. (2016). Physician Reimbursement: From fee-for-service to MACRA, MIPS and APMs. *Journal of Medical Practice Management, 31*(5), 266–269.

Mitka, M. (1998). A quarter century of health maintenance. *Journal of the American Medical Association, 280*(24), 2059–2060. doi:10.1001/jama.280.24.2059

Nelson, K. M., Helfrich, C., Sun, H., Hebert, P. L., Liu, C.-F., Dolan, E., . . . Hernandez, S. E. (2014). Implementation of the patient-centered medical home in the Veterans Health Administration: associations with patient satisfaction, quality of care, staff burnout, and hospital and emergency department use. *JAMA Internal Medicine, 174*(8), 1350–1358. doi:10.1001/jamainternmed.2014.2488

Nijagal, M. A., Shah, N. T., & Levin-Scherz, J. (2018). Both patients and maternity care providers can benefit from payment reform: Four steps to prepare. *American Journal of Obstetrics and Gynecology, 218*, 411.e1–411.e6. doi:10.1016/j.ajog.2018.01.014

Patient Protection and Affordable Care Act, 42 U.S.C. § 18001 et seq. (2010).

Porter, M. E. (2008). Value-based health care delivery. *Annals of surgery, 248*(4), 503–509.

Press, M. J., Rajkumar, R., & Conway, P. H. (2016). Medicare's new bundled payments: Design, strategy, and evolution. *Journal of the American Medical Association, 315*(2), 131–132. doi:10.1001/jama.2015.18161

Reinhardt, U. E., Hussey, P. S., & Anderson, G. F. (2004). US health care spending in an international context. *Health Affairs, 23*(3), 10–25. doi:10.1377/hlthaff.23.3.10

Resnick, M. J., Graves, A. J., Thapa, S., Gambrel, R., Tyson, M. D., Lee, D., . . . Penson, D. F. (2018). Medicare Accountable Care Organization Enrollment and Appropriateness of Cancer Screening. *Journal of the American Medical Association, 178*, 648. doi:10.1001/jamainternmed.2017.8087

Roberts, E. T., Zaslavsky, A. M., & McWilliams, J. (2018). The value-based payment modifier: Program outcomes and implications for disparities. *Annals of Internal Medicine, 168*(4), 255–265. doi:10.7326/M17-1740

Rosenthal, M. B., Frank, R. G., Li, Z., & Epstein, A. M. (2005). Early experience with pay-for-performance: from concept to practice. *Journal of the American Medical Association, 294*(14), 1788–1793. doi:10.1001/jama.294.14.1788

Ryan, A. M., Burgess, J. F., Pesko, M. F., Borden, W. B., & Dimick, J. B. (2015). The early effects of Medicare's mandatory hospital pay-for-performance rogram. *Health Services Research, 50*(1), 81–97. doi:10.1111/1475-6773.12206

Ryan, A. M., & Damberg, C. L. (2013). What can the past of pay-for-performance tell us about the future of value-based purchasing in Medicare? *Healthcare, 1*, 42–49. doi:10.1016/j.hjdsi.2013.04.006

Sandy, L. G., Bodenheimer, T., Pawlson, L. G., & Starfield, B. (2009). The political economy of U.S. primary care. *Health Affairs, 28*(4), 1136–1145. doi:10.1377/hlthaff.28.4.1136

Scamperle, K. (2013). The fee-for-service shift to bundled payments: Financial considerations for hospitals. *Journal of Health Care Finance, 39*(4), 55–67.

Starr, P. (1982). *The social transformation of American medicine.* New York, NY: Basic Books.

Tsai, T. C., Joynt, K. E., Wild, R. C., Orav, E. J., & Jha, A. K. (2015). Medicare's Bundled Payment initiative: Most hospitals are focused on a few high-volume conditions. *Health Affairs, 34*(3), 371–380. doi:10.1377/hlthaff.2014.0900

U.S. Government Accountability Office. (2011). Medicare: Private sector initiatives to bundle hospital and physician payments for an episode of care. Retrieved from https://www.gao.gov/products/GAO-11-126R

Van Herck, P., De Smedt, D., Annemans, L., Remmen, R., Rosenthal, M. B., & Sermeus, W. (2010). Systematic review: Effects, design choices, and context of pay-for-performance in health care. *BMC Health Services Research, 10*, 247. doi:10.1186/1472-6963-10-247

THE DNP PROJECT

II

12

THE DNP PROJECT—THE ESSENTIALS

TAMMY SPENCER

This chapter addresses the following DNP American Association of Colleges of Nursing (AACN) Essentials:

II. Organizational and Systems Leadership for Quality Improvement and Systems Thinking
III. Clinical Scholarship and Analytical Methods for Evidence-Based Practice 11
VI. Interprofessional Collaboration for Improving Patient and Population Health Outcomes
VIII. Advanced Nursing Practice

INTRODUCTION

The DNP project evaluates the DNP student's ability to apply academic knowledge gained through DNP coursework to a final scholarly project that reflects attainment of the DNP program outcomes and the Essentials of Doctoral Education for Advanced Nursing Practice (DNP Essentials; AACN, 2006). The AACN (2006) defines the final DNP project as "a tangible and deliverable academic product that is derived from the practice immersion experience and is reviewed and evaluated by an academic committee" (p. 20). The final DNP project incorporates leadership skills, system and organizational science, team building and the application and integration of evidence-based practice guidelines to practice (AACN, 2006). Gaps in evidence-based best practice guidelines are identified by the DNP student, who sees the opportunity for quality improvement (QI) and practice change as a means to improve patient-care outcomes. It is from these identified gaps that the DNP project is born, and QI science used to translate evidence-based best practice to the macro-, meso- and microorganization through techniques and tools gained by using QI and best practice models and approaches for process improvement. The final DNP project evaluates the student's development in seeing healthcare improvement through the lens of the broader healthcare system by being a change agent and leader to successfully improve patient-care outcomes in the practice arena.

The AACN DNP Essentials are necessary competencies for all DNP-prepared graduates and a successful DNP project (AACN, 2006). The extent and degree of nursing practice varies among students entering DNP programs, thus the degree to which the individual will meet the DNP Essentials will depend on the role the DNP student is ultimately planning for after attaining the DNP degree (AACN, 2006). Advanced practice nurses with many years of direct patient care will have far greater expertise in the clinical arena and thus be able to address patient-specific DNP Essentials in much greater depth in the DNP project than the novice advanced practice nurse with comparatively few clinical experiences (AACN, 2006).

One of the reccurring themes in any discussion around the essential elements of the DNP project is the focus on system leadership to transform practice in a variety of settings. Indeed, one of the main tenants of the DNP project is the disparity between evidence and practice, which triggers the opportunity to lead change. DNP students are educated to narrow the breach between current best practice guidelines and the implementation of these guidelines into the clinician's daily workflow (M. A. Brown & Crabtree, 2013). Regardless of the setting or project foci, the outcomes for the DNP project remain the same: translate evidence-based guidelines into practice. Flexibility in choosing a DNP project depends on the timeframe for project completion, the interests and practice expertise of the DNP student, and the needs of the organization in which the project is implemented (Kirkpatrick & Weaver, 2013). Ideas and benchmark data for the DNP project can be found by researching quality indicators for various clinical settings (Mayo, 2017). Table 12.1 presents several types of scholarly DNP projects from the National Organization of Nurse Practitioner Faculties (NONPF; 2007) along with potential DNP project outcomes provided by the author (NONPF, 2007).

THE DNP PROJECT: CONFUSION AND LACK OF CONSISTENCY

A lack of consistency in DNP programs regarding essential elements of the DNP project has been well documented (AACN, 2015; Dols, Hernandez, & Miles, 2016; Kirkpatrick & Weaver, 2013; Melnyk, 2013; Waldrop, Caruso, Fuchs, & Hypes, 2014). Because of the lack of consistent guidelines for the DNP project, a wide variety of project models and

TABLE 12.1 POTENTIAL OUTCOMES FOR VARIOUS TYPES OF DNP PROJECTS

Type of DNP Project	Potential DNP Project Outcome
Translate research into practice	Implement a new graduate nurse residency program to decrease burnout in new graduate nurses.
QI (care processes, patient outcomes)	Implement VAP bundles to decrease the percentage of patients with VAP in an intensive care unit.
Implement and evaluate evidence-based practice guidelines	Implement 3-hour and 6-hour sepsis bundles to increase antibiotic administration in an emergency department.
Analyze policy; develop, implement, evaluate or revise policy	Create and implement a discharge teaching policy to decrease postoperative length of stay in an ambulatory surgery center.
Design and use databases to retrieve information for decision-making, planning and evaluation	Design an electronic health record pathway for scheduling follow-up appointments to improve follow-up appointment adherence for postoperative urologic oncology patients.
Conduct financial analyses to compare care models and potential cost savings	Compare value-based models of care with insurer-based models of care to increase provider satisfaction in an outpatient internal medicine clinic.
Implement and evaluate innovative uses of technology to enhance or evaluate care	Educate students regarding the use of a exercise app to decrease the incidence of obesity in a high school health clinic.
Design and evaluate new models of care	Implement a value-based model of care to improve patient adherence to follow-up appointments in a primary care clinic.
Design and evaluate programs	Evaluate a system-wide osteoporosis screening program to improve osteoporosis screening rates in a large urban healthcare system.
Provide leadership of interprofessional or intraprofessional collaborative projects to implement policy, evaluate care models, and implement transitions	Implement a multidisciplinary "time out" policy to decrease wrong-site surgeries in the operating room.
Collaborate with researchers to answer clinical questions	Implement policies for indwelling urinary catheter insertion days with collaboration from nurse scientists in a subacute hospital.
Collaborate on legislative change using evidence	Create statewide educational resources to decrease the incidence of repeated substance abuse for nurses returning to practice following substance abuse treatment.

(continued)

TABLE 12.1 POTENTIAL OUTCOMES FOR VARIOUS TYPES OF DNP PROJECTS (*continued*)

Type of DNP Project	Potential DNP Project Outcome
Work with lay or professional coalitions to develop, implement, or evaluate health programs, such as health- promotion and disease-prevention programs for vulnerable patients, groups, or communities	Implement an evidence-based exercise program with the local community center to decrease depression in long term care residents.

QI, quality improvement; VAP, ventilator associated pneumonia.

Source: From Kirkpatrick, J. M., & Weaver, T. (2013). The doctor of nursing practice capstone project: Consensus or confusion? *Journal of Nursing Education, 52*(8), 437. doi:10.3928/01484834-20130722-01

methodologies exist. This lack of agreement leads to confusion regarding the competencies of the DNP-prepared nurse versus the baccalaureate-prepared and masters-prepared nurse, and difficulties in the evaluation of DNP projects (Waldrop et al., 2014). Although the DNP Essentials clearly define the underpinnings of the final DNP project, confusion exists for both DNP faculty and students in regard to the specific elements of the DNP Project (AACN, 2015; Zaccagnini & White, 2017). In addition, AACN does not address specific criteria to evaluate DNP projects. Fortunately, there are many high-quality guidelines for reporting QI projects (Roush & Tesoro, 2018; Box 12.1). A lack of clarity around the DNP project requirements, coupled with the increased growth of DNP programs and the ever-shifting healthcare system, prompted AACN's board of directors to create a DNP Implementation Task Force in 2014 to clarify and address important considerations in the preparation of DNP graduates (AACN, 2015).

BOX 12.1 Guidelines for Reporting Quality Improvement and Evidence-Based DNP Projects

Standards for Quality Improvement Recording Excellence (SQUIRE)
Standards for Reporting Implementation Studies (StaRI)
International Appraisal of Guidelines, Research, and Evaluation II (AGREE II)
International Council of Medical Journal Editors' (ICMJE)

Source: From Roush, K., & Tesoro, M. (2018). An examination of the rigor and value of final scholarly projects completed by DNP nursing students. *Journal of Professional Nursing, 34*, 437–443. doi:10.1016/j.profnurs.2018.03.003

American Association of Colleges of Nursing DNP Implementation Task Force

The recommendations from the DNP Implementation Task Force suggest program resources and a clarification of elements essential in educating DNP-prepared leaders to be effective change agents in process improvement (AACN, 2015). The DNP Implementation Task Force report uses the DNP Essentials as the bedrock for its recommendations, noting the DNP project should be synergistic with the eight principles outlined in the DNP Essentials (AACN, 2015). The curricular integration of the DNP Essentials culminates in the final DNP project, which incorporates organizational and systems leadership skills in the translation of knowledge into practice. In order to provide clarity and consistency in the final scholarly DNP project, the DNP Implementation Task Force provides specific recommendations regarding the elements of a DNP project.

DNP Implementation Task Force Recommendations for the DNP Project

Title: The culmination of the final DNP academic product should be entitled "DNP project" to separate the DNP project competencies from those in a PhD dissertation (AACN, 2015). Although the DNP project has been called many things, including *final project, dissertations,* and *capstone,* the term *DNP project* clearly reflects the implementation of clinical knowledge into the practice arena (AACN, 2015; Dols, Hernandez, & Miles, 2016; Nelson, Cook, & Raterink, 2013, p. 371).

Scholarly Project: The final scholarly DNP project must contain the same essential elements for all DNP students regardless of the academic degree (postbaccalaureate or postmasters) of the DNP student (AACN, 2015). Essential elements of the DNP project—planning, implementation, evaluation—remain unchanged from the original *AACN Position Statement on the Practice Doctorate in Nursing;* however, the product of the final DNP project relies on the creativity of the DNP student, and the clinical expertise the student brings to a DNP program (AACN, 2015). All eight DNP Essentials should serve as guideposts throughout the DNP project, but students are not required to show competency of all eight DNP Essentials as a part of the final DNP project (AACN, 2015).

The DNP Implementation Task Force indicates all DNP projects contain the following elements (AACN, 2015, p. 4):

a. Focus on change that improves healthcare outcomes, either through direct or indirect care.

b. Have a systems (micro-, meso-, or macro-level) or population/aggregate focus.

c. Demonstrate implementation in the appropriate arena or area of practice.

d. Include a plan for sustainability (e.g., financial, systems or political realities, not only theoretical abstractions).

e. Include an evaluation of processes and/or outcomes (formative or summative). DNP projects should be designed so that processes and/or outcomes will be evaluated to guide practice and policy. Clinical significance is as important in guiding practice as statistical significance is in evaluating research.

f. Provide a foundation for future practice scholarship.

Integrative and Systematic Reviews: A literature review is cited as an example of an acceptable DNP project in the DNP Essentials (AACN, 2006). However, the DNP Implementation Task Force does not support a systematic literature review for the DNP project (AACN, 2015). One reason for the DNP Implementation Task Force departure from the DNP Essentials in this particular area is that a systematic review does not allow for implementation of knowledge in the practice setting, which is a goal of the DNP-prepared advanced practice nurse (AACN, 2015).

Portfolios: A DNP portfolio showcases how the DNP student has applied each of the DNP Essentials to her or his final scholarly DNP project. DNP portfolios can be created using an online student tracking system, which has the ability for students to show individual examples of how they have met the DNP Essentials in the planning, implementation, and evaluation of the final DNP project. For example, the student may document how she or he collaborated with an interdisciplinary team by uploading meeting minutes into an online student tracking system as an example of meeting DNP Essential VI. Documentation of the application of leadership and process measures throughout the DNP program provides the student with tangible examples of the growth and development of his or her leadership skills; however, it is the recommendation of the DNP Implementation Task Force that the DNP portfolio should not be considered a DNP project (AACN, 2015). The DNP portfolio should be used as a means to evaluate student learning and reflection by faculty, and provide the opportunity for the student to integrate the DNP Essentials into her or his DNP project and ultimately assume the role of a leader in process improvement (AACN, 2015).

Group/Team Projects: In the spirit of interdisciplinary collaboration mandated in DNP Essential VI, group projects can serve as valuable learning experiences for DNP students. Barriers in the form of evaluation of individual student efforts are reflected in the hesitancy of many faculty to allow DNP group projects (AACN, 2015). Students participating in group projects should have clear, measurable guidelines for both the student and DNP project; these guidelines should be developed in tandem with faculty expectations at the onset of the DNP project (AACN, 2015). Each student in the group should be held accountable for sharing in the essential required elements of planning, implementation, and evaluation of the project. In addition, each student in the group should demonstrate a well-defined leadership role as part of the DNP project (AACN, 2015). For example, if a DNP group project entails the implementation of a hospital-wide sepsis protocol, each student may be assigned a leadership role implementing the sepsis protocol on a specific unit or with the infection control department in the hospital.

Dissemination of the DNP Project: Scholarly dissemination of project outcomes is expected of all DNP-prepared advanced practice nurses as DNP graduates translate research into practice to ultimately improve patient outcomes (DNP Essentials III). Dissemination of project outcomes may be in the form of publication in a journal, presentation at a nursing conference, grand rounds, or a stakeholder meeting (AACN, 2015). Faculty guidance and support are important in determining the appropriate avenue and audience for dissemination of the project outcomes, as many student are unfamiliar with the process for scholarly writing, presentation, or publication.

DNP Project Team: The *DNP Project Team* should replace any other name (such as *committee*) used in conjunction with the faculty and mentors who provide oversight to the DNP project (AACN, 2015, p. 5). The DNP Project Team should consist of (a) the DNP student as the team leader, (b) at least one doctorally prepared faculty member, and (c) one practice mentor (AACN, 2015). Depending on the project, other team members, including content practice experts, may be enlisted in an ongoing or sporadic manner (AACN, 2015). The role of the practice mentor is to help guide the DNP student in organizational processes measures, and provide onsite support during planning, implementation, and evaluation of the DNP project. The practice mentor should be knowledgeable in organizational policies, and ideally have expertise in the content area for the DNP project. Practice mentors are typically located in the practice environment versus academic environment, thus lending a unique lens to the DNP project by providing additional insight into organizational change (AACN, 2015; M. A. Brown & Crabtree, 2013).

Evaluation of the Final DNP Project: Faculty are responsible for evaluation of the DNP project, and may enlist advice or clarity from outside stakeholders in the review and application of the final scholarly project in meeting the DNP Essentials (AACN, 2015). DNP students are encouraged to seek advice from a variety of interdisciplinary team members throughout the DNP project; however, faculty are ultimately required to evaluate the student's ability to meet the goals of advanced nursing practice at the doctoral level using the DNP Essentials and the academic institution requirements as a template for achievement of DNP program outcomes (AACN, 2015).

A Digital Repository for DNP Final Projects: The DNP Implementation Task Force recommends a digital repository for DNP projects in order to have a central place for sharing project outcomes. The Sigma Theta Tau International Virginia Henderson International Library has created a central repository for scholarly DNP products but does not provide a complete index of peer-reviewed papers (Broome, Riner, & Allam, 2013). In a study reviewing 175 DNP-authored articles, almost 80% were published in practice-focused journals, with many DNP-prepared nurses being first author or publishing with interdisciplinary partners in practice and academic settings (Broome et al., 2013). These findings indicate DNP-prepared nurses are becoming leaders in dissemination of improvement processes, and are meeting the DNP Essential III and VI of dissemination and interprofessional collaboration to promote better patient outcomes (AACN, 2006; Broome et al., 2013). Future plans for a central repository for DNP pProject products continues to be a high priority in the national conversation of dissemination of DNP-lead process improvement successes (AACN, 2015).

Further Support of the DNP Implementation Task Force Recommendations

During the 2012 Committee on Institutional Collaboration DNP Invitational Conference, groups of deans and DNP program directors ($N = 120$) representing 116 institutions and three nursing organizations (Sigma Theta Tau, AACN, and the National League for Nursing) were asked to render their opinion on eight questions pertaining to the scope and critical elements of the DNP project (Kirkpatrick & Weaver, 2013). The findings from these dialogues among DNP leadership were synergistic with the DNP Essentials and the AACN DNP Implementation Task Force recommendations. Question two of the eight questions specifically asked about crucial elements of the DNP project: "What are key elements of the DNP project or capstone that contribute to acquisition and demonstration of the core competencies of the DNP graduate?" (Kirkpatrick & Weaver, 2013). A summary of the crucial points regarding the answer to question two are displayed in Box 12.2 (Kirkpatrick & Weaver, 2013). Other themes noted in the discussion for question two included the importance of "leadership development, functional knowledge of epidemiology and biostatistics, informatics, systems redesign, policy, and strong practice expertise" in the DNP program curriculum (Kirkpatrick & Weaver, 2013, p. 438).

THE KEY ELEMENT FOR SUCCESS IN THE DNP PROJECT: STAKEHOLDER BUY-IN

A *stakeholder* is defined as "a key individual or group of individuals who will be directly or indirectly affected by implementation of the EBP"

BOX 12.2 Key Elements of the DNP Project

- Understand systems and the systems change process to be an effective organizational and systems leader; able to assess the organizational system, culture, and the issue of interest.
- Use informatics to analyze systems and patient data and processes (ability to work with data sets).
- Clinical scholarship and analytical skills: Use critical thinking skills to identify the desired outcomes; use data to inform the clinical issue definition and to plan the project; monitor data, manage variation, and select variables based on clinic experience and data.
- Use translational application of evidence-based practice; understand quality improvement (QI) models and set QI priorities.
- Analyze the financial implications of the implementation.
- Implementf clinical practice expertise.
- Understand the theory and scientific underpinnings.
- Gain knowledge and apply it to public policy.
- Use interpersonal skills, emotional intelligence, and conflict negotiation while maintaining a self-awareness of style, strengths, and weaknesses.

Source: From Kirkpatrick, J. M., & Weaver, T. (2013). The doctor of nursing practice capstone project: consensus or confusion? *Journal of Nursing Education, 52*(8), 435–441. doi:10.3928/01484834-20130722-01

(Everett & Titler, 2006, p. 299). Stakeholders may or may not be members of the DNP project team, and may be positively or negatively affected by the DNP project. The influence and power of stakeholders in the positive adoption and sustainability of the evidence-based practice (EBP) cannot be underestimated. Barriers to stakeholder buy-in are numerous and include opposition to change, having doubts about the change, and lack of time (Becker, Renger, & McPherson, 2015). Consideration of many different types of stakeholders is key throughout the DNP project in order to ensure that (a) ethical practice is being conducted, (b) robust evaluation of the project is utilized by incorporating the perspective of many different stakeholders, and (c) the project has a good chance of having success in the organization since the "blind spots" have be identified through stakeholder input (Leviton & Melichar, 2016). Table 12.2 gives examples of the wide variety of stakeholders to be considered throughout the DNP project (Leviton & Melichar, 2016).

Everett and Titler (2006) created a series of eight useful questions to consider when recognizing stakeholders within the micro-, meso- and macroorganizational levels (Box 12.3). These questions are important for the DNP project team to consider in the planning stages of the project as

TABLE 12.2 EXAMPLES OF STAKEHOLDERS TO BE CONSIDERED THROUGHOUT THE DNP PROJECT

Stakeholder	Description
Program staff	Staff associated with the initiative, leadership, others accountable for program/project
Organizational leadership	Executives, board of directors, advisory boards
Program beneficiaries	Initiative beneficiaries, participants, clients, patients
Program researchers	Program/initiative eEvaluators
Contributors	Founders, donors, other founders and cofounders, collaborating organizations
Community groups	Community leaders, Community-based organizations, religious leaders, law enforcement, community service groups, business leaders
Experts	Expert consultants, evaluators of similar programs or initiatives, researchers, academics
Policy groups	Policy makers (local, state, federal), advocacy organizations, government agencies

Source: From Leviton, L. C., & Melichar, L. (2016). Balancing stakeholder needs in the evaluation of healthcare quality improvement. *BMJ, 25,* 803–807. doi:10.1136/bmjqs-2015-004814

they will prompt the DNP student to reflect on those individuals who will be critical to the adoption and sustainability of the change in practice. It is important that stakeholders be consulted as soon as a firm idea for the DNP project is solidified as stakeholders may want to play an essential role

BOX 12.3 Questions to Guide Stakeholder Identification

- How are decisions made in the practice areas where the EBP will be implemented?
- What types of system changes will be needed (e.g., electronic documentation systems)?
- Who is involved in the decision-making?
- Who is likely to lead and champion implementation of the EBP?
- Who can influence the decision to proceed with implementation of an EBP?
- What type of cooperation do you need from which stakeholders to be successful?
- Who is likely to facilitate sustainability of the change in practice?
- What system changes are necessary to sustain the change in practice?

Source: From Everett, L. Q., & Titler, M. G. (2006). Making EBP part of clinical practice: The Iowa Model. In R. F. Levin & H. R. Feldman (Eds.), *Teaching evidence-based practice in nursing.* (pp. 295–324). New York, NY: Springer Publishing Company.

in the implementation and evaluation of the project. Activities with stakeholders may include selecting evaluation methodology, defining project assumptions, and team member roles in the evaluation process (Leviton & Melichar, 2016). Stakeholders may only need broad, basic information about the project in order to feel informed, or they may want specific recognition in the evaluation of the results of the project to leverage their own personal organizational goals (Leviton & Melichar, 2016). All levels of involvement from stakeholders must be considered in the planning and implementation of the project.

Keeping stakeholders engaged throughout the DNP project requires purposeful and consistent communication. J. Brown (2010) recommends sharing what has been learned during project implementation, and acknowledging successes along the way. Coupling project outcomes to organizational or unit initiatives, missions, and goals and reporting project outcome measures to stakeholders to demonstrate project effectiveness is another effective tool for stakeholder buy-in (J. Brown, 2010).

Using The Iowa Model of Evidence-Based Practice to Promote Quality Care and Rogers's Diffusion of Innovation framework, a translation research model was developed to diffuse innovation of EBP in a social system such as a healthcare organization (Titler, 2007). Using this framework, several implementation strategies for EBP adoption are identified that may also be used in the context of stakeholder buy-in (Titler, 2007). Characteristics of the EBP, including the complexity of the EBP, the advantage of adopting the EBP to the organization, and the fit of the EBP to the organizations' mission and goals, affect its adoption into practice (Titler, 2007). A strategy to help with buy-in is to give clinicians a chance to review the EBP project and process measures and give feedback regarding how best to implement the EBP (Titler, 2007). By taking some ownership in implementation of the EBP, stakeholders are much more likely to promote and adopt the EBP.

The framework developed by Titler (2007) using Rogers's translation research model, also acknowledges communication as being vitally important in the adoption of EBP. Key stakeholders—defined as opinion leaders, change champions, and expert consultants—are important to consider in the implementation and adoption of the EBP (Titler, 2007). Opinion leaders are important stakeholders to consider as they are viewed by others as being competent, respected peers, and colleagues (Titler, 2007). Because others trust their judgment, opinion leaders are very effective in implementing and supporting broad organizational change. This is especially true in a multidisciplinary project such as the DNP project. Inviting discipline-specific opinion leaders to the multidisciplinary DNP project team can be a valuable asset in the adoption of the EBP (Titler, 2007). Change champions are individuals who are experts in the clinical environment and strong supporters of change (Titler, 2007). Having one or two "boots on the ground" change champions on the unit to promote

EBP change in a positive and enthusiastic way is invaluable to the project both for ongoing evaluation and adjustments when implementing the project. In addition, a change champion is identified as the "point person" who will answer questions from those individuals directly implementing the EBP. Change champions can serve as the "eyes and ears" of how well the implementation is going, and give valuable feedback to the project team to promote successful adoption of the EBP. Expert consultants who are external topic experts with expertise in the EBP and supporting literature, provide what is known as *academic detaining*, or educational outreach (Titler, 2007). Expert consultants can meet with the DNP project team to discuss evaluation tools and quality indicators associated with the EBP, and also help deflect any challenges or push back from organizational stakeholders regarding the project by using their in-depth knowledge of the topic (Titler, 2007). Expert consultants might also be used in the strategic planning of the project by identifying gaps between research and practice implementation.

Potential users of the EBP are also mentioned by Titler (2007) as important stakeholders in the positive adoption of EBP. Potential user strategies to promote adoption of the innovation include performing a gap analysis, monitoring the project during implementation, and encouraging use of the innovation before implementing the change (Titler, 2007). Adoption of the EBP is dependent on the motivation, learning style, and education of the potential user (Titler, 2007). Performance gap assessments highlight the gap in performance and areas for improvement related to the EBP topic (Titler, 2007). For example, a needs assessment may find nurses in a medical surgical unit practice hand hygiene 60% of the time when entering a patient's room. Audit and feedback involves watching how well individuals are implementing the EBP, and giving feedback throughout the implementation process to motivate individuals by highlighting a positive change in patient outcomes (Titler, 2007). Using the hand-hygiene example, the DNP project leader may report a 10% increase in hand hygiene on the medical surgical unit, and a 5% decrease in nosocomial infection rate following implementation of hand-hygiene reminders on the patient's door. And finally, users of the EBP will be more likely to incorporate it into their practice if they have used it for a period of time (Titler, 2007). Again using the hand-hygiene example, nurses are more likely to increase their hand-hygiene practices prior to entering a patient's room because they are accustomed to using hand hygiene in other situations throughout the day.

The organizational culture and readiness for change are important factors to consider in Titler and Rogers's Translation Research Model. Several elements may influence the right 'fit' between the EBP and successful organizational adoption. The "tension for change" is one such factor and involves situations within the organization that are intolerable for the staff (Titler, 2007, p. 30). If the EBP can resolve or at least decrease the intolerable situation, there is a much greater chance the EBP will be adopted (Titler, 2007). A good "fit" between the organizational structure and the EBP must also be considered. If the system and workflow are not synergistic with the EBP, it is less likely to be adopted (Titler, 2007). In addition, planning for the impact of the EBP can be a useful area to explore. If the EBP, and the implications of implementing the EBP are carefully planned utilizing key stakeholders, it is more likely to succeed (Titler, 2007). And finally, if strong adopters and dedicated time and resources to change are strategically placed in the organization and outnumber the naysayers, the EBP is much more likely to be adopted (Titler, 2007). In addition, if a means for effective evaluation is planned, the EBP is more likely to be successful (Titler, 2007).

As previously noted, much has been written about building stakeholder buy-in;, however, little has been identified in the literature about how to monitor buy-in (Becker et al., 2015). Continually monitoring buy-in is key to increasing efficiency, streamlining interventions necessary for change, and increasing support for the evaluation of the project (Becker et al., 2015). Monitoring buy-in in a practical and unobtrusive way may be a valuable approach for novice evaluators such as DNP students. Becker et al. (2015) created a unique and valuable tool for novice evaluators to gauge and monitor buy-in success (Table 12.3).

The tool includes four indicators of buy-in identified by the authors as being important to building and maintaining buy-in a variety of settings: (a) timely, respectful communication between subject matter experts (SMEs) and the evaluation team; (b) robust feedback from SMEs to evaluation team requests; (c) the ability of the evaluation team to work directly with project decision-makers; and (d) the degree to which others are willing to share resources in order to build a successful evaluation plan (Becker et al., 2015). Using these elements, a spreadsheet containing the four elements can be developed and buy-in monitored and tracked (see Table 12.3). The tool is cost-effective and simple to use, especially for novice evaluators, and it also provides documentation of key dates and times to ensure transparency (Becker et al., 2015). The authors acknowledge there is no one element for determining the extent of buy-in, but rather the tool works as a "visual accounting system," and also serves to remind and alert evaluators of potential problems throughout project implementation (Becker et al., 2015). The tool serves as a prompt for project members to meet with stakeholders to proactively thwart problems before they can occur or derail the project—this serves as a powerful reminder for novice process improvement evaluators to continually reflect on the evaluation process throughout the project (Becker et al., 2015).

TABLE 12.3 A TOOL TO MONITOR THE SUCCESS OF BUY-IN

	Indicator 1: Timeliness of evaluation team requests	Indicator 2: Quality of feedback to evaluation team requests	Indicator 3: Interaction with decision-makers	Indicator 4: Investment of in-kind contributions
Action step:	Response to email	Comments pertaining to member check	Approval for revised evaluation plan	Travel costs for leadership team meeting
Desired outcome:	Within 48 hours	Narrative reviewed and questions answered	Response from VP	50% of request
Date submitted:	July 15	August 1	September 3	November 9
Outcome & date:	No received response July 19	Yes, lengthy response of two paragraphs received August 4	Yes, response from VP on September 7	Yes, less than wanted but still received 25% on November 12

VP, vice president.

Source: From Becker, K. L., Renger, R., & McPheron, M. (2015). Indictors of buy-in to gauge evaluation success. *Evaluation Journal of Australia, 15*(2), 12–21. doi:10.1177/1035719x1501500203

THE DNP PROJECT: MODELS AND APPROACHES

A large majority of DNP projects center on QI initiatives or evidence-based practice projects and use the tools and techniques of QI models and best practice guidelines to implement change (Dols et al., 2016; Roush & Tesoro, 2018). These DNP projects focus on solving the identified problem through the use of an organized, systematic approach. Evaluation of the project outcomes, whether using a formalized model or a less rigid approach, may utilize statistical analysis, but other benchmarks, such as practice-specific quality measures, may be used for project analysis (Kirkpatrick & Weaver, 2013; Zaccagnini & White, 2017). Regardless of the model or approach used, the DNP Essentials serve as the "North Star" for the DNP project, guiding the DNP student through the essential leadership characteristics found when translating science into practice.

Several approaches and defined models have been used for successful DNP projects. Considerable overlap exists between these models and approaches, yet each represents a unique methodology for the DNP project. The DNP project leader is responsible for selecting the approach or model that best fits the project intention, population, and design. DNP project approaches and models are described in the text that follows.

Zaccagnini and White DNP Project Process Model

Zaccagnini and White (2017) developed a DNP model that outlines the essential characteristics of the DNP project. The model involves nine specific, well-defined steps of the DNP project, and provides a comprehensive approach from problem recognition to dissemination of project findings (Zaccagnini & White, 2017). The major benefit of the DNP Project Process Model comes with the identification of sequential, clearly defined steps necessary for a successful QI project. Specific resources and tools for each step are identified, along with practical tips and advice for implementation of each phase of the DNP project. The DNP Project Process Model is especially helpful for the novice QI practitioner, and can be applied to any setting.

Step I involves problem recognition, which is perhaps one of the more onerous pieces of the DNP project. Whether it is an individual clinician, organization, or regulatory body who has identified the problem, it is important to discuss the identified problem with the DNP project advisor and faculty member to ascertain appropriateness of the problem in terms of DNP project elements (Zaccagnini & White, 2017). In addition, the scope of the project must align with the timeframe for completion of the project as many times a project that requires initiation of multiple interventions with a large patient population becomes unwieldy (Zaccagnini & White, 2017). Focusing the project on a small improvement in practice with a well-defined patient population helps to ensure success when the inevitable barriers and setbacks arise during the project, and allows the DNP student to immerse him or hersel in the QI process. Once the project has been identified, it is important to align the project aims with the mission of the organization in which the project will be implemented in order to gain stakeholder support. A problem statement is developed in step I based on the identified problem, and a brief literature search is completed in order to support project implementation based on organizational practice gaps and national standards of care (Zaccagnini & White, 2017).

Step II involves conducting a needs assessment. The goal of a needs assessment is to systematically gather data from chart audits, patient surveys, organizational benchmark data or quality indicators to support the project, as well as identify what the current organizational practice *is,* versus what the current organizational practice *should* be (Zaccagnini & White, 2017). In addition to information gathered from internal and external sources, key stakeholders integral to the success of the project must be identified. An early assessment of available resources is also a vital component of step II, as a lack of financial support, adequate staff for the implementation of the project, or project supplies can create barriers to the implementation of project interventions (Zaccagnini & White, 2017). Clear, measurable outcomes must be defined in step II, although refinement of the outcomes may occur throughout the project and change depending on the success of the interventions (Zaccagnini & White, 2017). Finally, the formation of the DNP project team, led by the DNP student, and the scope of the project are identified in step II.

Step III involves the development of goals, objectives, and the mission statement of the project(Zaccagnini & White, 2017). *Goals* refer to generous statements that identify the anticipated outcomes of the project, where as *objectives* are very specific to the project. SMART objectives refer to the who, what, when, and where of the project using interventions that are specific, measureable, attainable, realistic and timely. These SMART objectives, first developed for the business sector, help to guide the project forward and allow for project evaluation (Doran, 1981). A mission statement outlining the purpose of the project and the methods utilized in the project is an optional element of step III as some DNP programs do not be require a mission statement for the DNP project (Zaccagnini & White, 2017).

Step IV commences when the DNP student is ready to begin the project interventions. Because the implementation of sustainable changes is often met with barriers and resistance, the use of a theoretical model to help guide change is needed (Zaccagnini & White, 2017). There are a plethora of middle range theories that are useful for guiding change (Smith & Liehr, 2018). It is up to the DNP project leader to find a theory that fits with the project context and goals, and speaks to the DNP student's own personal attitude toward change. A good theoretical model fit is invaluable in guiding the DNP student in her or his process improvement journey, and helps the DNP student to meet DNP Essential I.

Project management and budget allocation are important elements in step V (Zaccagnini & White, 2017). Breaking down the project into feasible and specific tasks with targeted dates for completion using a project timeline helps the DNP student to stay on track with project implementation. In addition, having a specific deadline for deliverables moves the project forward to completion by the specified project timeline. Step V incorporates the project management tools of steps I–IV (needs assessment, identification of specific goals and objectives, and problem identification; Zaccagnini & White, 2017).

Formulating clear outcomes, and choosing the correct tools to measure outcomes in the DNP project is the responsibility of the DNP project leader (Zaccagnini & White, 2017). Step VI speaks to the importance of measuring outcomes to provide evidence of change, and to support the need for QI (Zaccagnini & White, 2017). Measurement tools, whether quantitative,qualitative, or both, should be both reliable and valid, and congruent with the context of the DNP project goals and population (Zaccagnini & White, 2017). The creation of a logic model is a helpful tool to use to define appropriate outcome measures (Zaccagnini & White, 2017).

Step VII involves implementation of the project, as well as planning for closure of the project (Zaccagnini & White, 2017). Review of the project by the institutional review board or human subjects committee may be required to determine whether the project meets the requirements of a QI project versus a research project (Zaccagnini & White, 2017). During implementation of the DNP project, which may take several months to roll out, the DNP project leader must practice skills of effective communication and leadership in order to keep the project and its priorities in the forefront for the DNP project team (Zaccagnini & White, 2017). Stakeholder buy-in is essential to project success, as discussed earlier in this chapter. Barriers and setbacks will occur despite the best efforts of the DNP project leader, thus the DNP project leader must be flexible and nimble to develop alternative strategies with the DNP project team (Zaccagnini & White, 2017).

Steps VIII and IX are exciting points in the DNP project as they revolve around interpreting the data and disseminating results of the project (Zaccagnini & White, 2017). Descriptive statistical analysis is frequently used to interpret DNP project outcomes. It is important to remember to share project outcomes with stakeholders in the community who have served as mentors to guide the project to its completion (Zaccagnini & White, 2017). By doing so, the project is much more likely to be sustainable and the organization more likely to continue to support DNP students and DNP graduates. In addition, organizational leadership can become familiar with the role of the DNP graduate, and seek out guidance for future process improvements. Dissemination of project results through publication in scholarly journals and poster presentations at local or national conferences or other professional publications serves to enhance the body of nursing science, and provide a means for other providers to improve patient outcomes (AACN, 2015; Zaccagnini & White, 2017).

Table 12.4 illustrates the synergy among the DNP Essentials, the DNP Project Process Model, and the definition of a QI project. A DNP project checklist was created by the author utilizing these elements, and could be used by the DNP student while planning and implementing the DNP project, or by the DNP project evaluation committee to ensure the DNP model or project approach meets the DNP Essentials competencies and elements of QI (AACN, 2006; Cook & Lowe, 2012; Zaccagnini & White, 2017). The checklist (completed by the DNP student or the DNP evaluation committee) ensures the DNP project, which in this example uses the DNP Project Process Model developed by Zaccagnini and White (2017), is in alignment with attainment of the DNP Essentials. Any approach or model for the DNP project can be used in place of the DNP Project Process Model column.

The Institute for Healthcare Improvement Model for Improvement

The Institute for Healthcare Improvement (IHI) uses a unique approach to improving healthcare systems called the *science of improvement*. As an applied science, the science of improvement focuses on rapid, innovative improvement to spark subsequent insight about what changes promote improvement (IHI, 2018). The combination of expert knowledge combined with effective improvement methods and tools leads to rapid improvement

TABLE 12.4 SYNERGY AMONG DNP ESSENTIALS, DNP PROJECT PROCESS MODEL, AND DEFINITION OF QI

AACN DNP Essential Characteristic	DNP Essential	Zaccagnini and White DNP Project Process Model Step	Yes	No
Does the DNP project apply scientific concepts from nursing and other sciences to assess, implement, and evaluate new evidence-based processes to improve patient outcomes?	DNP Essential I: Scientific Underpinnings for Practice	IV	√	
Does the project use organizational and systems leadership skills (advanced communication skills, principles of business, budget analysis and health policy) to: • Ethically enhance patient safety and patient outcomes • Create care delivery approaches that are sustainable • Ensure accountability	DNP Essential II: Organizational and Systems Leadership for Quality Improvement and Systems Thinking	III, V	√	
Does the project translate, apply, and evaluate research into practice by: • Analyzing and applying current literature; defining outcomes • Designing processes that align with national benchmarks • Collecting data using standard/acceptable methods • Disseminating the findings to improve patient outcomes	DNP Essential III: Clinical Scholarship and Analytical Methods for Evidence-Based Practice	I, VI, VIII, IX	√	
Does the project use information systems/technology to evaluate healthcare practices, implement healthcare guidelines, and improve patient outcomes?	DNP Essential IV: Information Systems/Technology and Patient Care Technology for the Improvement and Transformation of Healthcare	II, VI	√	
Does the project use existing policy, or create new policy at the organizational, local, or international levels to align with the principles of patient advocacy and just culture in nursing?	DNP Essential V: Healthcare Policy for Advocacy in Healthcare	VI	√	

(continued)

TABLE 12.4 SYNERGY AMONG DNP ESSENTIALS, DNP PROJECT PROCESS MODEL AND DEFINITION OF QI (continued)

AACN DNP Essential Characteristic	DNP Essential	Zaccagnini and White DNP Project Process Model Step	Yes	No
Does the project include a multidisciplinary team in which the DNP student is the team leader with advanced communication and collaboration skills to analyze and employ system-wide change?	DNP Essential VI: Interprofessional Collaboration for Improving Patient and Population Health Outcomes	II, VII	✓	
Does the project acknowledge the environmental and cultural concepts of disease prevention and health promotion to promote and improve patient outcomes?	DNP Essential VII: Clinical Prevention and Population Health for Improving the Nation's Health	II, VI	✓	
Does the project apply advanced clinical practice skills to provide optimal care by: • Identifying gaps in clinical practice using a system-wide focused assessment • Mentoring and guiding other interdisciplinary team members through complex organizational transitions • Making connections among practice, organizational priorities, patient needs, and policy issues	DNP Essential VIII: Advanced Practice Nursing	II, VII	✓	
Does the project meet the definition of QI by: • Limited scope generalizability • Pre/post, nonrandomized methodology • Nonexperimental interventions delivered to all patients • Implementation of rapid-cycle changes that drive system improvement • Sustainability of the change will continue using tenants of organizational theory			✓	

Source: From American Association of Colleges of Nursing. (2006). The essentials of doctoral education for advanced nursing practice. Retrieved from http://www.aacnnursing.org/Portals/42/Publications/DNPEssentials.pdf; Cook, P. F. & Lowe, N. K. (2012). Differentiating the scientific endeavors of research, program evaluation, and quality improvement studies. *Journal of Obstetric, Gynecologic and Neonatal Research, 41*(1), 1–3. doi:10.1111/j.1552-6909.2011.01319.x

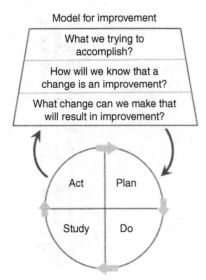

Model for improvement

FIGURE 12.1 Institute for Healthcare Improvement Model for Improvement.

Source: From Langley, G. L., Moen, R., Nolan, K. M., Nolan, T. W., Norman, C. L., & Provost, L. P. (2009). *The improvement guide: A practical approach to enhancing organizational performance* (2nd ed.). San Francisco, CA: Jossey-Bass.

(IHI, 2018). Based on the science of improvement first pioneered by W. Edwards Deming, the Model for Improvement was created by Associates for Process Improvement (API) as a simple tool used for improving quality, safety, and outcomes in patient care (Figure 12.1; IHI, 2018).

The Model for Improvement involves two parts: (a) creating project outcomes that answer three basic questions: "What are we trying to accomplish? How will we know that a change is an improvement? What changes can we make that will result in improvement?" and (b) using plan-do-study-act (PDSA) cycles to test rapid cycles of change (see Figure 12.1; IHI, 2018). Through multiple PDSA cycles, learning about what change has been most effective in accomplishing improvement is applied first to small systems and then to larger systems to improve health outcomes (IHI, 2018).

The Model for Improvement utilizes clinical science, systems theory, and a multidisciplinary team to approach QI (IHI, 2018). The project starts with a clearly defined aim and a measurement plan, and then initiates small PDSA cycles over a short period of time. As the PDSA cycles become more and more focused on what drives change, the PDSA cycles incorporate larger tests of change to initiate a system-wide approach to QI (IHI, 2018).

The Model for Improvement has seven simple steps: forming a team, setting aims, establishing measures, selecting changes, testing changes, implementing changes and spreading changes (IHI, n.d.). In addition to the broad steps, the Model for Improvement emphasizes the importance of developing a clear plan of how the project will be implemented, understanding systems using a process map, integration of behavioral and social sciences, and learning from events that cause variation in results (IHI, 2018).

The first step is establishing a multidisciplinary team. Team members vary according to the project and organization. A well-developed aim or project purpose, and the insight as to what systems will be impacted with the proposed change, are key to the improvement process (IHI, 2018). From this knowledge, a variety of team members who bring individual expertise and function in different parts of the project provide a broad spectrum of individuals who can implement change on a larger scale. For example, organizational leaders and informatics experts as well as direct patient-care providers are important team members for system-wide change from the macro- to the microlevel. Each team needs a team leader (the DNP student) to implement and coordinate the project, and who has an overall vision of the project goals and implementation (IHI, 2018). The team leader is also expected to have strong communication skills in order to inform and guide the team members using the knowledge gained with each PDSA cycle (IHI, 2018).

The next step in the Model for Improvement requires the project to have a clear aim statement. The aim statement should include the project population, have a specific and quantifiable outcome, and have an identified endpoint (IHI, 2018). The Model of Improvement refers to the Institute of Medicine's (now called the *National Academy of Medicine*) six overarching "Aims for Improvement" (safe, effective, patient-centered, timely, efficient, and equitable) as being the potential focus for developing the project aim statement (IHI, 2018).

Prior to implementing the project, establishing measures to confirm whether a change is occurring is an important next step in the Model of Improvement. All three types of measures should be included in the QI model: outcomes measures, process measures, and balancing measures (IHI, 2018). *Outcome measures* look at the overall project goals to improve the lives of patients and the broader community (IHI, 2018). *Process measures* are individual interventions created to improve system outcomes and keep the project focused to ultimately improve health outcomes and meet the goal of the outcome measures (IHI, 2018). *Balancing measures* are created to see whether improvement in one area causes unwanted consequences in another area (IHI, 2018). For example, a DNP project may have an outcome measure of decreasing sepsis in the oncology unit. Process measures might include implementation of a sepsis recognition algorithm. Balancing measures may include increased time for nurses to perform the algorithm, thus delaying care for other patients.

Selecting a change and testing changes, the next two steps in the Model for Improvement, starts with combining the concept of change with information about the project population: This sparks ideas from the project team for PDSA cycles (IHI, 2018). Testing change is reflected in the PDSA cycles—the project team plans for change, enacts change interventions, studies the results of the change interventions, and acts on what they have learned to modify and plan for the subsequent PDSA cycles in a short time frame (IHI, 2018). If the PDSA cycles result in change, continuing to refine and repeat PDSA cycles on a larger scale will hopefully result in system-wide improvement (IHI, 2018). It is important to track the PDSA cycles using a run chart to note when in the PDSA cycles project outcomes were improved.

Once the moment of insight has taken place, based on the numerous PDSA cycles, project leaders can leverage this knowledge and promote change on a system-wide scale (IHI, 2018). Steps six and seven of the Model for Improvement incorporate change on a larger scale. Incorporating larger system change may involve changing existing organizational culture and structure (IHI, 2018). Changes in policies, staffing, budgets, and workflow are a few of the processes that may be impacted by large-scale change, resulting in challenges with the implementation process. The project leader must exercise advanced practice skills in organizational leadership to keep the project on track. Continuing to use PDSA cycles at the broader system level is a helpful tool for successful spread, and may require the addition of more project team members to address previously un-explored areas of change (IHI, 2018).

The Model for Improvement provides a simple but effective improvement model that lends itself to the DNP project and effective integration of the DNP Essentials. The IHI website (www.ihi.org) provides robust QI resources in a variety of formats, and examples of QI projects using a variety of practice settings. In addition, the IHI website presents multiple examples of implementation of evidence-based practice interventions using the Model for Improvement in a variety of community and acute care health settings, both nationally and internationally.

Quality improvement collaboratives (QIC) often use a methodology similar to that used in the Model for Improvement, which has been shown to be an effective method for implementing change. Wells et al. (2018) conducted a systematic review of QICs; 220 studies met the QIC criteria with 64 chosen for inclusion. QIC criteria included the central elements of a clear aim; the use of QI methods; and engaging teams in structured, repetitive activities utilizing shared learning similar to the PDSA cycles found in the Model of Improvement. The authors found QICs were effective in reaching their stated aims, with 83% of the studies indicating improvement in one or more of the clinical processes and outcomes (Wells et al., 2018).

Enhances, Culmination, Partnerships, Implements, Evaluates: The EC as PIE Method

The EC as PIE (enhances, culmination, partnerships, implements, evaluates) method is an evidence-based practice method that mandates five robust elements be present in the DNP project (Waldrop et al., 2014). Although the EC as PIE method does not specify sequential, detailed steps for the project in a way that the Zaccagnini and White (2017) DNP Process Model and the IHI Model for Improvement (IHI, 2018) do, it does provide an outline of critical elements that culminate into one "pie," which supports the DNP Essentials (Figure 12.2).

The EC as PIE method can be used in the initial planning phase of the project, as the guiding template for the project itself, or as a framework for DNP project evaluation (Waldrop et al., 2014). Although the EC as PIE method distills the essential elements of the DNP project with the DNP Essentials, its broad guidelines may not provide enough detail for the DNP student looking for specific steps to follow in the DNP project. However, a lack of specific guidelines can also be a plus as it allows the DNP student flexibility to blend pieces from other process improvement models with the EC as PIE method to customize their approach to change.

The "enhance" element requires the DNP student to enhance end points of patient care, clinical practice outcomes, or health policy (Waldrop et al., 2014). The DNP student may acknowledge current healthcare systems as being valid vehicles for providing high-quality patient care but gaps in patient care may fuel the need for process improvement, and thus the DNP project can focus on enhancing certain elements of the healthcare system to improve patient outcomes (Waldrop et al., 2014). Conversely, the DNP project may initiate process improvements to replace the current model of patient care with a more evidence-based, effective model of care

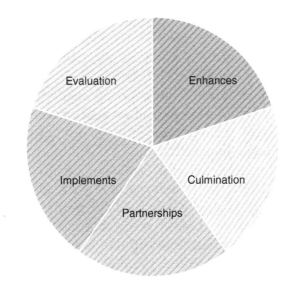

FIGURE 12.2 Enhances, culmination, partnerships, implements, evaluates: The EC as PIE Method.

Source: From Waldrop, J., Carusio, D. Fuchs, M. A., & Hypes, K. (2014). EC as PIE: Five criteria for executing a successful DNP final project. *Journal of Professional Nursing, 30*(4), 300–306. doi:10.1016/j.profnurs.2014.01.003

(Waldrop et al., 2014). Implementation and evaluation of crucial guidelines from new or existing healthcare policies may also serve to meet this element in the EC as PIE method (Waldrop et al., 2014).

Culmination of practice inquiry mandates that the DNP student demonstrate expertise in a specific area of practice and use this expertise, coupled with leadership skills, to be a change agent in the healthcare organization (Waldrop et al., 2014). The change must not end with the project itself, but rather be sustained by others in the clinical setting long after the DNP student has completed his or her DNP project. In addition, the change must be useful and convenient in the practice arena, and easily replicated by others (Waldrop et al., 2014).

The DNP project must formulate partnerships using a multidisciplinary, collaborative team approach. Healthcare does not take place in silos, but rather in a highly complex world of nuanced interprofessional teams and complex systems. The DNP student, using leadership skills acquired through the DNP curriculum, must cultivate partnerships with the patient, the healthcare system, and the individuals who create and implement health policy (Waldrop et al., 2014). As a DNP leader, these partnerships ultimately lead to change in our healthcare systems. All interprofessional partnerships have as their ultimate goal improving the patient's quality of life, with the patient's voice at the center of the proposed local or national change (Waldrop et al., 2014).

All DNP projects must implement evidence into practice. For baccalaureate- and master's-level degrees, it is enough to find and evaluate evidence. For the DNP project, it is the implementation and evaluation of the change that sets the doctorally prepared leader apart from the baccalaureate- and master's-prepared leader (Waldrop et al., 2014). The clinical change realized in the DNP project may not be generalizable, but has the potential to be reproduced and transferred to other practice settings (Waldrop et al., 2014). Many different tools, QI models, and evidence-based guidelines developed by researchers, professional organizations, or clinical experts can be used to implement change in practice.

And finally, the DNP student must evaluate how health practice, health policy, or patient care has been impacted by the DNP project (Waldrop et al., 2014). In order to achieve this, the DNP student may use patient data; national or organizational benchmark data; quality indicators specific to the practice setting and patient population, cost analyses, unit-based or organizational policy guidelines; or qualitative data (Waldrop et al., 2014). Although the ultimate goal of any DNP project is improving patient or system outcomes, DNP projects that do not show substantial change are not considered a failure (Waldrop et al., 2014). Indeed, improvements in patient health or organizational systems may not be reflected in outcome measures, but are apparent to the patient and the populations within the system (Waldrop et al., 2014).

The Iowa Model of Evidence-Based Practice to Promote Quality Care

The Iowa Model of Evidence-Based Practice to Promote Quality Care is an evidence-based, heuristic model designed to translate evidence into practice (Figure 12.3). The Iowa Model begins with identifying clues or triggers that are focused on a problem or on a need for knowledge or evidence catalysts for change, with the end result, the creation of purpose of the EBP project (Iowa Model Collaborative et al., 2017). Individuals then consider whether the identified problem or topic is a priority—a key to garner support for the project from administration, staff, and organizational leadership (Iowa Model Collaborative et al., 2017). A team is formulated, and a literature search is conducted, including research as well as nonresearch types of evidence (Iowa Model Collaborative et al., 2017). A critique of the literature and evidence-based guidelines is conducted by the team lead, which leads to the next decision point: Are there enough research and evidence-based guidelines to pilot the change in practice? If so, the Iowa Model describes conducting a pilot study similar to the PDSA cycles described in the IHI's Model for Improvement. Engaging patients and families in the pilot, as well as considering available resources and barriers are important additions to the recent revisions of the Iowa Model when planning and implementing the pilot study (Iowa Model Collaborative et al., 2017). If there is not enough evidence from the research to support change in practice, other types of evidence from expert opinion or case studies may be used to support a change in practice. After the evidence-based practice has been implemented in the practice setting, the Iowa Model uses implementation science and QI methods to constantly refine and sustain the change in the organization (Iowa Model Collaborative et al., 2017). Dissemination of results is the final step in the Iowa Model.

Although the Iowa Model does not specifically address the DNP project or DNP Essentials, it provides a practical and logical guide for implementation of research and evidence-based guidelines into practice to meet the DNP Essentials. Since 2001, the Iowa Model has been widely used in a variety of settings with "over 3,900 requests for permission to use the Iowa Model from clinicians, educators, administrators and researchers from all 50 states and 130 countries" (Iowa Model Collaborative et al., 2017, p. 175). The Iowa Model was revised in 2012 based on user feedback, changes in the healthcare system, and advances in patient-centered care (Iowa Model Collaborative et al., 2017). It has been successfully used in the academic and practice setting (Iowa Model Collaborative et al., 2017; Lloyd, D'Errico, & Bristol, 2016). The advantages of the Iowa Model are: (a) the model uses several different types of evidence (research studies, case studies, EBP guidelines) to support change; (b) the model stresses implementation and integration of EBP into quality indicators and performance improvement initiatives to help sustain change; (c) the model emphasizes change through a system-wide, organizational lens; and d) the model emphasizes

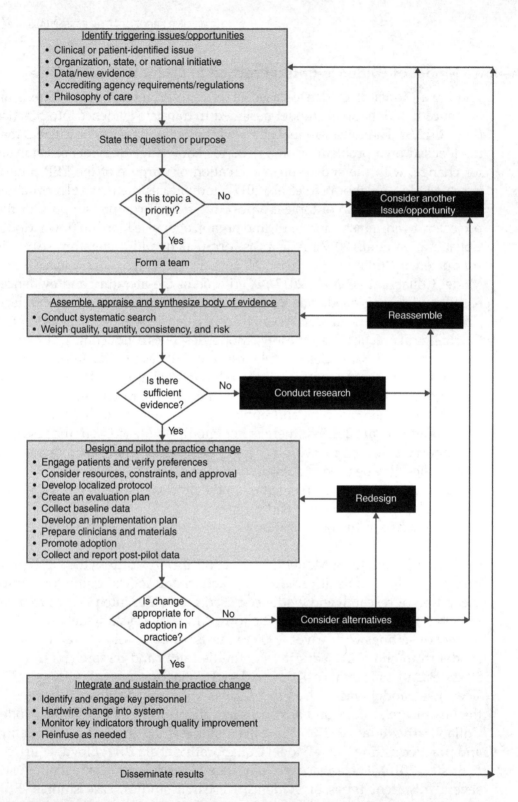

FIGURE 12.3 The Iowa evidence-based practice model to promote quality care.

Source: From The Iowa Model Collaborative, Buckwalter, K. C., Cullen, L., Hanrahan, K., Kleiber, C., McCarthy, A. M., . . . Tucker, S. (2017). Iowa model of evidence-based practice: Revisions and validation. *Worldviews on Evidence-Based Nursing, 14*(3), 175–182. doi:10.1111/wvn.12223. Reprinted with permission from the University of Iowa Hospitals and Clinics.

piloting the change on a small scale prior to organizational implementation (Iowa Model Collaborative et al., 2017; Titler, 2007). In addition, the model provides helpful feedback loops and decision points during the implementation process; these feedback loops and decision points serve as helpful guideposts for the novice DNP student navigating complex systems in his or her process improvement journey. A unique aspect of the model is the recommendation that the EBP be assimilated into job performance plans, allowing adoption of the EBP and ultimately an accepted standard of care within the organization (Titler, 2007).

Collaborative Practice Change Models

The number of postbaccalaureate DNP programs continues to grow nationally, thus many DNP students are entering the DNP program with very little clinical knowledge or awareness of the gap between evidence-based guidelines and current practice, much less possessing the skills to effectively implement change in a complex healthcare environment. M. A. Brown and Crabtree (2013) highlight the need for a paradigm shift in the DNP curriculum and suggest the development of collaborative practice change models through partnerships with academic and community agencies as a viable approach to DNP projects. Establishing partnerships with expert clinicians to guide and mentor DNP students in the final DNP project not only helps the agency to successfully implement change initiatives in the organization, but allows the student to have a "real-world" experience with expert staff and clinicians who can share their expertise in process improvement (M. A. Brown & Crabtree, 2013). Using the collaborative practice change model, a clinical area of interest is first identified by the student, or the agency provides a list of appropriate DNP project topics to the academic facility (M. A. Brown & Crabtree, 2013). Faculty and agency partners then match the student interest to the agency need, and provide agency mentors with guidelines for completion of the DNP project (M. A. Brown & Crabtree, 2013). Students have the unique advantage of mentorship from the agency staff and clinicians to build leadership and process improvement skills outlined in the DNP Essentials. Agency mentors may work with one student, or a group of students, to identify and facilitate the DNP project within the organization (M. A. Brown & Crabtree, 2013). As an added bonus, collaborative practice change models provide practical experiences that promote and market the DNP leader to organizations (M. A. Brown & Crabtree, 2013). DNP students become highly valued team members in financially strapped organizations working with vulnerable populations (M. A. Brown & Crabtree, 2013).

Collaborative practice models could be used as the primary model for the DNP project, or in conjunction with a QI model or evidence-based practice approach identified by the DNP faculty and DNP program curriculum. The downside of collaborative practice change models is the workload associated with partnering students with clinical agencies (M. A. Brown & Crabtree, 2013). In addition, orientation to the DNP project elements, QI methodology, and DNP Essentials requires purposeful education with identified agency mentors, and a commitment from the agency for ongoing collaborative partnerships in order to sustain the collaborative model for future DNP projects (M. A. Brown & Crabtree, 2013; Dols et al., 2016). M. A. Brown and Crabtree (2013) provide a framework for practice change proposals that might be used as a template by agency preceptors to guide and implement DNP projects.

CONCLUSIONS

The importance of the DNP project cannot be underestimated or understated. This chapter reviews the history of the development of the DNP project, and offers myriad valid, reliable, and widely used tools to structure a rigorous DNP project and garner stakeholder buy-in. The AACN DNP Essentials provide the bedrock of developing effective DNP projects. Practice doctorates prepare graduates for practice leadership as well as systems leadership. The DNP degree's cumulative academic requirement of the DNP project must be well designed, using a systematic approach that identifies clear connections to nursing practice. Completion of a well-designed DNP project prepares DNP graduates for their future work in practice and systems leadership.

Case Study

A.D. is an acute care nurse practitioner pursuing her DNP. She has finished her DNP coursework and is now ready to begin her DNP project. A.D. practices with a large hospitalist group that covers the oncology unit in a 300-bed academic medical center. A.D. has noticed an increase in central line-associated bloodstream infections (CLABSI) in the oncology unit patients with a central venous catheter (CVC) and decides this would be a great opportunity for process improvement. In a brief literature search, A.D. discovers a strong link between a lack of hand hygiene and bacteremia in oncology patients. She also finds new literature on prevention of CLABSI using EBP protocols and bundles. The oncology unit where she practices has a policy on central-line dressing changes that does not address the use of these new protocols or bundles for prevention of CLABSI.

A.D. formulates an outcome measure for her DNP Project: Increase hand hygiene of nurses by 20% when changing CVC dressings on oncology patients by May 14, 2018. Her process measures include educating the nurses on the oncology unit about the importance of good hand hygiene, educating the nurses about sterile technique when

(continued)

Case Study (*continued*)

changing a CVC dressing, and using reminders on bulletin boards posted in the nurse's break rooms and on patient doors to perform hand hygiene before and after the CVC dressing change.

A.D. formulates a team of nurses on the oncology unit to help implement the project. A.D. randomizes two groups for data collection: Group A consists of nurses who perform hand hygiene before and after central-line dressing change, and hroup B (control group), which consists of nurses who perform hand hygiene before the central-line dressing change only.

A.D. indicates to the nursing staff she will be presenting education on CVC dressing-change techniques and posting the reminders on the bulletin board and patient rooms on the unit on Thursday and collecting data on group A and group B on the following Friday, at which time the project will be completed. She compares the two groups using nondescriptive statistics.

Following data collection, A.D. sends an email to the nursing staff on the oncology unit indicating the project is completed, and thanks them for their time and energy. She reports her findings to the hospitalist group.

QUESTIONS

1. Complete the checklist in Table 12.4. What DNP Essentials are missing from this project?
2. Describe strategies to promote stakeholder buy-in missing in A.D.'s DNP project.
3. A.D.'s outcome measure is: Increase hand hygiene of nurses by 20% when changing central-line dressings on oncology patients by May 14, 2018. Based on A.D's original focus, is this an outcome measure or a process measure? What would be some balancing measures in this project?
4. List strategies to promote sustainability in this project.
5. What additional team members would be important to include in A.D's project?
6. After meeting with her advisor, A.D. needs to revise her DNP project. Using the information given, how would you revise A.D.'s project?

REFERENCES

American Association of Colleges of Nursing. (2006). The essentials of doctoral education for advanced nursing practice. Retrieved from http://www.aacnnursing.org/Portals/42/Publications/DNPEssentials.pdf

American Association of Colleges of Nursing. (2015). The doctor of nursing practice: Current issues and clarifying recommendations. Retrieved from http://www.aacnnursing.org/Portals/42/DNP/DNP-Implementation.pdf

Becker, K. L., Renger, R., McPherson, M. (2015). Indicators of buy-in to gauge evaluation success. *Evaluation Journal of Australasia, 15*(2), 12–21. doi:10.1177/1035719X1501500203

Broome, M. E., Riner, M. E. & Allam, E. S. (2013). Scholarly publication practices of doctor of nursing practice-prepared nurses. *Journal of Nursing Education, 52*(8), 429–434. doi:10.3928/01484834-20130718-02

Brown, J. (2010). Compliance effectiveness: How do we get there? *Journal of Health Care Compliance, 12*(4), 37–63.

Brown, M. A., & Crabtree, K. (2013). The development of practice scholarship in DNP programs: A paradigm shift. *Journal of Professional Nursing, 29*(6), 330–337. doi:10.1016/ j.profnurs.2013.08.003

Cook, P. F., & Lowe, N. K. (2012). Differentiating the scientific endeavors of research, program evaluation, and quality improvement studies. *Journal of Obstetric, Gynecologic and Neonatal Research, 41*(1), 1–3. doi:10.1111/j.1552-6909.2011.01319.x

Dols, J. D., Hernandez, C., Miles, H. (2016). The DNP project: Quandaries for nursing scholars. *Nursing Outlook, 65*, 84–93. doi:10.1016/j.outlook.2016.07.009

Doran, G. T. (1981). There's a S.M.A.R.T. Way to write management's goals and objectives. *Management Review, 70*, 35–36.

Everett, L. Q., & Titler, M. G. (2006). Making EBP part of clinical practice: The Iowa Model. In R.F. Levin & H.R. Feldman (Eds.), *Teaching evidence-based practice in nursing* (pp. 295–324). New York, NY: Springer Publishing Company.

Institute for Healthcare Improvement. (2018). Model for Improvement. Retrieved from http:// www.ihi.org/resources/Pages/HowtoImprove/default.aspx

Institute for Healthcare Improvement (n.d.). Science of improvement: How to improve. Retrieved from http://www.ihi.org/resources/Pages/HowtoImprove/Scienceof ImprovementHowtoImprove.aspx

Iowa Model Collaborative, Buckwalter, K. C., Cullen, L., Hanrahan, K., Kleiber, C., McCarthy, A. M., . . . Tucker, S. (2017). Iowa model of evidence-based practice: Revisions and validation. *Worldviews on Evidence-Based Nursing, 14*(3), 175–182.

Kirkpatrick, J. M., & Weaver, T. (2013). The doctor of nursing practice capstone project: Consensus or confusion? *Journal of Nursing Education, 52*(8), 435–441. doi:10.3928/01484834-20130722-01

Leviton, L. C., & Melichar, L. (2016). Balancing stakeholder needs in the evaluation of healthcare quality improvement. *BMJ Quality and Safety, 25*, 803–807. doi:10.1136/bmjqs-2015-004814

Lloyd, S. T., D'Errico, E., & Bristol, S. T. (2016). Use of Iowa model of research in practice as a curriculum framework for doctor of nursing practice (DNP) project completion. *Nursing Education Perspectives, 37*(1), 51–53.

Mayo, A. M. (2017). Time to define the DNP capstone project. *Clinical Nurse Specialist, 31*, 63–65. doi:10.1097/NUR.0000000000000287

Melnyk, B. M. (2013). Distinguishing the preparation and roles of doctor of philosophy and doctor of nursing practice graduates: National implications for academic curricula and health care systems. *Journal of Nursing Education, 52*(8), 442–448. doi:10.3928/01484834-20130719-01

Nelson, J. M., Cook, P. F., & Raterink, G. (2013). The evolution of a doctor of nursing capstone process: Programmatic revisions to improve the quality of student projects. *Journal of Professional Nursing, 29*(6), 370–380. doi:10.1016/j.profnurs.2012.05.018

Roush, R., & Tesoro, M. (2018). An examination of rigor and value of final scholarly projects completed by DNP nursing students. *Journal of Professional Nursing, 34*, 437–443. doi:10.1016/ j.profnurs.2018.03.003

Smith, M. J., & Liehr, P. R. (2018). *Middle range theory for nursing.* New York, NY: Springer Publishing Company.

Titler, M. (2007). Translating research into practice. *American Journal of Nursing, 107*(6), 26–33. doi:10.1097/01.NAJ.0000277823.51806.10

Waldrop, J., Caruso, D., Fuchs, M.A., & Hypes, K. (2014). EC as PIE: five criteria for executing a successful DNP final project. *Journal of Professional Nursing, 30*(4), 300–306. doi:10.1016/ j.profnurs.2014.01.003

Wells, S., Tamir, O., Gray, J., Naidoo, D., Bekhit, M., & Goldmann, D. (2018). Are quality improvement collaboratives effective? A systematic review. *BMJ Quality Safety, 27*, 226–240. doi:10.1136/bmjqs-2017-006926

Zaccagnini, M. E., & White, K. W. (2017). *The doctor of nursing practice essentials: A new model for advanced practice nursing.* (3rd ed.). Burlington, MA: Jones & Bartlett Learning.

13

USING AN EVIDENCE-BASED APPROACH TO DEVELOP A DNP PROJECT

JENNIFER DISABATO

This chapter addresses the following American Association of Colleges of Nursing (AACN) DNP Essentials:

III: Clinical Scholarship and Analytic Methods for Evidence-Based Practice
VI: Interprofessional Collaboration for Improving Patient and Population Health Outcomes
VIII: Advancing Nursing Practice

INTRODUCTION

This chapter outlines an evidence-based approach as a widely accepted method for DNP projects translating evidence into practice to improve outcomes for both patients and healthcare systems. It focuses both the novice DNP student and the practicing DNP graduate on establishing a solid foundation for a change project with a well-developed PICO (problem/patient, intervention/indicator, comparison, outcome) question and aim statement. Aspects of implementation, data collection and analysis, limitations and implications are also addressed. Attainment of a DNP degree culminates in a final sentinel project that demonstrates synthesis of knowledge and attainment of competency in The Essentials of Doctoral Education for Advanced Nursing Practice, detailed in previous chapters (American Association of Colleges of Nursing [AACN], 2006). The core elements in all DNP projects include a deliverable product upon which faculty can measure growth in the student's knowledge and expertise, and the use of evidence to inform and lead change to improve health outcomes for populations or healthcare systems (AACN, 2006). The AACN does not prescribe a single methodology for use in the DNP final project, but rather outlines potential options for demonstrating attainment of these skills. The project should ideally become the foundation for the student's subsequent scholarship as a doctorally prepared APRN (AACN, 2006; Brown & Crabtree, 2013; Kirkpatrick & Weaver, 2013).

Advanced practice nursing leaders have and will continue to occupy key positions in our healthcare system (Bleich, 2012). The DNP project can be seen as a practice implementation partnership between the academic and clinical and/or community setting to further advance nursing and healthcare science (Brown & Crabtree, 2013). A hallmark of the U.S. healthcare system is the rapidity with which change occurs and systems are required to adapt with flexibility, while maintaining safe environments for both patients and staff. With the current focus on data-driven decisions, patient-safety initiatives, transparency, population health and health equity, systems continue to increase in complexity. Frequent change is the norm, and there is a call for nurses, especially those in advanced practice roles, to lead interdisciplinary, evidence-based care (Committee on the Robert Wood Johnson Foundation Initiative on the Future of Nursing at the Institute of Medicine, Robert Wood Johnson Foundation, & Institute of Medicine, 2011).

The sheer volume of scientific reports and clinical research published in the medical literature has increased exponentially over the past two decades as use of the Internet evolved. Chronic illness or persistent conditions that are present in nearly half of the U.S. population are the leading cause of death and disability and are the costliest to the healthcare system. In addition, comorbidities are common in chronic illness, complicating the care of this population (Raghupathi & Raghupathi, 2018). Although published evidence about best practices for managing complex chronic illness exists, adoption by healthcare providers and systems is not consistent or uniform for myriad reasons (Sadeghi-Bazargani, Tabrizi, & Azami-Aghdash, 2014). Current evidence may be viewed as not being specific to a unique population or setting, or, given the sheer volume of publications, it is overwhelming to sift through so as to determine relevance. In other cases, clinical guidelines based on current evidence may be available to clinicians, but are not strictly adhered to, based on providers personal preference or historical practice (Fischer, Lange, Klose, Greiner, & Kraemer, 2016).

Inconsistent application and underutilization of established best practices in healthcare occurs for many reasons, including inadequate administrative support and staffing, poorly integrated systems, or other logistical issues (Fischer et al., 2016; Jun, Kovner, & Stimpfel, 2016). Often, historical precedent that does not match current or evolving needs leads to stagnation, until a group of invested individuals comes together to identify and plan change. Earlier chapters have explored various methodologies, including quality improvement, implementation science, and program evaluation, each of which may be chosen for a DNP final project. Successful projects, regardless of the methodology chosen, are the result of a clearly defined, well-thought-out query related to a clinical or system issue that impacts healthcare outcomes (Lloyd, D'Errico, & Bristol, 2016; Nelson, Cook, & Raterink, 2013).

Purpose of a DNP Project

The broad purpose of a DNP final project and subsequent foci of the nurse prepared with a practice doctorate is to change a current healthcare practice, process, or program for the better to enhance value to patients, healthcare providers, and/or micro and macro systems (Brown & Crabtree, 2013; Buchholz et al., 2013). DNP final projects may be focused on quality improvement of long-standing or new processes or protocols or on program evaluation to report outcomes, utilization, participation, or impact on cost or value. Unlike research, where the goal is to generate new knowledge on a subject, the DNP project applies what is currently known on the topic to the "living-breathing" clinical setting (Kirkpatrick & Weaver, 2013). As such, DNP projects may be derailed, or in some cases enhanced, by large system initiatives with unintended consequences, staff changes, or other unexpected developments. There are elements in the environment that the DNP student will have no power to control. It is within this milieu that the DNP student or graduate is challenged to lead an interdisciplinary team (Malloch, 2017; Montgomery, 2011; Polancich, Roussel, Graves, & O'Neal, 2017).

Regulatory requirements, coupled with point of care technology, mobile devices, electronic health record (EHR) enhancements, and telemedicine, are just some influences on the system that demand agility and team approaches to solve the end-user challenges that arise (Coiera, Ash, & Berg, 2016). As systems try to keep up in this environment, implementation of new procedures, processes, devices, care pathways, or patient engagement activities can be burdensome and lead to poor outcomes if changes are not planned and measured to determine whether they are effective and sustainable over time. A successful DNP project is first and foremost a planned approach to an identified problem or need. Key team members provide discipline-specific expertise. The best evidence on the topic is gathered, analyzed, and applied to determining new strategies, approaches, and/or tools to implement the change within the specific setting (S. T. Lloyd et al., 2016; Riner, 2015). Measurement of pre-determined clinical and process outcomes occurs at regular intervals over time beginning with baseline data prior to the interventions, and ongoing data tracking thereafter. If clearly defined steps in the process are overlooked or done poorly, the project can stall or worse yet, collapse.

Determining a Project Focus

Determining a focus area for the DNP project can be fraught with competing concerns. These include a student's desire to work on a long-standing interest or passion, the requirements set forth by the academic unit for completion, the availability and expertise of faculty mentors, and the time frames imposed from initiation through completion, which for most programs is generally between 12 and 18 months. Those who return for the DNP as post-master's students often have one or more challenging issues in their clinical practice appropriate for a project focus. Baccalaureate-to-DNP or MS students who are still early on their career paths may not. The DNP coursework focused on the final project guides the student through the steps and builds on core knowledge learned in earlier courses. Clear guideposts with evaluation elements integrated throughout the entire project, from initial identification through project implementation and final reporting and/or publication of outcomes, are essential.

Self-reflection on areas of clinical interest, expertise, and passion is important to the determination of a project focus. Current challenges, complaints, patient safety concerns, near misses, or other issues that lead to hallway discussions or staff discontent can also elucidate project foci. Complications with a new treatment protocol may be seen in a subset of clinic patients, raising the question why some patients do better than others. New clinical innovations often require a change in current processes to implement (Melnyk & Fineout-Overholt, 2015). Perhaps strategies used to educate patients in self-management vary depending on the expertise of the staff member providing it. If lack of consistency in patient teaching leads to return visits to the emergency department (ED), for example, would implementation of a consistent, evidence-based teaching, and follow-up protocol lead to more effective use of resources, avoid unnecessary phone encounters, and decrease costs?

Another consideration might be utilization of published national clinical care guidelines, or institutional care pathways or protocols. Institutional guidelines may lag behind newly published national best practices put forth by professional organizations and governing bodies (Fischer et al., 2016; Jun et al., 2016). In some settings, healthcare providers may be using outdated protocols as an individual choice, whereas others in the same clinical setting are implementing newer protocols, leading to lack of trust between providers and patients, who may find that the quality of their care depends less on their choice of setting, and more on which provider is caring for them.

DNP students and practitioners who are successful in project completion often have relationships with key stakeholders in the clinical area in which they intend to complete their DNP project, although this is not necessary. A balance of personal interest, system need, readiness to embrace change, and access to data to measure outcomes of the change are crucial to deciding a focus for the final project. Many students underestimate the degree of effort and length of time this initial problem identification phase requires.

Utilizing an Evidence-Based Approach

The development in the early 1990s of evidence-based medicine began the quest to bring more certainty to clinical decision-making through the incorporation of clinical epidemiology and health informatics (Sur & Dahm, 2011). Over time, the evolution to evidence-based practice (EBP) has changed clinical decision-making in healthcare and how we look at research outcomes as a basis for practice (Akobeng, 2005a; Fineout-Overholt & Johnston, 2005). Several EBP models have been developed and published since the early 1990s. Most are considered broadly applicable in healthcare, rather than focusing on a single discipline, like nursing or medicine. The use of EBP models has led to more timely translation of research into practice (Ciliska, DiCenso, Melnyk, & Stetler, 2015). Central to EBP is the development of a clearly written question that sets the foundation for a focused search of the literature to find related studies. Grading the level of evidence from higher level rigorous randomized controlled trials to lower level individual case reports determines the strength of the body of evidence and is followed by an analysis of whether the study is applicable to the proposed project question. This analysis of the literature is one leg of the EBP tripod. Incorporating the other two foundations—clinical expertise and patient/population preferences—the clinician using EBP can consider the current applicable evidence in the context of the setting of her or his project (Fineout-Overholt & Johnston, 2005; Fineout-Overholt & Stillwell, 2015; Johnston & Fineout-Overholt, 2005; S. T. Lloyd et al., 2016; Melnyk, Fineout-Overholt, Stillwell, & Williamson, 2010; Stillwell, Fineout-Overholt, Melnyk, & Williamson, 2010).

The APRN leader also considers a theoretical model or framework from which to apply the evidence to support changing practice. A theoretical foundation can be chosen from the discipline of nursing, a related social science, or be more specific to systems theories, depending on the focus of the project (Christenbery, 2011; Terhaar & Sylvia, 2016). Finally, applying evidence to change practice requires evaluation. How will the change be measured? Will there be more than one or several metrics? Where will the data be retrieved and who will determine how it is reported? Are there unintended consequences to the planned change that should be tracked in the form of a balancing measure? Measurement is essential, and using predetermined metrics, measured in consistent time intervals, it demonstrates whether progress is occurring, shows trends in data before and after interventions, and informs next steps in the planned change (R. Lloyd, 2010; Polancich, James, Miltner, Smith, & Moneyham, 2018; Riner, 2015).

Formulating a Well-Developed Question Using PICOT

The most widely accepted strategy for the first step of EBP, developing a question, is to use the acronym PICOT: population, intervention, comparison, outcome, and time frame (Akobeng, 2005b; Ciliska et al., 2015; Fineout-Overholt & Johnston, 2005; Fineout-Overholt & Stillwell, 2015). This first and most important step frames the project from initiation to completion. Questions that are clearly written, specific, and include all elements are the foundation for the subsequent literature search. This established structure for guiding a search of the existing evidence also helps determine whether the question is answerable as written, prompting further clarification of each element in PICOT, and possible rewriting of the question as existing evidence is reviewed and its applicability to the local problem evaluated. As the PICOT question is taking shape, key healthcare team members should be identified and approached about joining the project group. A project team represented by healthcare professionals from various disciplines and staff who are stakeholders in the outcome, including those for whom change may be seen in a negative light, is essential to understanding various perspectives and potential barriers (Sadeghi-Bazargani et al., 2014).

P = Population

The population that is the focus of the change project should be clearly identified. For example, in a pediatric ED, children diagnosed with pyelonephritis are noted to have had prior ED visits for symptoms of urinary tract infection (UTI) in the weeks preceding the current visit. In obtaining history from patients and families, it is unclear whether the prior UTI was treated appropriately. A DNP project in this scenario might focus on improving follow-up of urine culture results so that children with UTIs are treated with the correct antibiotic, or not treated if so indicated. The description of the population in this case should be specific: "Infants and children up to age 18 years discharged from a pediatric ED for whom a urine culture was obtained to evaluate for a possible UTI." One could even be more specific and define the type of urine culture (clean catch or catheterization). Because UTIs can be more difficult to diagnose in younger children, the population may be narrowed, for example: *Infants and children between birth and 5 years of age.*

I = Intervention

What will be done differently? What current practice or process will be impacted, replaced, or added to? Using this same example, perhaps the team determines that telephone follow-up with both the patient/family and the primary care provider in addition to the electronically sent lab results within 72 hours of ED discharge, is the most effective strategy to ensure appropriate treatment. Depending on the potential reasons for current ineffective follow-up, this intervention element of the PICOT question may focus on how the follow-up occurs (phone, text, email), to whom (family caregivers or primary care provider), or by when (within 48 hours of discharge from the ED).

C = Comparison

What is the proposed intervention being compared to? The comparison may be whatever the current practice is. In this example, the current practice may be that parents or caregivers are told to call their primary care provider within 3 days to find out whether any change in treatment is needed based on the result of the urine culture. The comparison in this example might be made more specific if there is an established, but generally ineffective method of communicating lab results, in place. For example, the team may decide that the issue is lack of knowledge on the part of the patient and family and decide to compare the intervention noted above with direct nursing phone calls to the caregiver's mobile phone 48 hours after discharge. These calls would include education on the importance of completing the antibiotic course, or stopping the antibiotics to avoid future resistance if the culture is negative, as well as checking on the child's status and reviewing symptoms that would require a return to the primary care office for further follow-up.

O = Outcome

What are the outcomes that should be measured to know whether the intervention made a difference? Consider what data are feasible to collect, where the data are housed (electronic system), and whether they are accessible. In this example, the patient outcome could be the prescribing the appropriate antibiotic (or none when the culture is negative). Another outcome could be the number of patients seen with a diagnosis of pyelonephritis who had a prior history of being seen in the ED with a UTI. The availability of reporting tools in current EHR systems allows for discrete data items to be collated in reports using diagnosis codes, unit, or clinic where the patient was seen, prior visits within a specific time window, and other data points. Outcomes in DNP projects are not a single measurement at one point in time, but rather viewed from before the project started, during the various cycles of change throughout the project, and ideally followed in an ongoing fashion after the project is finished to determine whether the desired outcomes are sustained. As reviewed in previous chapters, data are tracked using a run, or control chart. This allows milestones in the project to be labeled on the chart when they occur to see the impact various interventions had on the outcome.

T = Time

What is the time frame under consideration for the outcome? This can be stated as distinct dates, or in other terms like months, or quarters, and is usually future oriented. In this example, the time could be in the subsequent two quarters, or 6 months.

D = Digital

In 2015, Elias, Polancich, Jones, and Convoy proposed a new iteration of the PICOT question for the digital age, the PICOTD to further guide the DNP student in acquiring the requisite informatics competency. The authors argue that as digital resources are expanding constantly, the addition of this "D" includes the type of data gathered to evaluate the outcomes. Examples of this used by the authors relate to home-monitoring devices for many chronic illnesses. The format of this part of the question is suggested to be, "when looking at" and where the data are housed (Elias, Polancich, Jones, & Convoy, 2015). In the example being used, the "D" could be "when looking at positive urine culture results from the lab database. Another possibility might be "when looking at the number of patients admitted with pyelonephritis who also had a prior ED visit for suspected UTI from the admissions database."

Summary of the PICOT Elements

As suggested, the structured format of the PICOT question provides a platform for focused inquiry into the literature to gather research on a topic. The process of getting to a final question may be more fluid initially in that the question guides the literature search and the outcome of the search leads to further refinement of the PICOT question, and refines of the search. This melding of the question to better fit what is known on the specific topic of interest is consistent with the practice doctorate's focus on implementation science, which has a "real world" focus. It also further delineates the difference between the PhD focus on generating new knowledge that is generalizable, and the DNP focus on applying existing knowledge to a specific population in a specific setting (Kirkpatrick & Weaver, 2013; Velasquez, McArthur, & Johnson, 2017).

Ultimately, a well-written PICOT question focuses the DNP student on measurement. How are the outcomes (O) of the interventions (I) on the population (P) going to be measured? Reworking the PICOT question to reflect the current evidence guides the metrics chosen to determine the success of the interventions. Melnyk et al. (2010) developed six PICOT question templates for EBP projects focused on various aspects of healthcare, including (a) interventions or therapies, (b) prevention,

(c) prognosis or prediction, (d) diagnosis or diagnostic test query, (e) etiology, and (f) meaning (Melnyk et al., 2010). Finally, when reflecting on the PICOT question, the DNP student leader should consider the "why" of the change outcome. Why does it matter? Who is it important to? What is the hope for impact of the change? Will the project outcome have a direct impact on a day-to-day basis, or does it involve a broader, less apparent, but equally important goal? Keeping this "why" front and center can help the team avoid overlooking vital aspects of the proposed change.

CHOOSING A THEORETICAL MODEL AS A PROJECT FRAMEWORK

Advanced practice nurses utilize theoretical or conceptual frameworks to guide their practice with individual patients or populations, develop evidence-based inquiries, and describe and predict phenomena within their area of focus (Lor, Backonja, & Lauver, 2017). *Theory* is defined as a series of concepts, statements, propositions, and definitions that are interrelated. When applied to a project, a theoretical model helps organize knowledge and identify goals. A theoretical model can also help validate assumptions, and provide cohesive thinking about a practice, profession, or system (Lynch, 2014; Nielsen, 2016; Quinn, 2016). Integrating a theory from nursing or another related discipline in a DNP project is important because it provides a framework for connecting concepts inherent in professional APRN practice. A theoretical framework or model in a DNP project provides the means to think about how the work links to larger themes that impact practice, human behavior, and healthcare systems.

Choosing a theoretical model for a project is a crucial step in planning interventions to implement EBP. Begin with a clear understanding of the concepts that will be applied over the course of the project. Examples of concepts that might be identified include, but are not limited to, change, leadership, system functions, health behavior, innovation, social behaviors, self-determination, or motivation. There are many potential concepts, some more oriented toward biological processes, for example, symptom management, and others more focused on processes, human needs, or behavior change (Reed & Shearer, 2018). Once concepts are identified, seeking out published information about possible theoretical models, and how they have been applied in various settings will be useful to choosing a theoretical model. Once chosen, the project team should be included in discussion of the theory or framework, and it should be revisited throughout project implementation as needed. Conceptual models, theories, and frameworks applicable to improvement science were reviewed in earlier chapters.

USING LITERATURE TO SUPPORT THE DNP PROJECT

A thorough search of the literature to determine the current state of evidence specific to your PICOT question is the next step of the process. It is useful to develop a plan in advance for finding and reviewing published research on the PICOT question topic. Meeting with a trained medical librarian in your academic setting or clinical agency is key. If you cannot meet in person, many libraries offer live "chat" and other virtual opportunities to get assistance from library database experts.

Searching the Existing Research Literature

There are multiple databases available for searching the literature. The most recognized one is the U.S. National Library of Medicine's (NLM) PubMed (www.pubmed.gov). The Cochrane Review website is another place to look for supporting literature, focused on randomized controlled trials (RCTs; United States Cochrane Center, us.cochrane.org). The Cumulative Index of Nursing and Allied Health Literature (CINAHL) by EBSCO is another important database available (EBSCO Health, 2018). Health science library websites have links directly to these databases and gaining skills in how to use searchable terms and how to narrow the search can be accomplished through library assistance and/or online classes.

The PICOT question is the place to start identifying key words to search. Databases use indexing language based on key words. Individual key words can each be entered separately, and will lead to a large number of relevant studies. Tools provided by the search engine allow the key words to combine to further narrow the number of studies to a more manageable number. Narrow the search as much as possible initially, and then refine it further if needed. Limiting the search to English-only publications, a focused population by age (pediatrics or adults for examples), dates of publication (last 5–10 years), and journals published in the United States is useful.

Using the example PICOT question described earlier, related key words to search after putting in limits for patient age (pediatrics), past 5 years only, and English-only publications would be, *UTI, urine cultures, antibiotic therapy for UTI,* and *ED.* Once each of these searches is completed, the tools provided in the search engine will allow the key words to combine, for example, UTIs and urine cultures could be combined; and then narrowed further by adding *ED,* and then *antibiotic therapy.* Search strategies such as this one will substantially lower the number of related articles to choose for review. If done well, depending on the number of studies in the search that apply to the question and also the setting for the project, the PICOT question may need to be altered slightly during this process.

Developing an Evidence Table for Your PICOT

Each study determined to be applicable to the PICOT question in the search of titles and abstracts should be reviewed to determine whether they apply to the question. Once those studies that are not a fit are eliminated, developing an evidence table is an accepted method to organize and document the applicable research studies in a logical fashion for a more detailed review and analysis of applicability (Johnston & Fineout-Overholt, 2005; Melnyk et al., 2010). Across the top of a document, columns are created for the title of the article, including year and authors, theoretical framework, study design and variables, results, whether effect size was determined, and strength or quality of evidence. An additional column for strengths and limitations of the study may be helpful. An evidence table is an important step and keeps the information organized and easy to refer back to, which will be necessary throughout and also at the end of the project.

The strength or quality of each research study can be evaluated using standardized checklists for research review. This is separate from assigning a level of evidence. Methodologies that are more rigorous in terms of controlling for variation are deemed higher level studies. However, a study can be a lower level of evidence, based on the methodology employed, and be a sound and well-done study. Some studies at higher levels of evidence may be poorly conducted or reported with missing data and high dropout rates of participants that are not explained, or lack power analyses to determine the ideal number of subjects in each group to be able to conclude that the results are not the result of random chance. Studies that are lower level are not dismissed, but rather taken into consideration with two other key elements: (a) how well the study was conducted, and (b) the applicability of the study to clinical practice.

Levels of Evidence and Grading the Evidence

Assigning a level of evidence in a research study is a way of categorizing individual studies based on the level of rigor associated with the study methodology. For example, a prospective double-blind randomized controlled trial uses a more rigorous methodology than a retrospective chart review comparing two different treatments for a disease. Case reports or expert opinions from national committees or respected authorities are considered the lowest level of evidence (Akobeng, 2005b; Melnyk et al., 2010; Velasquez & Bonham, 2015). With the continuing evolution of EBP over the last two decades, and the subsequent growth of clinical practice guidelines (CPGs), there are now multiple appraisal tools for different types of evidence used in clinical practice (Melnyk et al., 2010).

A commonly used grading scheme has a I to IV ranking system with a total of six levels (Ia, Ib, IIa, IIb, III, and IV). Level Ia is a systematic review of RCTs, whereas level IV is evidence from expert committee reports or respected authorities. Once a level of evidence is assigned it can be graded A, B, C, or D as to the level of evidence it was based on with A grades based directly on level I studies and B grades based on level II studies with extrapolated evidence from level I studies, and so on (Fulk & Field-Fote, 2011; Melnyk et al., 2010). More recent, for example, in the Melnyk and Fineout-Overholt (2015) Level of Evidence Table, which grades studies from I to VII, a well-designed case-control or cohort study is considered a Level IV. Regardless of the grading scheme used, higher levels of evidence indicate greater randomization and control, and lower levels indicate a higher degree of variability, or outcomes based on fewer patients or cases.

Using a Reference Manager for the DNP Project

As the DNP project is conceived, initiated, and proceeds forward, the use of a web- or software-based reference manager is important for organizing references of evidence gathered, the theoretical model, and other literature related to the project. Because dissemination of the project outcomes is an expectation of the DNP scholar, having access to a system that organizes publications, and allows exporting of files from databases like PubMed for import into a reference management tool is essential. These tools have useful functions like creating a customized bibliography based on the required publishing style, such as the American Psychological Association style, for example. In addition, they provide access to search engines for full text, allow annotation of articles, and citations to be integrated directly into a document. These tools improve accuracy, help avoid plagiarism, and save time. One Internet-based service, EndNote Web (www.myendnoteweb.com) is a free web-based account that has the capability to synchronize with program software.

Applying the Evidence to the DNP Project

After critical appraisal of the chosen studies, applicability of each study to the patient population and unique clinical setting is evaluated. Considerations might include costs and or the availability of a particular treatment, tool, or personnel, or other practical aspects that will need to be considered (Laibhen-Parkes, 2014). When EBP is applied to individuals, patient preferences are considered during the discussion with the healthcare provider. When EBP is applied to a population of patients, the concept of patient preference is considered more broadly. There may be patient satisfaction surveys or anecdotal feedback from patients or other groups that intersect with the clinical issue. Repeated patterns observed in a group of patients may point to unstated preferences or knowledge deficits. In the example used previously, poor rates of follow-up with primary care after ED visits may have been the topic of discussions in other venues.

Applying the evidence to the project allows the team to discuss how to move toward a more evidence-based approach to the specific challenge identified for change. The evidence may point to current practices in the clinical setting that are out of date or applied differently based on provider or staff historical preferences. This is where having a team in place with individuals from the different disciplines or aspects of the project that include those who may be the most resistant to change is vital. Often times, applying the evidence leads to a discussion about creating new or updating existing policies or procedures. Care pathways and guidelines often come out of this process to help standardize practice across a clinical setting.

At this point, during project meetings led by the DNP student or practitioner, discussions should be shifting to writing a project aim statement and identifying subaims, and defining the project outcomes that will be measured upon implementation. The Institute for Healthcare Improvement defines the aim statement in the following framework: "What is the problem? Why is it important? What are we going to do about it?" (Institute for Healthcare Improvement, 2018c). The aim statement also includes the elements of how much change is expected and by when. As project outcomes are agreed upon and defined, a plan for exactly what data will be gathered, where the data are stored, who will be responsible for obtaining them, how the data will be reported, and in what intervals (monthly or quarterly are most common) should be formulated (Ciliska et al., 2015; Institute for Healthcare Improvement, 2018c; Melnyk et al., 2010). The DNP project should begin moving forward with a focus on small cycles of change as described in previous chapters. Improvement science strategies will break these interventions into small feasible cycles, which then provide information for the next small change.

Often the application of the evidence to the project is best understood through the review, discussion, and integration of nationally accepted CPGs from a professional specialty organization. The guidelines generally incorporate the existing evidence, but may be outdated or positioned for revision, so they do not negate the need for a formal search of the evidence. They do, however, provide a framework for care pathways for specific and common clinical challenges (Jun et al., 2016). Going back to the example used in the PICOT question, the evidence search may yield studies related to treatment of UTIs and risk of pyelonephritis, or UTIs and the likelihood of a positive urine culture based on the presenting symptoms. There may also be a practice guideline from a pediatric urology society about treatment of UTI. The team would review and discuss all of these and consider where current practice could be changed in a small way, and gather feedback to inform further project steps and interventions.

DATA COLLECTION AND REPORTING

Healthcare enterprises today collect data for a variety of purposes, including as part of required reporting for state and federal agencies. Having a clinical informatics specialist from the clinical area on the team is very helpful throughout the project, but particularly in the beginning, and as a consultant when needed throughout. Measurement is tied to predetermined and carefully defined outcomes. Once an aim statement has been formulated, the next step is to decide what will be measured throughout the project, where to find the data to measure, how to use or create a report for the data so that the output clearly indicates whether the changes implemented are having the intended effect (Institute for Healthcare Improvement, 2018c; R. Lloyd, 2010).

Outcome Measure

Generally, the primary outcome measure of the project is an important indicator as to whether identified patient outcomes are improved or unintended outcomes are decreased (Institute for Healthcare Improvement, 2018b). Using the example from the PICOT question, the outcome measure for a project focused on follow up of urinary cultures from the ED to ensure that antibiotics were being prescribed appropriately to avoid future pyelonephritis, might be a monthly report generating data from the medical records with the diagnostic code for pyelonephritis from the ED over a specified time period. The data report from the medical record could be designed to also pull retrospective ED visit diagnostic codes and urine cultures sent within a specified time interval associated with the medical record number of the patient with a diagnosis of pyelonephritis. Visit dates and pharmacy prescribing records could also be included in the reporting schema.

Process Measures

Process measures are also predetermined and defined. These metrics specifically relate to the aspects of the project that involve processes that are changed during implementation (Institute for Healthcare Improvement, 2018b). Usually students identify two or three process measures. In the example used, one process measure may track the number of calls made by a follow-up nurse to inform of culture results, compared with the number of cultures sent. Another measure might be whether there was a follow-up visit with the primary care center. Decisions about process measures will vary based on the systems and ability to gather data with relative consistency. Despite the existence of robust medical record systems, many students still have an element of their project that requires going through data or charts by hand, for at least a portion of the data gathering. This may not be sustainable after the project, but may be necessary during the implementation phase.

Balancing Measures

When one aspect of care is chosen for a change or improvement project, or a new program is developed, it is not uncommon for other aspects of care to shift as well. Sometimes this shift can lead to an unexpected or even negative outcome (Institute for Healthcare Improvement, 2018b). For example, if one of the interventions in an improvement project includes an educational intervention by nurses in a clinic setting that will take 5 minutes of time at the beginning of the visit during patient check in, an appropriate balancing measure may be tracking whether the time to do the education impacts another aspect of the nurses workflow, for example, medication prescription review. The balancing measure in this case would be tracking levels of incomplete medication reconciliation at the same time the completion of the educational intervention was measured.

Collecting Data Using Standardized Accepted Methods

Collection of data requires a careful selection of instruments or tools with which to measure and report outcomes. This aspect of the project is driven by all aspects of the project leading up to it, including the PICOT question, the evidence search, the project aims and subaims, and the measures chosen. Because project outcomes are used by the systems where the project takes place, and can be reported internally and externally to monitor patient care, the data collected and method of reporting must be reliable, rigorous, and consistent (Velasquez & Bonham, 2015). The type of data being measured will drive the methods of collection. For example, in a clinical project focused on improving outcomes in a chronic illness, a lab value drawn in routine clinic visits may be part of a monthly report from the lab for a population of patients. Projects that are focused on improving process flow may use time stamps in the electronic medical record (EMR) reported as time checked in, time in the exam room, time checked out to evaluate clinic flow. In a program evaluation, level of knowledge may be measured by a 10-item survey administered before and after the program implementation.

The use of existing valid and reliable instruments is recommended over developing one unique instrument for the project. Instrument development is the purview of those with a strong research background who have had formal coursework on this skill. Use of a valid and reliable tool to measure an outcome may require permission from the instrument developer, so this should be considered in advance. Instruments commonly used in DNP projects may be those established to report symptoms in chronic illnesses, like depression, diabetes, and recurrent headache as examples. Using readily available online survey tools like SurveyMonkey™ (www.surveymonkey.com) is common, especially in unique diagnosis-specific specialty clinic settings. However, the process of developing a survey is complex and requires expertise and work with faculty or other available resources in the students' program in advance to design questions and to structure the survey so that it acquires data that tracks the desired outcomes.

The EHR continues to evolve as a reporting tool. As in all reporting, the information that comes out of a report is only as good as the careful design of the report itself. Examples of discrete elements that may be pulled into an EHR report include data from flow sheets like vital signs, patient responses to questions, nursing assessment elements, timing of interventions, medication administration, and numerous other elements. In projects that involve indirect care or larger system program evaluation, depending on the project foci, data may be retrieved from human resources (HR) databases specific to employee characteristics, quality, and safety reporting databases, or procedure logs as some examples. The data experts in the organization where the project is being done will help determine how to access data, who is in charge of running reports, and the degree to which a report can be customized to look at data specific to the project.

Reporting of data should be consistent over time to pull the same data elements at every time interval, whether weekly, monthly, or quarterly. Once reports are established, the use of a run chart allows changes in the data to be clearly seen over a longitudinal time line so that trends are easily visualized and numbers that fall well outside the upper and lower limits can be discussed with the team to determine whether the variation is an outlier or a pattern indicating that change is not occurring as planned. This then alerts the team to further discuss aspects of the project implementation that may be causing the variation, and determine a plan to address further adjustments in the interventions (Institute for Healthcare Improvement, 2018a). Healthcare systems today are required to report quality outcomes data on a routine basis, and this important aspect of the DNP project should be coordinated and integrated with the existing reporting to add value to existing reports.

ANALYZING THE PROJECT RESULTS

Once the plan for collecting data is in place and functioning, analysis of the results is best organized based on the project aim statements. Statistical analysis used in EBP is about measuring differences in group outcomes, before, during, and at an established endpoint for the student to complete the project, even though tracking and reporting of the data will in many cases continue after the student graduates. Measurements of the size of the effect of the interventions are done using statistical procedures based on the level of data specific to the independent variables (the interventions) and the dependent variables (the outcomes). Descriptive statistics for describing a population uses percentages, frequency distributions, and may include a z-score, which describes the number of standard deviations the data are from the mean. Correlating independent variables with specific outcomes also describes the population in more detail.

Inferential statistical tests compare *pre-* and postintervention groups, and in DNP projects the use of nonparametric tests is common, as they do not assume a normal distribution of the population. Nonparametric tests include chi-square (more than two groups), or the Fisher's exact test for two groups. Other tests applied to infer an impact of an intervention are based on whether the level of data is ordinal, interval, or ratio level. The goal is to determine whether a desired outcome has occurred because of the interventions, or just by chance random occurrence. This is done by hypothesis testing that assumes there will be no difference (null) between the standard population and those being evaluated for improvement (patients or program participants, for example). The "null" hypothesis compares a known standard value to the value of the test population using an alpha or p value set in advance. The standard accepted p value of equal to or less than .05 (5%) is the probability of rejecting the null hypothesis (that no change has occurred) when change actually did occur. The *t*-test is another statistical test commonly reported in DNP projects. One-tailed *t*-tests are more common than two-tailed tests because the change is expected to be in one direction rather than a change in either direction (Magyary, Whitney, & Brown, 2006; Melnyk et al., 2010). Guidance on the choice of statistical test from a nursing research center within the academic program is important to thorough consideration of the data and methods of reporting results that are clear, concise, and documented in applicable software or computer programs.

In addition to the statistical analysis, a narrative description of the data analysis is essential. The narrative explains the statistical tests or procedures chosen, and summarizes unique aspects of the results. For example, if interventions in a project are designed to improve the patient experience with clinic flow in several clinics, and one of the clinics is being remodeled, the narrative might explain why or how the data outcomes of the measure used to report the patient experience for this one area were impacted. The project team has hands-on experience in the clinical setting and can propose logical explanations for why results were or were not anticipated by the team. It is incumbent on the DNP student to avoid making assumptions about the outcomes. Objective consideration of the project results will inform further steps and guide additional changes or interventions.

Meaning of Statistical and Clinical Significance

Outcomes of the DNP project can be understood with both reporting of statistical significance as determined by the alpha or *p* value, and clinical significance within the setting or organization where the project takes place. Achieving statistical significance is not always expected in DNP projects, in part because the length of time available to measure interventions is limited by the academic calendar and coursework completion dates. When others look at the results and consider whether the interventions might be useful in their unique setting, they will consider how similar their setting is from the setting described in terms of population, processes, scope, and myriad other factors. This is ultimately how the practice doctorate uses EBP to lead change and improve outcomes, then reports the outcomes to further add to the literature to guide others who will repeat the cycle (Crabtree, 2013).

Statistical Tests in EBP: Risk, Odds, and Reduction of Harm

EBP uses other measures of reporting outcomes called *measures of association*. Relative risk or risk ratios indicate the probability that an event will happen to an individual. This is done using risk ratios and is calculated by the risk of people in the intervention group who experience an outcome divided by the risk of people in the control group (those not exposed to the change or improvement, for example, prior to when the project interventions began). Odd ratios are another measure of association and report the chance of an event occurring compared to the chance of the event not occurring (Akobeng, 2005c). Odds ratios are commonly reported in DNP clinically focused projects. They are calculated using a 4-by-4 table and the odds of the event in the intervention group happenng is divided by those in the control group to report the odds that the event will occur (Buchholz et al., 2013; Polancich et al., 2018). For example, in a project focused on reporting the likelihood that screening for depression occurs in every encounter prior to the patient being put in the exam room, the odds ratio computed from the raw data can tell you the odds that the patient will be screened after the front desk staff were educated about screening processes, compared with before the education.

Measures of clinical effectiveness help give context to the risk calculations. These measures are the number needed to treat (NNT) and number needed to harm (NNH). These calculations give context to the clinical impact. Relative risk numbers may seem high, so put them in the context of the number of patients who need to be treated to prevent one adverse outcome or achieve one positive outcome. NNH reports the number of people who would have to undergo an intervention that would result in one added patient being harmed compared with those who did not receive the intervention (Polancich et al., 2018). The statistical measures chosen for the DNP project will depend on the PICOT question, aim statement, interventions, and outcomes being examined. The reporting of outcomes in statistical terms is essential in a terminal degree program, even when the outcomes may not be generalized to broader populations. The rigor associated with reporting statistical measures utilized in a DNP project is important to evolving nursing science and practice, and adds to its reliability for interdisciplinary applicability (Crabtree, 2013).

Implications of the Project: Practice and Systems

Final DNP projects should be considered in the context of the implications to the specific setting; the larger system the setting is a part of and the profession of nursing and other healthcare disciplines. Students should think of this aspect "why does this matter?" from the focused perspective of the patient, individual, or system involved as well as the broader healthcare lens (Fuller, Palmer, & Kramlich, 2013). In the example used earlier, proper treatment with antibiotics for a UTI in a child will improve comfort and prevent missed school days, and avoidance of pyelonephritis will preserve kidney health and eliminate the risk of sepsis, which is life-threatening. For the system, having fewer patients return to the ED due to inadequate treatment of a UTI may improve care for other ill patients in the ED by not taking provider time away from those in most need. Another implication of proper prescribing in this example is that it serves as a way to teach parents about the importance of judicious use of antibiotics to avoid the risk of an adverse drug effect for their child, but also the development of resistant strains of bacteria for which we have fewer treatment options in the healthcare system.

Clarifying Project Limitations

All projects have limitations in their design, implementation, and reporting, and also their wider applicability. In complex systems, clinical or administrative examples of limitations include everything from staff changes in the middle of a project, to roll out of new medical record systems that change how a data report looks. Other limitations may be related to work flow that changes because of elements outside the control of a project team, or new initiatives that take time away from those involved in implementing the project. Another limitation may be word of mouth among patients about a new process that leads them to determine a work around if they are unfamiliar or unhappy with the change. The project team, led by the DNP student, should discuss these challenges on an ongoing basis at regular intervals throughout the project to address them as they come up and report the findings in the context of the limitations.

Disseminating the Project

Becker, Johnson, Rucker, and Finnell (2018) reported on dissemination of findings through publication across cohorts of post-master's DNP graduates and noted that there has been an upward trend in the publication of quality-improvement publications over time, and that the time to publication is beginning to decrease (Becker et al., 2018). Dissemination of findings is part of the DNP Essentials in that program graduates are required to generate deliverable scholarly products that improve practice, patient outcomes, and healthcare systems (AACN, 2006; Melander, Hampton, Hardin-Pierce, & Ossege, 2018; Terhaar & Sylvia, 2016). Given that this is an expected outcome, many programs include both a presentation of the scholarly project to faculty, peers, and interprofessional colleagues and a publishable manuscript as final project course deliverables. In addition, faculty advisors play a role in co-publishing, guiding students as to the appropriate journal selection for their work, and encouraging students to set time aside to make this step of the project completion a priority. Other avenues of dissemination include specialty conferences seeking abstracts for presentations and participation on hospital, local, regional, and national professional organization committees where the scholarship can be sustained and built upon (Crabtree, 2013). In larger academic systems, there may be small-project grant funding opportunities offered by quality improvement or patient safety departments to further spread the initiatives that were successful to other areas of the organization. Professional nursing associations also offer small research grants and will consider quality-improvement or program evaluation proposals for award funding.

CONCLUSIONS

It is incumbent upon the nursing doctorate scholar, whether a student or an experienced practitioner to disseminate her or his scholarly work, through publication and/or presentation to national professional organizations as well as regional and local educational forums. Successful completion and dissemination of a DNP project translates evidence into practice and further supports the Institute for Healthcare Improvements' Triple Aim of improving the patient experience, improving population health, and reducing healthcare costs (Swensen, Pugh, McMullan, & Kabcenall, 2013). Nurses prepared with the practice doctorate are well prepared to lead change and improve the health of the nation as essential members and leaders of interdisciplinary teams.

Case Example

A DNP-prepared urgent care (UC) provider, J.C., returns from a national conference where evidence-based strategies for managing superficial skin abscesses (SSA) for a new CPG were presented. In his UC center, he is aware that there is a significant variability in how his colleagues treat SSA. Some prescribe broad-spectrum antibiotics, and recommend follow-up with a primary care provider in 5 to 7 days. Others perform an incision and drainage (I&D) procedure with culture, and may or may not prescribe antibiotics. In addition, these superficial skin lesions are referred to as abscess, furuncle, or boil, so it is not always clear what is being treated. One focus of the newly published guidelines is to reduce the overprescribing of antibiotics. For many cases of SSA, the guidelines recommend I&D and no antibiotics. With his awareness of a recent organizational initiative focused on antibiotic stewardship, J.C. discusses his thoughts about the new CPG with his unit director and is given the go ahead to put together a team to explore a quality improvement initiative to implement the new guidelines.

With the experience gained from completing a DNP project as a student there, J.C. arranged a meeting that included provider colleagues, nurses, a pharmacy representative, a Quality-improvement department lead, and an infectious disease specialist. After J.C. reviewed the conference presentation and the new guidelines, the group agreed to move forward with the initiative and invited a clinical application systems (CAS) analyst to join the group to guide the retrieval of data from the EHR. The group determined that they should each discuss their ideas for this project with others in the department individually to gather anecdotal impressions and identify possible champions who could join their team. The pharmacist and CAS analyst agreed to focus on identifying the various diagnostic names and codes for these lesions and gather baseline data on the number of patients who presented to the UC center monthly for the past 6 months, whether antibiotics were prescribed, and/or an I&D procedure with culture was performed. Simultaneously, J.C. led others in development of a PICO question to guide a literature search. The PICO question they agreed on was as follows:

P: Adult UC patients with a diagnosis of SSA
I: Does implementation of standardized definitions with treatment algorithms (CPG)
C: Compared with the current practice
O: Decrease the number of inappropriate prescriptions for antibiotics when they are not indicated

In searching the current literature, J.C. finds a systematic review and several level I and II evidence research articles on the treatment of SSA. The group developed an evidence table to determine the studies' applicability to the PICO question, and the strength of the evidence.

The group meets again to review the baseline data pulled from the EHR for the past 6 months, and to discuss the PICO question and literature table. They also discussed input they had received from staff about the proposed project and where barriers to change may exist, and decided to invite a few more individuals to join their team. They plan a three-pronged education approach, including adding short teaching sessions after staff meetings, monthly emails, and posters about the project in common staff

(continued)

Case Example (*continued*)

areas. The CAS analyst works with some of the providers to develop an order set for the EHR that follows the CPG and guides providers in clinical decision-making. A primary outcome measure of antibiotic prescriptions through the order set was determined and several process measures related to frequency of I&D procedures and unplanned patient return to the ED for the same diagnosis were identified.

The team creates run charts for the measures and refines the monthly data they are pulling from the EHR. The team meets monthly to discuss any issues or concerns and after 6 months with J.C., they analyze the results for each outcome, comparing the data from the preintervention (education and implementation of bundled orders in the EHR) to the postintervention time interval. They determine that using both descriptive and nonparametric inferential statistical tests on the data will determine whether there was statistical significance in addition to the clinical significance they have observed with improved adherence to the national CPG. They plan dissemination of their project findings internally in their network of UC centers, and discuss implementation of the improvements across the organization in other urgent or acute care settings.

QUESTIONS:

1. What elements of this case example address DNP Essential VI: Interprofessional Collaboration for Improving Patient and Population Health Outcomes?
2. What is the value of gathering and plotting monthly data on the measures chosen for the project on a run chart? Why not just pull the data 6 months after the interventions and compare it with the baseline data?
3. Once the pre- and postdata are available, J.C. uses descriptive statistics to describe the population and inferential statistical tests to help determine whether the interventions were the reason for the improvement or whether improvement was a chance occurrence. What DNP Essential does this step in the project reflect?
4. How can J.C. further achieve DNP Standard III: Advancing Nursing Practice with this project?

REFERENCES

Akobeng, A. K. (2005a). Evidence in practice. *Archives of Disease in Childhood, 90*(8), 849–852. doi:10.1136/adc.2004.058248

Akobeng, A. K. (2005b). Principles of evidence based medicine. *Archives of Disease in Childhood, 90*(8), 837–840. doi:10.1136/adc.2005.071761

Akobeng, A. K. (2005c). Understanding measures of treatment effect in clinical trials. *Archives of Disease in Childhood, 90*(1), 54–56. doi:10.1136/adc.2004.052233

American Association of Colleges of Nursing. (2006). *The essentials of doctoral education for advanced nursing practice*. Washington, DC: Author.

Becker, K. D., Johnson, S., Rucker, D., & Finnell, D. S. (2018). Dissemination of scholarship across eight cohorts of doctor of nursing practice graduates. *Journal of Clinical Nursing, 27*(7–8), e1395–e1401. doi:10.1111/jocn.14237

Bleich, M. R. (2012). Leadership responses to the future of nursing: Leading change, advancing health IOM report. *Journal of Nursing Administration, 42*(4), 183–184. doi:10.1097/NNA.0b013e31824ccc6b

Brown, M. A., & Crabtree, K. (2013). The development of practice scholarship in DNP programs: A paradigm shift. *Journal of Professional Nursing, 29*(6), 330–337. doi:10.1016/
j.profnurs.2013.08.003

Buchholz, S. W., Budd, G. M., Courtney, M. R., Neiheisel, M. B., Hammersla, M., & Carlson,
E. D. (2013). Preparing practice scholars: teaching knowledge application in the Doctor of
Nursing Practice curriculum. *Journal of the American Association of Nurse Practitioners, 25*(9),
473–480. doi:10.1002/2327-6924.12050

Christenbery, T. L. (2011). Building a schematic model: A blueprint for DNP students. *Nurse
Education, 36*(6), 250–255. doi:10.1097/NNE.0b013e3182333f85

Ciliska, D., DiCenso, A., Melnyk, B. M., & Stetler, C. (2015). Models to guide implementation
and sustainability of evidence-based practice. In B. M. Melnyk & E. Fineout-Overholt (Eds.),
Evidence-based practice in nursing and healthcare (3rd ed.). Philadelphia, PA: Wolters Kluwer
Health.

Coiera, E., Ash, J., & Berg, M. (2016). The unintended consequences of health information technology revisited. *Yearbook of Medical Informatics, 25*(1), 163–169. doi:10.15265/IY-2016-014

Committee on the Robert Wood Johnson Foundation Initiative on the Future of Nursing at the
Institute of Medicine, Robert Wood Johnson Foundation, & Institute of Medicine. (2011). *The
future of nursing: Leading change, advancing health*. Washington, DC: National Academies Press.

Crabtree, K. (2013). Capstone project: Development, implementation, evaluation and dissemination. In S. Ahmed (Ed.), *DNP education, practice and policy: Redesigning advanced practice roles
for the 21st century*. New York, NY: Springer Publishing.

EBSCO Health. (2018). *The cumulative index to nursing and allied health literature*. Ipswich, MA:
EBSCO Health

Elias, B. L., Polancich, S., Jones, C., & Convoy, S. (2015). Evolving the PICOT Method
for the Digital Age: The PICOT-D. *Journal of Nursing Education, 54*(10), 594–599.
doi:10.3928/01484834-20150916-09

Fineout-Overholt, E., & Johnston, L. (2005). Teaching EBP: asking searchable, answerable clinical
questions. *Worldviews on Evidence-Based Nursing, 2*(3), 157–160. doi:10.1111/j.1741-6787.2005.
00032.x

Fineout-Overholt, E., & Stillwell, S. B. (2015). Asking compelling clinical questions. In B. M.
Melnyk & E. Fineout-Overholt (Eds.), *Evidence based practice in nursing and healthcare* (3rd
ed.). Philadelphia, PA: Wolters Kluwer Health.

Fischer, F., Lange, K., Klose, K., Greiner, W., & Kraemer, A. (2016). Barriers and strategies in
guideline implementation—A scoping review. *Healthcare (Basel), 4*(3), 36. doi:10.3390/
healthcare4030036

Fulk, G., & Field-Fote, E. C. (2011). Measures of evidence in evidence-based practice. *Journal of
Neurologic Physical Therapy, 35*(2), 55–56. doi:10.1097/NPT.0b013e31821ba134

Fuller, V., Palmer, D., & Kramlich, D. (2013). The scholarship supporting leadership, organizations, and systems as they adopt evidence-based practice. In S. Ahmed (Ed.), *DNP education,
practice and policy: Redesigning advanced practice nursing roles for the 21st century*. New York,
NY: Springer Publishing .

Institute for Healthcare Improvement. (2018a). *Run and control charts*. Cambridge, MA: Author.

Institute for Healthcare Improvement. (2018b). Science of improvement: Establishing measures. Retrieved from http://www.ihi.org/resources/Pages/HowtoImprove/Scienceof
ImprovementEstablishingMeasures.aspx

Institute for Healthcare Improvement. (2018c). Science of improvement: Setting aims.
Retrieved from http://www.ihi.org/resources/Pages/HowtoImprove/Scienceof
ImprovementSettingAims.aspx

Johnston, L., & Fineout-Overholt, E. (2005). Teaching EBP: "Getting from zero to one." Moving
from recognizing and admitting uncertainties to asking searchable, answerable questions.
Worldviews on Evidence-Based Nursing, 2(2), 98–102. doi:10.1111/j.1741-6787.2005.05006.x

Jun, J., Kovner, C. T., & Stimpfel, A. W. (2016). Barriers and facilitators of nurses' use of clinical
practice guidelines: An integrative review. *International Journal of Nursing Studies, 60*, 54–68.
doi:10.1016/j.ijnurstu.2016.03.006

Kirkpatrick, J. M., & Weaver, T. (2013). The doctor of nursing practice capstone project: Consensus
or confusion? *Journal of Nursing Education, 52*(8), 435–441. doi:10.3928/01484834-20130722-01

Laibhen-Parkes, N. (2014). Evidence-based practice competence: a concept analysis. *International Journal of Nursing Knowledge, 25*(3), 173–182. doi:10.1111/2047-3095.12035

Lloyd, R. (2010). Understanding The Model for Improvement and PDSAs: Worksheets. Retrieved from http://www.ihi.org/IHI/Improvement

Lloyd, S. T., D'Errico, E., & Bristol, S. T. (2016). Use of the Iowa Model of Research in Practice as a curriculum framework for doctor of nursing practice (DNP) project completion. *Nursing Education Perspectives, 37*(1), 51–53.

Lor, M., Backonja, U., & Lauver, D. R. (2017). How could nurse researchers apply theory to generate knowledge more efficiently? *Journal of Nursing Scholarship, 49*(5), 580–585. doi:10.1111/jnu.12316

Lynch, V. A. (2014). Enrichment of theory through critique, restructuring and application. *Journal of Forensic Nursing, 10*(3), 120–121. doi:10.1097/JFN.0000000000000042

Magyary, D., Whitney, J. D., & Brown, M. A. (2006). Advancing practice inquiry: Research foundations of the practice doctorate in nursing. *Nursing Outlook, 54*(3), 139–151. doi:10.1016/j.outlook.2006.03.004

Malloch, K. (2017). Leading DNP professionals: Practice competencies for organizational excellence and advancement. *Nursing Administration Quarterly, 41*(1), 29–38. doi:10.1097/NAQ.0000000000000200

Melander, S., Hampton, D., Hardin-Pierce, M., & Ossege, J. (2018). Development of a rubric for evaluation of the DNP portfolio. *Nursing Education Perspectives, 39*(5), 312–314. doi:10.1097/01.NEP.0000000000000381

Melnyk, B. M., Fineout-Overholt, E., Stillwell, S. B., & Williamson, K. M. (2010). Evidence-based practice: Step by step: The seven steps of evidence-based practice. *American Journal of Nursing, 110*(1), 51–53. doi:10.1097/01.NAJ.0000366056.06605.d2

Melnyk, B. M., & Fineout-Overholt, E. (2015). Making the case for evidence-based practice and cultivating a spirit of inquiry. In B. M. Melnyk & E. Fineout-Overholt (Eds.), *Evidence-based practice in nursing and healthcare* (3rd ed.). Philadelphia, PA: Wolters Kluwer Health.

Montgomery, K. L. (2011). Leadership redefined: Educating the doctorate of nursing practice nurse leader through innovation. *Nursing Administration Quarterly, 35*(3), 248–251. doi:10.1097/NAQ.0b013e3181ff38bc

Nelson, J. M., Cook, P. F., & Raterink, G. (2013). The evolution of a doctor of nursing practice capstone process: Programmatic revisions to improve the quality of student projects. *Journal of Professional Nursing, 29*(6), 370–380. doi:10.1016/j.profnurs.2012.05.018

Nielsen, A. (2016). Concept-based learning in clinical experiences: Bringing theory to clinical education for deep learning. *Journal of Nursing Education, 55*(7), 365–371. doi:10.3928/01484834-20160615-02

Polancich, S., James, D. H., Miltner, R. S., Smith, G. L., & Moneyham, L. (2018). Building DNP Essential Skills in Clinical Data Management and Analysis. *Nurse Education, 43*(1), 37–41. doi:10.1097/nne.0000000000000411

Polancich, S., Roussel, L., Graves, B. A., & O'Neal, P. V. (2017). A regional consortium for doctor of nursing practice education: Integrating improvement science into the curriculum. *Journal of Professional Nursing, 33*(6), 417–421. doi:10.1016/j.profnurs.2017.07.013

Quinn, B. L. (2016). Using theory integration to explore complex health problems. *Advances in Nursing Science, 39*(3), 235–243. doi:10.1097/ans.0000000000000126

Raghupathi, W., & Raghupathi, V. (2018). An empirical study of chronic diseases in the United States: A visual analytics approach. *International Journal of Environmental Research and Public Health, 15*(3). doi:10.3390/ijerph15030431

Reed, P. G., & Shearer, N. B. C. (2018). *Nursing knowledge and theory innovation: advancing the science of practice* (2nd ed.). New York, NY: Springer Publishing.

Riner, M. E. (2015). Using implementation science as the core of the doctor of nursing practice inquiry project. *Journal of Professional Nursing, 31*(3), 200–207. doi:10.1016/j.profnurs.2014.11.002

Sadeghi-Bazargani, H., Tabrizi, J. S., & Azami-Aghdash, S. (2014). Barriers to evidence-based medicine: a systematic review. *Journal of Evaluation in Clinical Practice, 20*(6), 793–802. doi:10.1111/jep.12222

Stillwell, S. B., Fineout-Overholt, E., Melnyk, B. M., & Williamson, K. M. (2010). Evidence-based practice, step by step: Asking the clinical question: A key step in evidence-based practice. *American Journal of Nursing, 110*(3), 58–61. doi:10.1097/01.naj.0000368959.11129.79

Sur, R. L., & Dahm, P. (2011). History of evidence-based medicine. *Indian Journal of Urology, 27*(4), 487–489. doi:10.4103/0970-1591.91438

Swensen, S., Pugh, M., McMullan, C., & Kabcenall, A. (2013). *High impact leadership: Improve the health of populations, and reduce costs*. Cambridge, MA: Institute for Healthcare Improvement.

Terhaar, M. F., & Sylvia, M. (2016). Scholarly work products of the doctor of nursing practice: one approach to evaluating scholarship, rigour, impact and quality. *Journal of Clinical Nursing, 25*(1–2), 163–174. doi:10.1111/jocn.13113

Velasquez, D., & Bonham, E. (2015). The clinical practice project: planning to publish. *Journal of the American Association of Nurse Practitioners, 27*(8), 420–425. doi:10.1002/2327-6924.12226

Velasquez, D., McArthur, D. B., & Johnson, C. (2017). Doctoral roles in knowledge generation. In P. Reed & N. B. C. Shearer (Ed.), *Nursing knowledge and theory innovation*. New York, NY: Springer Publishing Company.

FINDING EVIDENCE TO IMPROVE PROCESSES

REBECCA S. GRAVES

This chapter addresses the following American Association of Colleges of Nursing (AACN) Essential:

IV   Information Systems/Technology and Patient Care Technology for the Improvement and Transformation of Healthcare

INTRODUCTION

Properly searching the literature for evidence for a DNP scholarly project calls for a high level of effort and precise documentation. It requires care and deliberation in choosing the terms for the search and the selection of databases. During their graduate studies and later through continuing-education classes and conferences, librarians spend considerable time learning how to search. The National Network of Libraries of Medicine (NNLM) offers courses on expert search strategies and searching effectiveness and experts in evidence-based searching share knowledge in online forums. Searching well is not a quick or easy task and it is recommended that the DNP-prepared leader reach out to a librarian for assistance. The Institute of Medicine (IOM; 2011) *Standards for Systematic Reviews* explicitly states the importance of working with a librarian. Although this chapter ooks at effective and efficient search techniques to allow for the DNP-prepared nurse to perform such tasks, it is imperative that a librarian be included in such an undertaking.

The question at hand drives the search and terms that should be chosen. The question also drives the choice of studies to include and exclude from the analysis. It behooves the scholar to take time to focus the question to ensure that the question being asked is a foreground question instead of a background question. Background questions are typically general, and often begin with *how, what, why, who,* or *where.* These are basic knowledge questions such as how to the treat ...? or what is the prognosis for ...? Background questions are best answered by textbooks or reviews. Foreground questions are specific and can follow the PICOT (P = population/problem, I = intervention, C = comparison, O = outcomes, T = time, if appropriate) format. When seeking answers for answers regarding a particular intervention in relation to a particular problem within a defined population, foreground questions are unparalleled.

If the question does not concern treatment or interventions, consider these alternate versions of PICO:

Diagnosis
P – Patient
I – Test
C – Standard test
O – Outcome

Prognosis
P – Patient
I – Prognostic factors
C – Absence of prognostic factor
O – Outcome (ex., mortality)

Risk/etiology/harm
P – Patient
I – Risk factor
C – Absence of risk factor
O – Outcome

SEARCH TERMS

Once the question is clarified, the next step is to develop the list of search terms using PICOT to set up the term sets. The following term sets are derived from the example: *Are compression garments effective in reducing lymphedema after breast cancer therapy?*

P: Lymphedema and breast cancer
I: Compression garments
C: No set

O: Reduction or prevention of swelling
T: No set

Depending on the topic, within each term set there may be a few or multiple terms. This is because there are some terms that have many synonyms and alternate spellings. For example, if the search is focused on the topic of stroke, there are only a few terms for this: *stroke, cerebrovascular accident (CVA)*, or *brain vascular accident*. On the other hand, if the search is focused on an intervention such as use of online apps to assist patients, then there will be many search terms: *online, Internet, social media, social networks, cell phones, smart phones, text messages, Facebook, Twitter*, and so on. . Depending upon the time frame of the search, that is, what years are covered, there may be a need to include terms that have fallen out of use in order to retrieve older articles. Terms from the literature review may provide insight into the development of the list.

For the previous PICOT example, the basic terms sets might look like: P: *lymphedema, lymphodema, lymphoedema, edema, oedema, elephantiasis, swelling*; C: *compression garment, compression garments, support hosiery, support hose, compression stockings, compression stocking, pressure garment, pressure garments, compression sleeve, compression bandaging, compression bandage, compression bindings*. Would it be simpler to search *compression* alone instead of adding in *garment, hose, sleeve*, and so on? Yes, searching *compression* alone would retrieve all of the phrases; however, it would also retrieve articles on chest compression and data compression. Searching requires a balance between being comprehensive and specific. If one is too comprehensive, then the results are full of "noise" or irrelevant results; if too specific, the results will be highly relevant, but it is likely useful articles will have been missed. Finally, there is not always a set of terms for each aspect of PICOT. If the question does not include a comparator, then there will be no term set for "C." Likewise, terms for outcomes can sometimes be broad and therefore not useful in the search. Not all questions include a time element and so have no terms or limits for "T".

Keyword Searching

Although technology is moving toward using natural language, most databases are still best searched using a combination of keyword searching and subject searching. *Keyword searching*, sometimes called *text word searching*, refers to searching for significant terms within the article itself or within content-rich fields of the citation, such as the title and abstract. In the field of healthcare, article titles are typically descriptive and specific. Therefore, searching the key terms in the title field usually retrieves many highly relevant citations. Abstracts cover the main points of the article and also offer a rich field to search. Most databases, by default, search the title and abstract fields, along with subject-heading fields.

There is a difference between searching for keywords within a citation, or record of an article, and within the full text. When the keywords are unique, the preferred strategy is to search the full text of an article, as the title or the abstract will not contain complete information. The drawbacks to full-text searching are as follows: Not all databases allow the full text to be searched. Text searching can result in irrelevant results if the terms are in the list of conditions or interventions excluded from the study. One should be cautious when using the *AND* operator during search of full text. Terms combined with *AND* can be far apart from each other; and the farther apart, the less likely the terms will pertain to each other. For more details on how to combine terms when searching full text, see the Operators section.

Subject Searching

Subject headings are terms that are tagged to the article by indexers. These headings are part of a controlled vocabulary that is overseen and managed by the organization in charge of the database. For example, the MEDLINE (Medical Literature Analysis and Retrieval System Online) database (www.nlm.nih.gov/bsd/medline.html) is maintained by the U.S. National Library of Medicine. The subject headings used in MEDLINE are called *MeSH*. Each year, the staff at the National Library of Medicine review the MeSH headings, adding or changing terms as needed based upon changes in the fields of health and medicine. The subject-heading vocabularies reflect their disciplines, so a term in a nursing database might be different from terms in a medical database, and again different in a database for sociology. MeSH offers the subject headings "compression bandages" and "stockings, compression" whereas CINAHL (Cumulative Index to and Allied Health Literature) subject headings offer "compression garments" or "compression therapy" or "elastic bandages."

Why is this important? In a database with a strongly controlled vocabulary, such as MEDLINE or CINAHL, using subject headings gives more power to the search. As noted, some topics can be described by many terms. The subject heading for a topic, such as lymphedema, will be tagged to a citation regardless of whether the author uses *lymphodema, lymphoedema, edema,* or *oedema*. In this way, using the subject heading for the topic results in a broader search than only doing a keyword search on lymphedema.

Another way in which subject terms can result in a broader search is by using the explode feature, which includes more specific subject headings in a search. In many databases, the subjects are arranged in a hierarchy from general to specific. Often, the more specific terms are relevant to the search. For example, the MeSH subject heading, "breast cancer lymphedema," is more specific than "lymphedema." Both are relevant to the example search.

The explode feature allows all terms to be included in the search. This is especially helpful when there are multiple subject terms. The PubMed interface automatically explodes the subject terms. CINAHL and Ovid MEDLINE allow for the choice.

Conversely, subject headings also allow the person searching to narrow the search by selecting subheadings and by restricting the subject heading to a major concept in the article. *Subheadings* are terms that can be attached to subject terms. Common ones are *complications, diagnosis, economics, epidemiology, etiology, mortality, prevention and control, therapy*. Selecting one or more subheadings narrows the subject down. For example, using the subject heading "compression bandages" with the subheading "complications" will only find articles that discuss the complications arising from the use of compression bandages. Restricting a subject heading to be a major topic means that only those articles will be retrieved where that term or concept is a significant theme of the article.

The drawbacks to subject headings are the time it takes the headings to be tagged to citations, an absence of available subject headings for every topic, and a lack of strong controlled vocabularies in some databases. For these reasons, it is recommended that the search also include keywords to allow for the retrieval of citations that do not have a subject heading or have not been tagged.

SEARCH TOOLS

Operators

Search terms, whether subject headings or keywords, can be combined with the Boolean operators *AND/OR/NOT* or proximity operators such as *ADJ, NEAR,* or *Within.* PICOT partners well with Boolean operators. Generally, *OR* is used to combine the terms within each segment of PICOT. That is, all the terms that can be used to describe the P of the question will combined with *OR* and is written as: *lymphedema OR lymphodema OR lymphoedema OR edema OR oedema OR elephantiasis.* Combine the different segments of PICOT together with *AND.* For example: (*lymphedema OR lymphodema OR lymphoedema OR edema OR oedema OR elephantiasis*) *AND* (*compression garment OR compression garments OR support hosiery OR support hose OR compression stockings OR compression stocking OR pressure garment OR pressure garments OR compression sleeve OR compression bandaging OR compression bandage OR compression bindings*). Note that parentheses are used to group each term set so that the computer program knows to solve for the OR before combining the sets with AND. This process can be likened to the "order of operations" in math (Figure 14.1).

When terms are searched using AND, the terms do not need to be close together or even in the same field unless specified. This type of broad search

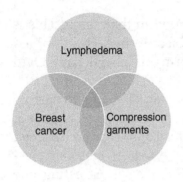

FIGURE 14.1 Visual representation of search terms for the PICOT example, "Are compression garments effective in reducing lymphedema after breast cancer therapy?"

can result in a high number of irrelevant results, especially when searching the full text of an article. One way to decrease the irrelevant results is to search by exact phrase. In most databases, the terms can be searched as an exact phrase by placing them in quotation marks. Searching using the exact phrase eliminates those citations in which the terms are present but that are not related to each other. Some databases, like PubMed, do not allow for true phrase searching.

Proximity searching can be used when an exact phrase is too tight or specific and AND is too broad. Proximity searching is a way to search for two or more words that occur within a certain number of words from each other. The proximity operators are composed of a phrase or a letter (ADJ or W) and a number (to specify a number of words). This technique is especially helpful when searching the full text, but, again, does not work in all databases. Common proximity operators are: *ADJ, Within, Near*. All three allow the search terms to be in either order and within a specified number of words from each other. A general rule of thumb is to set adjacency at three or five words if the terms are to be in the same sentence, 15 if they are to be in the same paragraph.

Parent* ADJ3 Report = finds *parent OR parents OR parental* within three words of *report*
Economic Near/5 Impact = finds *economic* within five words of *impact*
Economic W/15 Impact = finds *economic* within 15 words of *impact*.

Truncation and Wild Cards

A keyword may have multiple suffixes or various spellings. Truncation and wild-card characters save time by allowing the placement of a character at the end of the word instead of typing all the word variations combined with *OR*. The common wild-card character is the question mark (?) and allows for 0–1 characters. For example, *nurse?* will return *nurse OR nurses OR nursed*. It will not return *nursery*. The asterisk is the common truncation character and, depending upon the database, allows from five to an unlimited number of characters. For example, *neoplas** will return: *neoplasm OR neoplasms OR neoplastic OR neoplasia*.

Field Searching

Each database is made up of records, which are in turn made up of fields, most of which can be searched either together or separately. Field searching allows one to specify where in the record the keywords are to be found. Common fields in databases are: source (journal title), publication date, tTitle (article), authors, author affiliation, abstract, subject headings, author keywords. Subject-heading searches by definition are field searches of the subject-heading field. By default, most databases search the "term rich" fields of title, abstract, and subject terms. For most searches this works well. If the search needs to be narrowed, the selection of a specific field, such as title or abstract, can be chosen. Limiting the search to the title field can be useful when running pilot searches to test out search terms. Generally, such a search will bring back a smaller number of relevant results providing a small pool to check for how well the term works to retrieve articles on the topic. However, for this same reason, it is not recommended to only search one field, such as the title, as this will result in missing key articles in which the term was in the abstract or subject-heading field.

Filters

Filters can be selected to narrow the search by age, language, publication type (e.g., randomized controlled trials [RCTs], clinical trials, comparative studies, etc.). Many databases provide filters for a quick way to narrow the search. Which filters are available is up to the database provider. Filter terms are tagged to articles by indexers along with subject headings. Again, this takes time and newer articles may not yet have been tagged. For comprehensive searches, more than just the filter should be used to avoid missing articles. For example, when searching on a topic relating to children in MEDLINE, narrow the search by selecting the filter *age: child: birth – 18 years*. This will limit the articles to those on children. For a comprehensive search, supplement the prefiltered search with the addition of a set of age terms such as: *child OR children OR toddler OR teenagers OR adolescents OR teen*. This method retrieves citations that have not yet been tagged with the filter for age. Finally, combine the two age sets—the filtered set and the keyword set—with *OR*:

1. Overweight.mp. OR OVERWEIGHT/
2. Limit 1 to "all child (0 to 18 years)"

3. (Child or children or infant* or toddler* or teenagers or adolescents or teen).mp.

4. 1 AND 3

5. 2 OR 4

RESEARCH METHODOLOGY SEARCH FILTERS

Searching for articles on the project topic or using the PICOT question is just the beginning of the search process, and in order to find the highest level of evidence, further steps must be taken. The next step is to narrow the search to "research articles," that is, the evidence. This can be done by employing filters, subject terms, and keywords. Some databases, such as CINAHL and MEDLINE, have filters that can be checked to limit the search to specific article types such as RCTs or comparative studies. Subject headings can be employed, such as the MeSH terms *cohort studies, longitudinal studies, or retrospective studies* to narrow the search even further. Finally, the addition of a set of research methodology terms can be placed in the search, such as: *random* OR clinical trial OR study*.

Significant research has been done on which terms are best for retrieving research articles, both for quantitative and for qualitative research (Booth, 2016; DeJean, Giacomini, Simeonov, & Smith, 2016). McMasters University and the Joanna Briggs Institute are leaders in this area (Guyatt, Rennie, Meade, Cook, & American Medical Association, 2015; Jordan, Lockwood, Munn, & Aromataris, 2019). The research from these institutes details the best keyword and subject terms to use in searching broken out by type of question—therapy, diagnosis, prognosis—and by type of search—broad (sensitive) or narrow (specific).

LEVELS OF EVIDENCE

Although the search for the highest level of evidence is the goal, one must take into account factors, such as cost, time, or ethical considerations, before choosing to include the study. For example, an RCT would not be appropriate to use in a project testing the efficacy of parachutes. An RCT is a study design that randomly assigns participants into an experimental group or a control group. As the study is conducted, the only expected difference between the control and the experimental groups is the outcome variable being studied. Yet, these studies are not always appropriate when, for example, it is unethical to randomly expose people to toxins or to withhold treatment. Another study design, called *cohort studies*, is used when one or more samples (called *cohorts*) are followed prospectively or retrospectively, recording their exposure to certain risk factors to find clues to the possible causes of disease. Cohort studies, as well as longitudinal studies, can be filled with unknown variables or confounders, so the outcomes are correlations rather than causes. Yet, as cohort studies often have a less restricted pool of participants, they might be more inclusive and representative of the patients and populations in the project.

When deciding on the desired level of evidence for a project, one needs to judge the question being asked against the strength of a particular methodology. For example, if the PICOT request is on prognosis, the search should include cohort studies. If the PICOT is focused on therapy, RCTs are the methodology of choice as they can show which therapy causes an improvement in the disease. Thus, the appropriate level of evidence for the DNP project really depends on the question being answered in a particular study.

Systematic reviews are ranked highly. A *systematic review* can be defined as an appraisal and synthesis of all types of primary research papers using a rigorous and clearly documented methodology in both the search strategy and the selection of the studies. Systematic review methodology is explicit and precise and aims to minimize bias, thus enhancing the reliability of the conclusions drawn. A high-quality systematic review is often described as the most reliable source of evidence to guide clinical practice and is an excellent resource for a DNP-led project.

Pyramids are a common way of imagining the levels of evidence, with systematic reviews at the top followed by RCTs, cohort studies, with expert opinion at the bottom (Figure 14.2 for an example). The idea of showing levels of evidence in the shape of a pyramid comes from the fact that opinions are plentiful, but RCTs are far more rare.

Many evidence ranking systems have been devised over the years to assist healthcare providers in ranking the evidence. A few examples are SORT (strength of recommendation taxonomy), GRADE (grading of recommendations assessment, development, and evaluation), Oxford Centre for Evidence-Based Medicine (OCEBM) Levels of Evidence, and JBI (Joanna Briggs Institute) Levels of Evidence. The JBI Levels of Evidence (Jordan et al., 2019) has the benefit of being divided by question—effectiveness, diagnosis, prognosis, economic evaluation, and meaningfulness. Within each of these categories, it ranks the evidence based on appropriateness to the question, then based on the use of experimental or observational design. One common rating system for the hierarchy of evidence used in nursing is *Evidence-Based Practice in Nursing & Healthcare: A Guide to Best Practice* by Melnyk and Fineout-Overholt (2018).

The choice of level of evidence will depend on the needs of the project as defined by the question or the project lead and team members. Regardless of which ranking system is used and which level of evidence is decided on, the quality of research must still be evaluated. The DNP-prepared nurse is

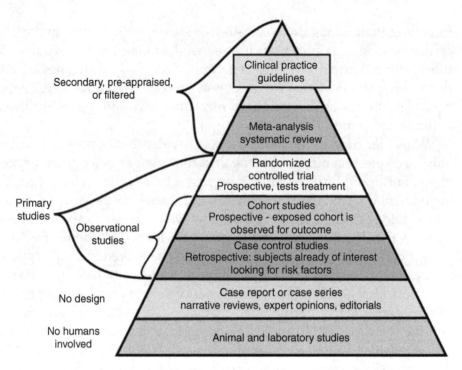

FIGURE 14.2 Levels of evidence represented by a pyramid.

experienced with appraising the methodology and asking questions. such as Did the authors use an appropriate sample size?How many patients did they lose to follow-up? Were the cohorts sufficiently comparable? This process of evaluating the quality of the research is known as *critical appraisal*. Critical appraisal is the process of carefully and systematically assessing the outcome of scientific research (evidence) to judge its trustworthiness, value, and relevance in a particular context. There are numerous tools and worksheets on this topic such as *The User's Guide to Medical Literature* (Guyatt et al., 2015).

DATABASES

When accessing a systematic review for a DNP-led project, it is very important to note not only the name of the database where the systematic review was obtained, but also the name of the vendor. A vendor is the company that does the setup, install, and maintains the database so there may be some differences in the database when it is set up by different vendors (see Table 14.1 for examples).

There are many databases available and many of them have a particular focus. Most people are familiar with CINAHL and MEDLINE. CINAHL is a major database in the nursing field and has robust indexing

TABLE 14.1 A SHORT LIST OF HEALTH SCIENCE DATABASES

Database	Coverage	Materials	Vendor
CINAHL— Cumulative Index of Nursing & Allied Health Literature	Nursing, allied health, biomedicine, and healthcare	Journals; also includes dissertations, books	**EBSCO**
MEDLINE/PubMed	Biomedicine and health; portions of life, behavioral, and chemical sciences, and bioengineering	Journals, online books; citations may include links to full text from PubMed central	**National Library of Medicine** – PubMed EBSCO Ovid ProQuest
Scopus	Medicine; health, life, and physical sciences; engineering and computing (Includes Embase and MEDLINE)	Journals, books, conference proceedings	**Elsevier**
Embase	Medicine, healthcare, pharmacology	Journals, conference abstracts	**Elsevier** EBSCO Ovid ProQuest
PsycINFO	Behavioral and social sciences, especially psychology and related fields	Journals, dissertations, books	**American Psychological Association** EBSCO Ovid ProQuest
ERIC— Education Resources Information Center	Education	Journals, reports, conference papers	**U.S. Dept. of Education** EBSCO Ovid ProQuest
LILACS—Latin-American and Caribbean System on Health Sciences Information	Health sciences literature of Latin America and Caribbean	Journals, thesis, books, conference papers, reports	**BIREME**
Cochrane Database of Systematic Reviews	Cochrane systematic reviews in healthcare	Journals	**Cochrane** EBSCO Ovid
PROSPERO	Prospective register of systematic reviews	PROSPERO protocol records	**National Institutes for Health Research (a part of Britain's National Health Service)**

of nursing theories and models. CINAHL also tends to have better index-ing for psychosocial issues that are not as well covered elsewhere. This indexing makes it easier to find articles on specific theories and topics in CINAHL, where they might be missed in another database such as MEDLINE or Scopus.

MEDLINE, whether searched through PubMed, Ovid, or another inter-face, is considered the premier health sciences database, but does not have the coverage for nursing and allied health issues that is seen in CINAHL. It has strong coverage of the biomedical fields and, as mentioned, excellent indexing through use of the MeSH headings.

It is important to search more than one database. Different journals are indexed by different databases. Although some of the larger journals are covered by multiple databases, there are many journals that are only covered by one or two databases. To make sure that the majority of rel-evant articles are included in the search, it is important to not only know where a particular journal is indexed, but also which databases cover the journals that exist in that field of study. Searching only one database will likely result in missed data (Bramer, Rethlefsen, Kleijnen, & Franco, 2017; Lawrence, 2008).

Some databases index only journal articles, whereas others include dis-sertations, book chapters, and conference proceedings. Knowing what type of material is to be included in the project will factor into the decision on the database to use. Librarians can provide more information on additional databases, what they cover, and the search features they offer.

GREY LITERATURE

Grey literature is defined as documents or publications not controlled by commercial publishers or commercial databases. Common grey literature publication types include reports, working papers, governmental docu-ments, white papers, and evaluations.

To find the grey literature, one can search library catalogs, university repositories, dissertations abstracts, the World Health Organization, clini-cal trial registries, and PROSPERO (an international prospective register of systematic reviews). To find conference proceedings, check the websites, and publications of the host organizations. Often, they will post an archive of the paper and poster abstracts from past conferences.

Clinical trials registries can be a source, not only of trials in progress, but of trials that have been completed. ClinicalTrials.gov is a database of both privately and publicly funded research. The database is maintained by the National Library of Medicine. The World Health Organization also has a list of international clinical trial registries (www.who.int/ ictrp/en).

DOCUMENTING THE SEARCH

Document the steps of the literature search by keeping track of the details. All team members on the project should discuss the search process at the initiation of the project and keep track of individual efforts. Rebuilding the searches from memory is a next-to-impossible task and saving citations in a scatter-shot fashion can lead to having to taking additional time to find them again through searching or hunting through the files. Having a plan in place ahead of time will allow the work to go more smoothly and lead to a better product.

Oftentimes a text document, such as one created in MS Word or Google Documents, works well to document the steps of the literature search. A project team decision of all of the terms that will be included in the search as well as the ones decided against, can be included in this document. The full search strategy includes all of the terms and the fields used, including the Boolean and Proximity operators. Also, the names of the databases that are searched, the names of the vendors, as well as any limits on years, language, and so on should be documented. Dating the start of the search, and each subsequent search, is helpful. All of this information will allow other researchers to replicate the search in the future.

Considering the journal where the project may be published, as well as authorship, should be discussed early in the process and agreed upon by all project team members. Many journals require that a search guideline be followed and the project team needs to be aware of this. Some schools may have specific search guidelines that the DNP student must follow. The EQUATOR (Enhancing the QUAlity and Transparency Of health Research) network has a registry of guidelines for reporting research from case reports to quantitative or qualitative systematic reviews.

Bibliographic managers, such as Zotero or EndNote, are commonly used when reports are written. These programs allow multiple users to search and easily save citations, as well as insert the references into a document in a chosen format, such as that used by the American Psychological Association (APA).

PRISMA (Preferred Reporting Items for Systematic Reviews and Meta-Analyses) is an evidenced-based set of items for reporting systematic reviews and meta-analyses. PRISMA focuses on the reporting of reviews evaluating randomized trials, but can also be used as a basis for reporting systematic reviews of other types of research, particularly evaluations of interventions. The PRISMA checklist provides an outline of all of the items that should be included in a report.

The PRISMA flow diagram allows for the documentation of the steps of the review from the database searches through the steps of screening and excluding studies (Figure 14.3).

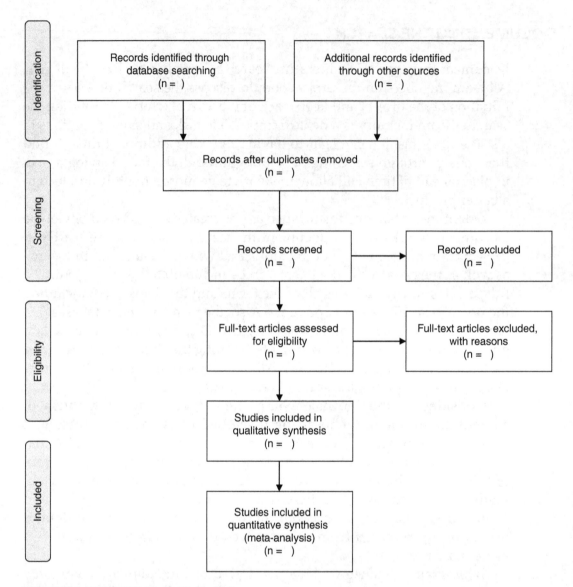

FIGURE 14.3 PRISMA 2009 flow diagram.

PRISMA, Preferred Reporting Items for Systematic Reviews and Meta-Analyses.

Source: From Moher, D., Liberati, A., Tetzlaff, J., Altman, D. G., The PRISMA Group. (2009). Preferred Reporting Items for Systematic Reviews and Meta-Analyses: The PRISMA statement. *PLoS Medicine*, 6(6), e1000097. doi:10.1371/journal.pmed.1000097

For more information, visit www.prisma-statement.org.

Evidence synthesis tools, such as CADIMA and Covidence, have been created for the systematic review process. Covidence was created in collaboration with the Cochrane Collaboration and requires a fee for use. CADIMA is open access, that is, free to use at the time of this writing, and is maintained by the Julius Kühn-Institut. Both programs not only allow the download of citations, but also guide authors through the review process,

TABLE 14.2 EXAMPLES OF COLUMNS IN A TABLE OF EVIDENCE

Biblio-graphic citation	Study type	Number of participants	(P) Patient characteristics	(I) Intervention	(C) Comparison	(O) Outcomes	(T) Time, length of study/ follow up	Level of evidence	Other (comment, funding source, etc.)

Source: From National Institute for Health and Care Excellence. (2014). *Interim methods guide for developing good practice guidance.* London, UK: Author. Retrieved from https://www.nice.org.uk/process/pmg15/chapter/appendix-c-examples-of-evidence-tables

facilitate the review of citations by multiple reviewers, and assist with analyis of results.

BUILDING AND USING AN INTERVENTION TABLE

One of the most important steps in writing the final project is showing the strength and rationale of the evidence that was chosen for use in the project. A tables of evidence is simply a chart that showcases the key characteristics of a study and allows for easy examination of those characteristics across studies. The columns can vary depending on school, organization, or personal choice.

Table 14.2 provides an example of the structure of a table of evidence based on guidelines from the National Institute for Health and Care Excellence (NICE, 2014). Although the number of patients or participants could go under the "(P)— Patient characteristics" column, many researchers find it useful to have this information broken out. The next five columns cover PICOT. If a section is not relevant, mark it "not applicable" or "not described" if the information was not provided. The final column can be used to capture the comments or to note who funded the study so determinations can be made about possible bias.

CONCLUSIONS

Finding the evidence is a key piece of a DNP scholarly project and the PICOT question is a key determinate in how the literature search will be done. There are many databases to use to search for the evidence. Each database offers unique tools for searching such as subject headings, field searching, filters, and the use of Boolean and Proximity operators. Being aware of the various tools and enlisting the assistance of a librarian assits in creating a better project.

A search of the literature requires many steps, thus, having a plan for documenting and recording these steps makes the process go more smoothly. Using the PRISMA Checklist and intervention tables assists in documenting the search process at the level that is required for evidence-based initiatives and reports that will drive patient care.

Case Study

Headache is a common complaint among pediatric patients (Wöber-Bingöl, 2013). Screen use—smartphones, tablets, computers—is also common among children and teens and has been linked with headache (Rideout, Foehr, & Roberts, 2010; Torsheim et al., 2010). Yet, many patients resort to television to relax. What does the evidence show regarding headaches in children and screen use?

QUESTIONS

1. What is one possible PICOT question based upon the case study?
2. What databases should be searched and why?
3. What search terms could be used to find the evidence? How could the search term sets be combined?
4. What study types would work for this case?

REFERENCES

Booth, A. (2016). Searching for qualitative research for inclusion in systematic reviews: A structured methodological review. *Systematic Reviews, 5*(1), 74. doi:10.1186/s13643-016-0249-x

Bramer, W. M., Rethlefsen, M. L., Kleijnen, J., & Franco, O. H. (2017). Optimal database combinations for literature searches in systematic reviews: A prospective exploratory study. *Systematic Reviews, 6*(1), 245. doi:10.1186/s13643-017-0644-y

DeJean, D., Giacomini, M., Simeonov, D., & Smith, A. (2016). Finding qualitative research evidence for health technology assessment. *Qualitative Health Research, 26*(10), 1307–1317. doi:10.1177/1049732316644429

Guyatt, G., Rennie, D., Meade, M., Cook, D., & American Medical Association (Eds.). (2015). *Users' guides to the medical literature: A manual for evidence-based clinical practice* (3rd ed.,). New York, NY: McGraw-Hill Education Medical.

Institutes of Medicine. (2011). Finding what works in health care: Standards for systematic reviews. Retrieved from http://www.nationalacademies.org/hmd/Reports/2011/Finding-What-Works-in-Health-Care-Standards-for-Systematic-Reviews.aspx

Jordan, Z., Lockwood, C., Munn, Z., & Aromataris, E. (2019). The updated Joanna Briggs institute model of evidence-based healthcare. *International Journal of Evidence-Based Healthcare, 17*(1), 58–71. doi:10.1097/xeb.0000000000000155

Lawrence, D. W. (2008). What is lost when searching only one literature database for articles relevant to injury prevention and safety promotion? *Injury Prevention: Journal of the International Society for Child and Adolescent Injury Prevention, 14*(6), 401–404. doi:10.1136/ip.2008.019430

Melnyk, B. M., & Fineout-Overholt, E. (2018). *Evidence-based practice in nursing & healthcare: A guide to best practice* (4th ed.,). Philadelphia, PA: Lippincott Lilliams & Wilkins.

Moher, D., Liberati, A., Tetzlaff, J., Altman, D. G., The PRISMA Group. (2009). Preferred Reporting Items for Systematic Reviews and Meta-Analyses: The PRISMA statement. *PLoS Medicine, 6*(6), e1000097. doi:10.1371/journal.pmed.1000097

National Institute for Health and Care Excellence. (2014). *Interim methods guide for developing good practice guidance.* London, UK: Author. Retrieved from https://www.nice.org.uk/process/pmg15/chapter/appendix-c-examples-of-evidence-tables

Rideout, V. J., Foehr, U. G., & Roberts, D. F. (2010). *Generation M²: Media in the lives of 8- to 18-Year-olds.* Menlo Park, CA: The Henry J. Kaiser Family Foundation. Retrieved from https://www.kff.org/other/report/generation-m2-media-in-the-lives-of-8-to-18-year-olds/

Torsheim, T., Eriksson, L., Schnohr, C. W., Hansen, F., Bjarnason, T., & Välimaa, R. (2010). Screen-based activities and physical complaints among adolescents from the Nordic countries. *BMC Public Health, 10*(1), 324. doi:10.1186/1471-2458-10-324

Wöber-Bingöl, C. (2013). Epidemiology of migraine and headache in children and adolescents. *Current Pain and Headache Reports, 17*(6), 341. doi:10.1007/s11916-013-0341-z

15

COST ANALYSIS IN DNP PROJECTS

AMY J. BARTON | PAMELA JONES

This chapter addresses the following American Association of Colleges of Nursong (AACN) DNP Essentials:

II Organizational and Systems Leadership for Quality Improvement and Systems Thinking
III Clinical Scholarship and Analytical Methods for Evidence-Based Practice

---

INTRODUCTION

The Institute for Healthcare Improvement (IHI) developed the Triple Aim in 2008 as "a statement of purpose for fundamentally new health systems that contribute to the overall health of populations while reducing costs" (Stiefel & Nolan, 2012, p. 2). The Triple Aim consists of improving population health, improving the patient experience of care, and reducing per capita cost. Subsequently, the Triple Aim was adopted by the U.S. Department of Health and Human Services National Quality Strategy as well as the Centers for Medicare & Medicaid Services (CMS). Considering all three facets together allows for determination of the cost-effectiveness and value of healthcare. Despite the movement toward the Quadruple Aim, adding the goal of improving work life for providers (Bodenheimer & Sinsky, 2014), IHI remains committed to the Triple Aim because all of the elements of the framework focus on patients (Feeley, 2017).

The importance of understanding principles associated with the cost of healthcare and its relevance to DNP can be found in *The Essentials of Doctoral Education for Advanced Nursing Practice* (AACN, 2006).

The second Essential, Organizational and System Leadership for Quality Improvement and Systems Thinking, clearly describes the role of the DNP (AACN, 2006):

- "DNP graduates have the ability to evaluate the cost effectiveness of care and of economics and finance to redesign effective and realistic care delivery strategies" (p. 10).

- "Advanced nursing practice requires political skills, systems thinking, and the business and financial acumen needed for the analysis of practice quality and costs" (p. 10).

- "The DNP program prepares the graduate to analyze the cost-effectiveness of practice initiatives accounting for risk and improvement of healthcare outcomes" (p. 11).

Thus, the purpose of this chapter is to prepare the DNP with the basics of cost analysis within the context of the Triple Aim.

Budget Basics

Before considering a cost analysis, it is essential to first understand the components of a budget. The budget consists of two major categories: income and expenses. *Income* is funding that flows into an organization. Within a healthcare environment, this is revenue generated from patient-care activities. Within an educational environment, it may be student tuition. *Expenses* tend to be divided into two large categories: personnel and operating. Personnel costs are the salary and benefits for each individual attributed to the project, prorated for the appropriate amount of time spent on the project. Personnel are generally listed in terms of a full-time equivalent (FTE). Each FTE constitutes 2,080 work hours over the course of a year. It is easy to remember when you consider that a person working 0.2 FTE is working 1, 8-hour day per week. Someone working 5 days is then 1.0 FTE, and the remaining increments can be calculated from there.

Operating expenses include a variety of categories that may be necessary to complete the project. These might be medical supplies, office supplies, lease costs for space, advertising materials, utilities, legal expenses, and so on. It is helpful to obtain a copy of a budget within your organization to understand the categories used before projecting financial needs for a project.

A few additional concepts concerning the budget are important: direct and indirect costs as well as fixed and variable costs. *Direct costs* are those that can be easily assignable to a project. Patient supplies that are charged specifically to a patient are an example. Indirect costs are those that are not necessarily attributable to a specific process. Utility costs within an organization are an example of these. *Fixed costs* are those that do not change regardless of the intensity or use of a product or process. For example, depreciation of equipment is a fixed cost that occurs over time. *Variable costs* are those that change with activity level. For example, printing costs of materials vary by the quantity produced.

Finally, it is important to understand the budget cycle of the organization, which is often referred to as its *fiscal year*. Many organizations operate on a July 1st to June 30th fiscal year. The federal government operates on an October 1st to September 30th fiscal year. In some organizations, the fiscal year and calendar year are the same.

COST-ANALYSIS MODELS

Cost analysis is based on economic theory and several models have been applied to healthcare. These include (Goodman, 2014):

- *Cost-of-illness analysis:* This approach determines the economic impact of an illness or condition (typically on a given population, region, or country) for example, cardiovascular disease, low birth weight, obesity, including treatment costs associated with the condition.
- *Cost-minimization analysis:* This approach compares alternatives with similar outcomes to determine which intervention costs less.
- *Cost-effectiveness analysis (CEA):* This approach compares monetary costs to quantitative health outcomes such as reduced mortality or morbidity.
  - *Cost–utility analysis (CUA):* This approach is a form of CEA that compares monetary costs to outcomes important to the patient such as quality-adjusted life years.
  - *Cost–consequence analysis:* This approach is a form of CEA that presents costs and outcomes separately and distinctly, without aggregating or weighting them. It leaves the decision regarding which outcome is better to the reader.
- *Cost–benefit analysis (CBA):* This approach compares monetary costs and benefits.
- *Budget-impact analysis (BIA):* This approach is typically used at the policy level and determines the impact of implementing or adopting a particular practice or policy on a specific budget. This might include adding particular drugs to a formulary.

TIME-DRIVEN ACTIVITY-BASED COSTING

A method for cost analysis for improvement work, fairly new to healthcare, is time-driven activity-based costing (TDABC). A recent systematic review demonstrated applicability to healthcare to efficiently apply costs to processes (Keel, Savage, Rafiq, & Mazzocato, 2017). TDABC applies principles of process mapping from industrial engineering and activity-based costing from accounting. Improvement teams that use this method start by identifying events that occur within the care cycle of interest. Once the high-level events are identified, they drill down and map out the process for each event. The process maps detail all clinical and administrative steps that occur within the process of care (Kaplan et al., 2014).

Kaplan and Norton (2001) have developed a framework for strategic management that helps us understand internal and external perspectives of a project or organization. Like most strategic initiatives, they build on the mission and vision of an organization or initiative. Their scorecard is built on those important mission-driven matters at the heart of the project. This approach to strategic management can serve as an effective tool for any industry or discipline.

Taking care to clearly define and understand the heart of your project or business—the mission and vision—the next steps to be taken when using the balanced scorecard, a performance management tool that tracks activity performance and outcomes (Kaplan & Norton, 2001), is to consider four perspectives that can influence strategic management through goals aligned with each perspective: financial, customer (patients), internal business processes, and organizational learning and growth. The financial perspective incorporates fiscal and productivity goals. Is the project or initiative profitable and how do we know our efforts are productive? The customer perspective (in our industry the patient) helps us to understand whether what we are doing or the service we offer supports the needs and wants of a patient (customer). When addressing the internal business perspective, we are establishing goals and/or objectives that area focused on the delivery of the service and our ability to do so. Finally, when taking into consideration an organization or project's learning and growth perspective, the balanced scorecard helps to understand how the organization's strategy is growing knowledge—primarily knowledge of its employees and their motivation to deliver goods and services.

Activity-based costing involves the finance staff who develop a "dollar-per-minute capacity cost rate for each clinical resource involved in the care cycle" (Kaplan et al., 2014, p. 403). An equation demonstrating the calculation is provided:

$$\frac{\text{total cost incurred by provider organization to make each resource available to the patient}}{\text{estimated total capacity (measured in hours or minutes) during which each resource is available}}$$

Variables considered in the numerator:

• Personnel costs: Compensation (salary and benefits); plus cost of office space, technology, supervision, training, and other indirect expenses

- Space and equipment costs: Depreciation, rental expense, utilities, consumable supplies, maintenance, and repairs

Variables considered in the denominator:

- Personnel capacity: Total clinical time available for work minus the time not available due to vacations, holidays, training, education, research, meetings, and breaks during the day
- Space and equipment capacity: Total budgeted time available during normal working hours minus maintenance and schedule down time

For each process step, the following calculation occurs:

dollar – per-minute capacity cost × time spent by each resource = cost of resources

The cost of any consumable supplies is added to the cost of resources. Finally, costs for all process steps are totaled to give the TDABC estimate of total costs.

EXEMPLARY CASE STUDY

In 2016, the Health Resources and Services Administration (HRSA) awarded a 2-year grant to the University of Colorado College of Nursing.[a] The purpose of this project was to integrate interprofessional and collaborative care models of behavioral health services into routine nurse-led primary care delivered in vulnerable and underserved populations across the life span. The practice site was a federally qualified, nurse-managed health center (FQHC) and faculty practice of the University of Colorado College of Nursing (CU), which serves a low-income population in the Denver metropolitan area. The intent of the project was to improve healthcare outcomes that are the result of a primary care model of care that is fully integrated with behavioral health support. The activities aligned with the CMS focus on the updated Triple Aim: (a) better care, (b) smarter spending, and (c) healthier people. This project was designed to increase access to an integrated care delivery model for behavioral health issues in underserved patients, enhance care coordination, and use

[a] This project was supported by the Health Resources and Services Administration (HRSA), of the U.S. Department of Health and Human Services (HHS) under grant number UD7HP30261 ACE: Access, Care Coordination, & Evidence-Based Practice to Enhance Integration of Behavioral Health in Primary Care for $998,591. This information or content and conclusions are those of the author and should not be construed as the official position or policy of, nor should any endorsements be inferred by HRSA, HHS or the U.S. government.

evidence-based tools to facilitate diagnosis and treatment of behavioral health problems within primary care.

The first goal was to improve access to nurse-led quality behavioral health services and included the establishment of an expanded behavioral health team and development of protocols/systems to support care integration. In addition to the expanded care team and support systems, communication strategies were developed to increase patient awareness of the model of care and analyses were conducted to establish possible bundled payment options for payer's consideration.

The patient-care team is composed of a psychiatric mental health nurse practitioner, a registered nurse care coordinator, a case manager, and a psychiatric consultant. A core study team and a resource team supported the patient-care team. Both assisted the care team to function as an integrated system, communicate effectively, and apply the philosophy of team-based care for their patients.

The project established a vision, personality, culture, and desired consumer experience that reflected the benefits of holistic nurse-led integrated healthcare. These qualities were incorporated into a grass-roots communications plan that targeted community agencies and organizations that support vulnerable populations. The marketing strategies employed included printed brochures, presentations to community boards and representatives, and website information. The messaging was focused on educating the consumer on what integrated behavioral health is and how this model of care can improve one's health.

The overall goal of this study was to ascertain the potential for nurse-led integrated behavioral and primary healthcare to cost-effectively improve a patient's health status with particular emphasis on improving depression status. The approach used to determine success involved monitoring changes in depression screen scores from the initial screen and throughout the patient's care process. In addition to monitoring depression screen scores, utilization of healthcare services was monitored to gage an understanding of the cost impact of the care team. Utilization data collected included things like number and type of visits/patient, the amount of support provided by the care manager and the case manager, care codes billed for services delivered to patients, and so on. These data were then analyzed to establish a bundled price that is based upon a care cycle delivered by the integrated team. The tool utilized to perform this analysis is TDABC. This approach to pricing (bundling) measures cost over the cycle of care (Porter & Kaplan, 2016). Key to understanding the impact of the care model was the cost of direct patient care and nonclinical services that were part of the integrated care team.

Over a period of 18 months, the care team provided services to 177 patients. Table 15.1 shows the data used to understand impact and cost of the care model.

TABLE 15.1 UTILIZATION DATA FOR INTEGRATED CARE STUDY

Average primary care visits per patient	4
Average behavioral health visits per patient	4
Average primary care service codes billed	9
Average psychiatric nurse practitioner care codes billed	6
Percenatge of improvement using posttraumatic stress depression screen	26
Percentage of improvement using Hamilton Depression Rating Scale screen	41
Percentage of improvement using the Bipolar Depression Rating Scale screen	50
Average number of case management minutes per patient	82
Average number of care coordination minutes per patient	97

The average clinical charge per patient visit was $261, or a total of $2,089 in clinical charges per patient during his or her cycle of care. In addition to direct-care charges, we analyzed the number of case management minutes per patient at a cost of $2.17 per minute and added this cost to the total cost of the cycle of care. The average case management cost per cycle of care was $177.94 per patient. We then added case management costs to clinical charges and arrived at an average bundled rate of approximately $2,267 per patient's cycle of care. We compared total clinical charges plus care management costs per patient under this model of care to reimbursement we would expect from Medicaid for advanced practice nursing care. Results are listed in Table 15.2.

To better understand the true impact of this project and the notion of integrating behavioral and primary care health services in a nurse-led practice, we analyzed this initiative through the use of a strategic management framework called the *balanced scorecard* (Kaplan & Norton, 2001). So how might the balanced scorecard help us to understand if a clinical service is successful in meeting its mission and vision? Let us apply the Balanced Scorecard perspectives to our case study.

Vision and Strategy—The integrated behavioral and primary healthcare project sought to establish a new unique approach to caring for both the emotional and physical health needs of a patient through a nurse-led interprofessional model of care. The vision was to deliver a set of

TABLE 15.2 COMPARISON OF BUNDLED CHARGE VERSUS EXPECTED MEDICAID PAYMENT

Bundled charge	Medicaid payment	Difference
$2,267	$2,707	$440 savings with bundled charge

Note: The primary payment source in this FQHC is Medicaid, paid through an encounter rate of $225.54 reimbursement per visit.

clinical services based upon the basic tenets of nursing care where support is provided to the whole person in a highly collaborative manner. The strategy was to establish a well-defined process of care the ensured cost-effective highly collaborative services that improved the health status of patients.

The financial perspective incorporated two goals:

- Establish a bundled payment option for payer reimbursement that represents a time-based cost of care.
- Incorporate integrated care team costs, such as care management support, that is not reimbursed by health insurance.

The customer (patient) perspective also comprised two goals:

- Successful delivery of the nurse-led integrated model of care, which results in improved healthcare status
- Patient's increased understanding of the value of the integrated model of healthcare services

Delivery of this new model of care required changes in internal business processes through three primary goals:

- Establishment of a dedicated interprofessional care team consisting of a primary care nurse practitioner, psychiatric mental health nurse practitioner, registered nurse, and care manager
- Development and implementation of care workflow to ensure consistent application of the model of care for each patient
- Monitoring of key operations variables to determine the impact of the care model

The learning and growth perspective goals included:

- The interprofessional integrated model of care contributed to the provider team's ability to collaborate in a way that improved cost and quality of care.
- The integrated model of care has applications in other clinical service areas across the healthcare spectrum.

By applying Kaplan and Norton's balanced scorecard to this project, we are able to refine our strategic thinking about how to implement our model and we have an effective tool to track our progress. Furthermore, Kaplan and Norton suggest the balanced scorecard is a useful tool if "collaboration and consensus are achieved." Figure 15.1 illustrates how such a

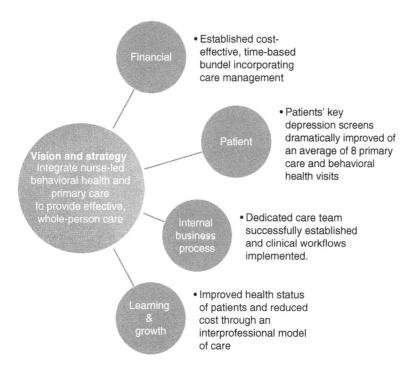

FIGURE 15.1 Study results seen through the multiple lenses of the balanced scorecard.

management tool can help us understand and improve our efforts in comprehensive interprofessional nurse-led patient care initiatives.

An important feature of Kaplan and Norton's balanced scorecard is the natural and critical nature of collaboration across the perspectives—this collaboration is key to success in any organization or strategic project initiative. Ironically, the importance of collaboration across the whole is an important feature in nursing theory and nursing leadership.

CONCLUSIONS

There are two themes that can be consistently found throughout the exemplary case study project and the financial worth of the DNP—the strategic positive impact on the status of the patient's health and the related positive financial outcome directly associated with the integrated interprofessional nurse-led team. The alignment of the balanced scorecard and nursing philosophy is remarkable and is well demonstrated through the integrated health project example. The philosophy of care utilized in the DNP profession results in two important improvement outcomes: health status and cost of care—two key factors in the IHI Triple Aim.

Case Study

D.B. is a clinic manager pursuing a DNP in health systems. She works with a low-income, aging population and is concerned that the health education literature available at the clinic often misses its mark. She is interested in a more comprehensive approach to patient education and discovered the evidence-based health literacy toolkit (Agency for Healthcare Research and Quality [AHRQ], 2015) while searching online. This looks like the perfect solution for her clinic, but she wants to get a sense of how much implementation of the toolkit might cost. D.B. also wants to get a sense of what the project launch might cost. The basic steps of the time-driven activity-based costing process are defined as follows:

　　Time-Driven Activity-Based Costing

1. Identify events that occur within the care cycle of interest. D.B. is defining her "care cycle" as the first three steps outlined in the toolkit: forming a team, creating a health literacy improvement plan, and raising awareness (AHRQ, 2015). D.B. will chair the task force, with support from her boss, the cinical director. She has selected a nurse practitioner, medical assistant, a receptionist, and a patient to join the group.
2. Create a process map that details all clinical and administrative steps that occur within the process of care. D.B. is using a simple flow diagram (Figure 15.2).

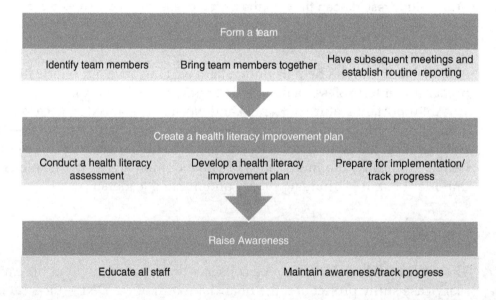

FIGURE 15.2 Flow diagram of clinical and administrative steps in process of care.
Source: From Agency for Healthcare Research and Quality. (2015). *Health Literacy Universal Precautions Toolkit* (2nd ed.). Rockville, MD: Author. Retrieved from http://www.ahrq.gov/pro-fessionals/quality-patient-safety/quality-resources/tools/literacy-toolkit/healthlittoolkit2.html

3. Consider the balanced scorecard (Kaplan & Norton, 2001; Figure 15.3).
　　a. Financial (fiscal and productivity goals)
　　b. Customer

(continued)

Case Study (*continued*)

c. Internal business perspective
d. Organizational learning and growth

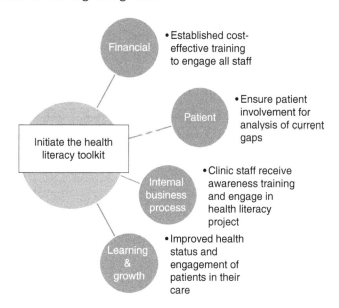

FIGURE 15.3 Application of Kaplan and Norton's balanced scorecard.

4. Identify costs.

$$\frac{\text{total cost incurred by provider organization to make each resource available to the patient}}{\text{estimated total capacity (measured in hours or minutes) during which each resource is available}}$$

a. Numerator
   i. Personnel: Compensation (salary and benefits; technology, training)
   ii. Space and equipment (consumable supplies, depreciation)
b. Denominator
   i. Personnel capacity (total time available to meet)
   ii. Space and equipment capacity

dollar – per-minute capacity cost × time spent by each resource = cost of resources

In order to determine costs, D.B. works with the financial manager for basic salary and benefit information for the members of her team (Table 15.3).

Materials are estimated at $500, projecting the total cost for the launch of the Health Literacy initiative to be $3,937.98. Determining total capacity, in this example, requires calculating the total amount of administrative time available. Capacity is more pertinent when calculating costs for clinical examples. Because a small amount of administrative time is projected, the projected cost is appropriate for this example.

(*continued*)

Case Study (*continued*)

TABLE 15.3 HEALTH LITERACY PROJECT BUDGET – 3 MONTH PROJECT

Health Literacy Project Budget

Personnel	Annual Salary	Benefits	Compensation	Meetings	Needs Assessment	Planning	Training	Track Progress	Grand Total
		25%		4 hours/ month x 3 months	4 hours team/1 staff	4 hours	1 hour	6 hours/ year	
D.B.	$60,000	$15,000	$75,000	$432.69	$150	$150		$225	
NP	$90,000	$22,500	$112,500	$649.04	$225	$225			
MA	$35,000	$8,750	$43,750	$252.40	$87.50	$87.50			
Receptionist	$37,500	$7,500	$37,500	$216.35	$75	$75			
Patient									
All staff	$470,000	$117,500	$587,500		$293.75		$293.75	$335	
Totals				1,550.48	$831.25	$537.50	$293.75		$3,437.98

MA, medical assistant; NP, nurse practitioner.

(continued)

Case Study (*continued*)

QUESTIONS

1. In selecting the task force, D.B. selected a nurse practitioner, medical assistant, receptionist, and patient. Is anyone missing?
2. What tools are available to describe the process of care?
3. D.B. identified staff time, training, and materials as the key costs. Are there others?

REFERENCES

Agency for Healthcare Research and Quality. (2015). *Health Literacy Universal Precautions Toolkit* (2nd ed.). Rockville, MD: Author. Retrieved from http://www.ahrq.gov/professionals/quality-patient-safety/quality-resources/tools/literacy-toolkit/healthlittoolkit2.html

American Association of Colleges of Nursing. (2006). The essentials of doctoral education for advanced nursing practice. Retrieved from http://www.aacnnursing.org/Portals/42/Publications/DNPEssentials.pdf

Bodenheimer, T., & Sinsky, C. (2014). From Triple to Quadruple Aim: Care of the patient requires care of the provider. *Annals of Family Medicine, 12*(6), 573–576. doi:10.1370/afm.1713

Feeley, D. (2017, November 28). The Triple Aim or the Quadruple Am? Four points to help set your strategy. Retrieved from http://www.ihi.org/communities/blogs/the-triple-aim-or-the-quadruple-aim-four-points-to-help-set-your-strategy

Goodman, C. S. (2014). *HTA101: Introduction to health technology assessment: V. Economic analysis methods*. Bethesda, MD: National Library of Medicine (US); Retrieved from https://www.nlm.nih.gov/nichsr/hta101/ta10107.html

Kaplan, R., & Norton, D. (2001). *The strategy-focused organization: How balanced scorecard companies thrive in the new business environment*. Brighton, MA: Harvard Business School Press.

Kaplan, R. S., Witkowski, M., Abbott, M., Guzman, A. B., Higgins, L. D., Meara, J. G., . . . Feeley, T. W. L. (2014). Using time-driven activity-based costing to identify value improvement opportunities in healthcare. *Journal of Healthcare Management, 59*(6), 399–412. doi:10.1097/00115514-201411000-00005

Keel, G., Savage, C., Rafiq, M., & Mazzocato, P. (2017). Time-driven activity-based costing in health care: A systematic review of the literature. *Health Policy, 121*(7), 755–763. doi:10.1016/j.healthpol.2017.04.013

Porter, M., & Kaplan, R. (2016). How to pay for health care. *Harvard Business Review, 94*(7–8), 88–100.

Stiefel, M., & Nolan K. (2012). *A guide to measuring the Triple Aim: Population health, experience of care, and per capita cost*. IHI Innovation Series white paper. Cambridge, MA: Institute for Healthcare Improvement. Retrieved from http://www.ihi.org/resources/Pages/IHIWhitePapers/AGuidetoMeasuringTripleAim.aspx

THE DNP PROJECT DELIVERABLES: SUSTAINABILITY AND SPREAD

NOREEN HEER NICOL | SHARON SABLES-BAUS

This chapter addresses the following American Association of Colleges of Nursing (AACN) DNP Essentials:

Essential II: Organizational and Systems Leadership for Quality Improvement and Systems Thinking

Essential III: Clinical Scholarship and Analytical Methods for Evidence-Based Practice

Essential IV: Information Systems/Technology and Patient Care Technology for the Improvement and Transformation of Healthcare

Essential V: Healthcare Policy for Advocacy in Healthcare

Essential VI: Interprofessional Collaboration for Improving Patient and Population Health Outcomes

INTRODUCTION

The focus of this chapter is the sustainability and spread of evidenced-based projects within healthcare organizations. For sustainability and spread to occur, the choice and timing of the project must be weighed against the criteria of value to the organization, alignment with organizational goals, and compatibility with other ongoing evidence-based initiatives, such as nurse residency programs.

An evidenced-based project, including those led by a DNP-prepared nurse or DNP student, must integrate several components together with "a plan for sustainability," as outlined by the AACN DNP Essentials (AACN, 2004). Sustaining and spreading desired practices are fundamental prerequisites for the delivery of high-quality care in the appropriate healthcare arenas. A project will be most successful in sustaining change when it aligns with the unit or organization's mission, vision, and values. Knowledge alone does not translate into behavior, and dissemination of evidence alone does not lead to spread of consistent, sustained practice. The DNP professional must ensure that (a) the new project proposal aligns closely with the organization's philosophy and mission and (b) there are resources to promote sustainability and spread. For the project to be significant, the DNP professional must assess the workplace capacity to engage in, sustain, and/or spread the project.

QUALITY HEALTHCARE

Healthcare has no shortage of evidence-based practice (EBP) innovations; however, bridging the gap and then sustaining/spreading the fix has become a priority for the nation's top healthcare service organizations over the past two decades. Research supports the link between implementation of EBP and the provision of high-quality, safe, and cost-effective care, but because tremendous variability in EBP implementation persists throughout the United States, there remain concomitant gaps in healthcare quality (Berwick, 2003; National Academies of Sciences, Engineering, and Medicine [NASEM], 2018).

The DNP professional is familiar with the fundamental documents that have influenced EBP and quality-related work across healthcare service organizations over the past two decades. The Institute of Medicine (IOM) has produced two landmark reports on quality and safety in healthcare. *To Err Is Human* (Institute of Medicine [IOM], 2000) broke the silence surrounding healthcare errors and their consequences. The report found that adverse events in healthcare are the product not of flawed people but rather of flawed systems that need improvement. The second report, *Crossing the Quality Chasm: A New Health System for the 21st Century* (IOM, 2001a), called for a quality-driven redesign of the American healthcare system, informed by overarching principles. The 2001 report provided (a) a set of performance expectations for the 21st-century healthcare system, (b) a set of 10 new rules to guide patient–clinician relationships, (c) a suggested organizing framework to better align incentives inherent in payment and accountability with improvement in quality, and (d) key steps to promote EBP and strengthen clinical information systems. As a result of this work, six urgently needed "aims for improvement" in healthcare in America were identified: safety, effectiveness, patient-centeredness, timeliness, efficiency, and equity (IOM, 2001a).

A third report, *Envisioning the National Health Care Quality Report* (IOM, 2001b), was done at the request of the Agency for Healthcare Research and

Quality (AHRQ). This mandated report by Congress provides an assessment of the quality of the healthcare delivery in the United States. The latest addition to the quality-related corpus as generated by the U.S. government is *Crossing the Global Quality Chasm: Improving Health Care Worldwide* (NASEM, 2018). The authors of this study explore the global impacts of poor-quality healthcare; they recommend ways to improve quality while expanding universal health coverage, particularly in low-resource areas. Together, the four reports comprise a framework for U.S.-based/worldwide quality- and safety-related work in healthcare, including building knowledge on sustainability and spread of EBP.

There is a great effort needed to inform key stakeholders about the innovations and discovery in healthcare that are worthy of implementation (Long, 2003). These stakeholders are found within healthcare environments and include patients and families, frontline staff, entire healthcare teams, unit managers, department directors, executive groups of healthcare service organizations, insurance partners, policy makers, and researchers. Nurses influence all of these key stakeholder groups and are positioned to take on this role. Leaders of organizations and healthcare systems can embrace DNP graduates as professionals who are able to inform consumers of worthy evidenced-based care innovations (AACN, 2006) and possess abilities and knowledge of strategies that maintain an EBP culture (Melnyk, Gallagher-Ford, Long, & Fineout-Overholt, 2014).

SUSTAINABILITY AND SPREAD THROUGHOUT THE SERVICE ORGANIZATION

Despite years of work related to dissemination and implementation of evidence-based recommendations across many environments and industries (including healthcare), significant challenges critical to sustainability and spread remain (Berwick, 1991, 2003). The exemplary work of the Institute for Healthcare Improvement (IHI) promulgates EBP strategies for implementing and sustaining exemplary healthcare initiatives. Five organizational factors are widely acknowledged as vital to patient quality and safety: (a) medical education reform, (b) care integration, (c) restoring joy and meaning in work and ensuring the safety of the healthcare workforce, (d) patient/consumer engagement in healthcare, and (e) transparency across the continuum of care (Leape et al., 2009). The National Patient Safety Foundation's Lucian Leape Institute (LLI) convened expert roundtables to address each of the five factors so as to examine obstacles to implementation, to assess potential for improvement, to identify potential implementation partners, and to issue recommendations for action. Reports of the recommendations from these roundtables were published between 2010 and 2015. Current members of the LLI (now based at the

Institute for Healthcare Improvement) assessed progress made since 2009 and identified ongoing challenges. The IHI states that

> For more than 25 years, we have partnered with a growing community of visionaries, leaders, and frontline practitioners around the globe to spark bold, inventive ways to improve the health of individuals and populations. Together, we build the will for change, seek out innovative models of care, and spread proven best practices. To advance our mission, IHI is dedicated to optimizing health care delivery systems, driving the Triple Aim for populations, realizing person- and family-centered care, and building improvement capability. The IHI has developed IHI's white papers as one means for advancing our mission. The ideas and findings in these white papers represent innovative work by IHI and organizations with whom we collaborate. The white papers are designed to share the problems IHI is working to address, the ideas we are developing and testing to help organizations make breakthrough improvements, and early results where they exist. (Scoville, Little, Rakover, Luther, & Mate, 2016, p. 2)

The IHI commissioned a white paper by Dr. Juran titled "Sustaining Improvement," which presents a framework that healthcare organizations can use to sustain improvements in the safety, effectiveness, and efficiency of patient care. The paper is grounded in the Juran Trilogy, which espouses the importance of seeking out the voice of the customer; determining what to measure and deciding upon performance goals; and then refining, reinventing, or repairing what is not working. This trilogy improvement cycle is presented as (a) quality planning, (b) quality control, and (c) quality improvement (QI). Dr. Juran is frequently cited in literature on Total Quality Management (TQM) as well as in Lean Six Sigma trainings and certification courses (Juran & Godfrey, 1999; Scoville & Little, 2014; Scoville et al., 2016). In addition, the white paper he authored references current literature that healthcare organizations can use to sustain evidence-based improvements in the safety, effectiveness, and efficiency of patient care.

An example project from the IHI with substantial resources dedicated to aligning sustainability and spread within healthcare service organizations is the 5 Million Lives Campaign (IHI, 2008. The 5 Million Lives Campaign was developed to support improvement of medical care in the United States, significantly reducing levels of morbidity (illness or medical harm such as adverse drug events or surgical complications) and mortality. IHI quantified this aim and set a numeric goal: They asked hospitals participating in the campaign to prevent five million incidents of medical harm over the 2-year period from December 12, 2006 through December 9, 2008. The how-to guides associated with this campaign remain timely, informative resources for all professionals committed to sustaining and spreading quality initiatives. The following definitions of sustainability and spread from the 5 Million Lives Campaign are straightforward: *sustainability* entails locking in the progress or holding the gains that hospitals (or any service organization) have made already and continually building on them; *spread* entails active dissemination of best practices and knowledge about every intervention and implementing each intervention in every available care setting to which it is appropriate.

Multiple initiatives focused on achievement of sustainability in the healthcare environment exist, yet the definitions of sustainability and spread are not universally agreed upon. An organizing principle that can be considered speaks to sustainable development occurring over interconnected environmental, economic, and social domains, allowing for change that meets the needs of the present without compromising the ability to meet the needs of the future. The one constant measure is that organizational commitment is necessary for project sustainability and spread to occur. DNP graduates proficient in QI and program evaluation methodologies appreciate that creating, sustaining, and spreading change at the organizational and policy levels is complex. Changes in organizational arrangements, organizational and professional cultures, and financial structures that support practice may need to be evaluated and or enhanced in order to provide the structure necessary to support EBP projects.

The eight DNP Essentials (AACN, 2006) ensure graduates have the knowledge and skill set to incorporate approaches that influence project sustainability and spread within/among healthcare service organizations (AACN, 2006). To be specific, DNP professional graduates, having met Essential II in their school programs (a) have the ability to evaluate the cost-effectiveness of care and (b) use principles of economics and finance to redesign effective and realistic care delivery strategies. In addition, DNP graduates are knowledgeable in methods of organizing care so that emerging practice problems and the ethical dilemmas derived from evolving diagnostic and therapeutic technologies are recognized and acted on, thereby ensuring the sustainability and spread of evidence.

KEY COMPONENTS OF SUSTAINABILITY

A national initiative led by IHI, the 5 Million Lives Campaign, shares six key components of sustainability, or ways of holding the gains (www.ihi.org/IHI/Programs/Campaign) that can be utilized by a DNP graduate leading an evidence-based project. They are: (a) supportive management structure; (b) structures to "foolproof" change; (c) robust, transparent feedback systems; (d) shared sense of the systems to be improved; (e) culture of improvement and a deeply engaged staff; and (f) formal capacity-building programs (IHI, 2008).

Supportive Management Structure

When choosing a project, recognize that a supportive management structure at every level of the organization is the one of the most important properties of sustainability; it is fundamental to achieving all of the other five key organizational components for sustaining improvements. Everyone in the healthcare organization needs to be on board and supportive of the project, including the people in the boardroom and the C-suite as well as physicians, nursing staff, and all healthcare service teams. Everyone needs to view the desired change as important.

Not all healthcare organizations prioritize quality and safety. A 2016 descriptive study of 276 chief nursing executives (CNEs) showed that although CNEs believe that EBP results in high-quality care, it is ranked as a low priority with little budget allocation (Melnyk et al., 2016). The National Database of Nursing Quality Indicators™ (NDNQI®) is the only national nursing database that provides quarterly and annual reporting of structure, process, and outcome indicators to evaluate nursing care at the unit level. It has been described in one cross-sectional descriptive study that was published in 2018 that more than one-third of the hospitals are not meeting NDNQI performance metrics, and nearly one-third of the hospitals fail to meet national core-measures benchmarks (e.g., falls and pressure ulcers) (Melnyk et al., 2016). Due to these concerning results, a DNP-led project that aligns with improving NDNQI performance is typically met with enthusiasm.

Diffusion of Innovation (DOI) theory, developed by E. M. Rogers in 1962, explains how, over time, an idea or product gains momentum and diffuses (or spreads) through a specific population or social system. The end result of this diffusion is that people, as part of a social system, adopt a new idea, behavior, or product (Rogers, 2004). In a special communication published in the *Journal of the American Medical Association* in 2003, Dr. Berwick suggests three clusters of influence on the rate of diffusion of innovations within an organization: the perceptions of the innovation, the characteristics of the individuals who may adopt the change, and contextual and managerial factors within the organization (Berwick, 2003). He also detailed three potential rate-limiters for intraorganization innovation diffusion: (a) the perceptions of the innovation, (b) the characteristics of the individuals who may adopt the change, and (c) contextual and managerial factors within the organization. In addition, Berwick made seven recommendations to accelerate the rate of diffusion of innovations within an organization: (a) find sound innovations, (b) find and support "innovators," (c) invest in "early adopters," (d) made early adopter activity observable, (e) trust and enable reinvention, (f) create slack for change, and (g) lead by example (Berwick, 2003). He posits that successful diffusion depends on how an organization sees its innovators, early adopters, and the interface between the early adopters and the early majority. Knowing that a supportive management structure is necessary for the sustainability and spread of worthy evidence is knowledge that cannot be overlooked by the DNP clinician when beginning a project.

Structures to "Foolproof" Change

Designing an organizational structure that supports innovative teams can have a big influence on the sustainability and spread of evidenced-based projects. Having a trained quality- or process- improvement professional on the project team can provide the support and experience to allow for success. Engaging the electronic medical health record experts on a project team can provide assistance for the development of new processes for charting, placing orders or evidence-based guidelines. For service organizations using electronic medical records or electronic reporting activities, innovations need to be worked into information technology systems as early as possible to avoid duplication and potential resistance to process. Care team members can become very dissatisfied if they are asked to do things twice, such as record data or responses in multiple places in the electronic health record. Likewise, when trying a new supply or device, the item needs to be available to the user at the same time as any normal supply or device would be obtained. For example, if a new care item is being tested in an area that receives supplies in a "kit," the kit needs to have all required items to complete the process. Patient and family members serve as invaluable members of the project team, sharing what matters most: how the care provided affects them personally. Even if the organizational structure is not such that this work is easily promoted, the DNP clinician can compensate by putting together intraprofessional project teams.

Robust, Transparent Feedback Systems

Transparency to all stakeholders is key to sustainability and spread. A successful project will have a formal measurement system that provides data and compares results, either to internal targets or national standards. Stakeholders must be able to easily access and track process indicators (e.g., through screensaver slide shows, bulletin boards, emails, printed scorecards for patients/families, and/or internal and external web presence). Channels must be opened for blame-free inquiry with predictable follow-up and results; this will enable staff to gain trust in the management system. The DNP graduate is skilled in process mapping, as well as putting data into run and control charts to keep the organization informed of project progress.

Shared Sense of the Systems to Be Improved

All stakeholders must (a) share an understanding of the processes and systems that they are seeking to improve and (b) be clear about their unique roles in pursuing the sought-after improvements. Clearly articulated community goals create a galvanizing community purpose. Capturing incremental progress and providing tools that map the entire process will also allow for group celebration and heighten the sense of meaningful productivity. The map and measurement tools need to be clear and available for reference and evaluation. A DNP professional can use many tools for developing a shared sense of the system or process to be improved such as driver diagrams, process-mapping tools, or flow charting. Begin the project's goal-setting process by seeking to understand the overarching strategic goals. An aim statement with measurable and time-sensitive goals provides the template for the improvement initiative.

Culture of Improvement and a Deeply Engaged Staff

Healthcare has joined many other industries (e.g., the military and the airline industry) in committing to the value of teamwork (Salas, Sims, & Burke, 2005). Contributions of highly skilled and knowledgeable individuals from multiple professions are required to succeed in today's complex, multitiered healthcare environment. In order to accomplish the IOM mandate for safe, timely, effective, efficient, equitable, and patient-centered care in a complex environment, healthcare professionals must function in highly collaborative teams. DNP professionals are well positioned to lead such teams due to their advanced preparation in the interprofessional dimension of healthcare as well as practicum experiences facilitating collaborative teams (AACN, 2004; Greiner & Knebel, 2003). Team structure, function, and communication play an important role in supporting patient and clinician productivity and safety. The operating room (OR) was one of the first arenas to embrace broadly the concept of team process, and while team training has been shown to improve OR performance, continued team training is required to sustain improvement in OR culture (Forse, Bramble, & McQuillan, 2011).

In committed environments, everyone can articulate the organization's major QI activities, explain his or her individual roles, and feel invested in outcomes. All staff view quality and safety work as part of their career and daily commitments. The staff believe that they have a stake in continually enhancing performance in any given intervention area. The organization shares a sense of pride about performance and improvement skill, and many stakeholders enjoy their work in these areas. Individual job descriptions and performance evaluations can be created to include attention to QI, process improvement, program evaluation, and other EBP skills. As more and more DNP-educated nurses join the workforce, the culture of improvement should also improve and the number of deeply engaged staff should increase.

Formal Capacity-Building Programs

The sustainability-seeking organization makes training of executives, managers, and staff a high priority, building skill in appropriate fiscal or clinical disciplines. Hiring, training, mentoring, or succession planning with quality skills in mind builds strength and continuity.

The DNP professional can ensure successful diffusion of innovations by being mindful of the three clusters of influence, especially seeking feedback about how early innovations were viewed, as well as being an expert communicator about the innovation. Organizations that value quality have in place (a) clear accountability systems for tracking and openly reporting performance of care outcomes, (b) local champions who are supported by senior-level staff, and (c) boards and executives who both celebrate success and support needed improvements. These organizations will typically have mechanisms for open and frequent communication about the diffusion. Moreover, organizations across the country have begun to motivate staff/teams through bonuses and incentives (e.g., offering bonuses for teams that meet and exceed quality thresholds and targets).

SPREADING CAMPAIGN INTERVENTIONS TO ALL LOCATIONS

In healthcare, it is vitally important that participating service organizations plan to sustain and spread improvements to which they are committed. When priorities shift, it seems that hard-won improvements are lost and staff revert to the "way we have always done it" or worse yet to the "way we want to do it because we can." Overall, the goal with spread is to ensure that the change reaches every part of the organization. Developing a plan for spread involves the following three steps (IHI, 2008): (a) laying a foundation for spread (i.e., sending a clear message, designating an executive sponsor, appointing a day-to-day leader, establishing a spread team, sharing results of successful pilots), (b) developing an initial plan for spread (i.e., establishing an aim, utilizing existing organizational structure, developing a communication plan, building/supporting a measurement system), and (c) refining the plan.

The need to gain a greater understanding of the factors that influence long-term sustainment and spread of QI initiatives continues. The goal is to promote organizational ability to sustain worthy EBPs over time, help improve future interventions, and increase the value of these project investments. A recent qualitative study in addiction facilities isolated four important themes related to long-term sustainment of QI practices consistent with broader discussions of sustainability and spread (Stumbo, Ford, & Green, 2017). The four themes that lead to sustainability were as follows: (a) finding alignment between business- and client-centered practices, (b) engaging staff early in QI process, (c) integrating data into monitoring practices and identifying a data champion, and (d) devoting adequate organizational human resources to sustainment. In addition, the study authors found (consistent with other literature) four corollary factors among agencies that did not sustain practices: (a) lack of evidence of impact on business practices led to discontinuation, (b) disengaged staff and lack of organizational capacity during the implementation period led to lack of sustainment, (c) no data integration into overall business practices and no identified data champion, and (d) high staff turnover (Stumbo et al., 2017).

Another large mixed-methods study (Cranley et al., 2018) showed QI-project sustainability requires ongoing staff and leadership engagement. The study emphasized the need for (a) strategies to support QI-project leaders (e.g., opportunities for leadership coaching), (b) education and coaching for involved staff, (c) dedicated time for QI activities, and (d) acknowledgment/celebration of small wins to increase visibility of the work and foster an ongoing commitment to sustaining improvements (Cranley et al., 2018). Both of these studies lend support to the tenets positioned in this chapter.

Planning for spread begins with the choice of a worthy, evidenced-based project, and this choice must be evaluated and reevaluated constantly (Massoud et al., 2006; Melnyk et al., 2018). The scope and reach of spread are based on the aims and goals of the initial project. The initial plan should set the groundwork for reaching all the appropriate units or departments with all the project interventions. After successful implementation of a change for a pilot population or an entire unit, the team can spread the changes to other parts of the organization or to other organizations. During the pilot, the hope is that great strides in testing and implementing can point to specific recommendations for unique departments or units. All stakeholders must engage to fully implement a spread plan. Further research is needed into the factors that may facilitate sustainability and spread beyond the initial microsystem into which the intervention was introduced.

Improvement teams often take missteps when it comes to successfully sharing and spreading improvement ideas in their organizations (Figure 16.1; Haraden & Resar, 2017). IHI faculty Carol Haraden and Roger Resar developed the "Seven Spreadly Sins" to give teams practical tips for overcoming challenges that impede spread. It identifies the "sin" and then provides the quick "practical tips for successful sharing." These practical measures can help further shape project plans.

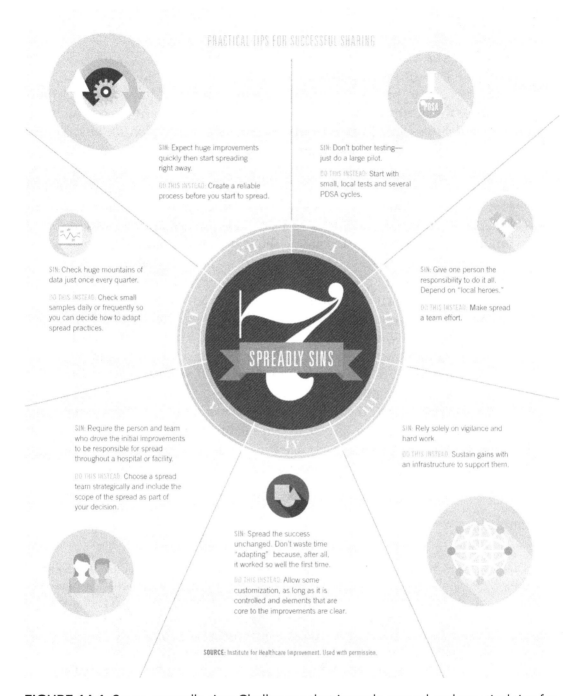

PRACTICAL TIPS FOR SUCCESSFUL SHARING

SIN: Expect huge improvements quickly then start spreading right away.

DO THIS INSTEAD: Create a reliable process before you start to spread.

SIN: Don't bother testing— just do a large pilot.

DO THIS INSTEAD: Start with small, local tests and several PDSA cycles.

SIN: Check huge mountains of data just once every quarter.

DO THIS INSTEAD: Check small samples daily or frequently so you can decide how to adapt spread practices.

SIN: Give one person the responsibility to do it all. Depend on "local heroes."

DO THIS INSTEAD: Make spread a team effort.

SIN: Require the person and team who drove the initial improvements to be responsible for spread throughout a hospital or facility.

DO THIS INSTEAD: Choose a spread team strategically and include the scope of the spread as part of your decision.

SIN: Rely solely on vigilance and hard work

DO THIS INSTEAD: Sustain gains with an infrastructure to support them.

SIN: Spread the success unchanged. Don't waste time "adapting" because, after all, it worked so well the first time.

DO THIS INSTEAD: Allow some customization, as long as it is controlled and elements that are core to the improvements are clear.

SPREADLY SINS

SOURCE: Institute for Healthcare Improvement. Used with permission.

FIGURE 16.1 Seven spreadly sins: Challenges that impede spread and practical tips for successful sharing.

Source: From Haraden, C., & Resar, R. (2017). *Seven spreadly sins.* Retrieved from http://www.ihi.org/resources/Pages/Tools/IHISevenSpreadlySins.aspx; Reprinted from www.IHI.org with permission of the Institute for Healthcare Improvement.

CONCLUSIONS

Sustaining and spreading changes that advance the quality of healthcare is essential to improve patient, client, or population outcomes. The DNP professional can play a critical role in the success or failure of such outcomes at the healthcare organization and system levels. At the project level, the DNP professional project must include a specific plan for sustainability. A specific plan for sustainability should be a required step in all projects. Falling back on the old, easy, or preferred way is a waste of resources and is antithetical to implementing QI processes and change. At the system level, functioning of the system will either enhance or suspend quality efforts. However, individual participation in the system is essential to influence such initiatives. Changing the system is the most effective route to improvement. To be specific, the service organization that changes the way of delivering care or operating to produce improved outcomes will see more quality outcomes. These desired changes must be maintained and spread to sustain the improvements. Trying to fit an orphan project (i.e., one that does not clearly align with the institution's or leadership's target interests) into an organization lends itself to unsustainability and lack of spread.

Future healthcare will be well served as DNP professionals embrace the concept of becoming the expert within the organization to ensure spread and sustainability of desired outcomes. As such, the DNP professional will always be seated at any healthcare leadership table to (a) ensure that every approved care strategy is used and evaluated, (b) sustain and spread desired outcomes, and (c) improve patient care quality and safety.

Case Study

A DNP-prepared nurse works in a large inner-city hospital. The hospital has been supportive of implementing evidence-based projects and has put systems into place that support such initiatives. It has been noted that the length of stay for inpatients with a diagnosis of dysphagia is longer than in comparison hospitals. This nurse, P.G., is asked to introduce a nationally recognized, interdisciplinary dysphagia competency framework to guide care for these patients with the outcome measure of decreasing the length of stay. P.G. is able to lead a translation project promoting dysphagia as vital for patient safety.

QUESTIONS

1. How will the organization share progress on the dysphagia project?
2. How should P.G. begin this project? What are the initial steps to ensure sustainability and spread?
3. How would P.G. develop a shared sense of the need for such a project?

REFERENCES

American Association of Colleges of Nursing. (2004). AACN position statement on the practice doctorate in nursing. Retrieved from https://www.aacnnursing.org/News-Information/Position-Statements-White-Papers/Practice-Doctorate

American Association of Colleges of Nursing. (2006). AACN position statement on the essentials of doctoral education for advanced nursing practice. Retrieved from https://www.aacnnursing.org/Portals/42/Publications/DNPEssentials.pdf

Berwick, D. M. (1991). Controlling variation in health care: A consultation from Walter Shewhart. *Medical Care, 29*(12), 1212–1225. doi:10.1097/00005650-199112000-00004

Berwick, D. M. (2003). Disseminating innovations in health care. *Journal of the American Medical Association,, 289*(15), 1969–1975. doi:10.1001/jama.289.15.1969

Cranley, L. A., Hoben, M., Yeung, J., Estabrooks, C. A., Norton, P. G., & Wagg, A. (2018). Scopeout: Sustainability and spread of quality improvement activities in long-term care—a mixed methods approach. *BMC Health Services Research, 18*(1), 1–10. doi:10.1186/s12913-018-2978-0

Forse, R. A., Bramble, J. D., & McQuillan, R. (2011). Team training can improve operating room performance. *Surgery, 150*(4), 771–778. doi:10.1016/j.surg.2011.07.076

Greiner, A. C., & Knebel, E. (Eds.). (2003). *Health professions education: A bridge to quality*. Washington, DC: National Academies Press.

Hammer, M. (2002). Process management and the future of Six Sigma. *MIT Sloan Management Review, 43*(2), 26–32. doi:10.1109/emr.2002.1167284

Haraden, C., & Resar, R. (2017). *Seven spreadly sins: IHI tool*. Retrieved from http://www.ihi.org/resources/Pages/Tools/IHISevenSpreadlySins.aspx

Institute for Healthcare Improvement. (2008). 5 Million lives campaign. getting started kit: Rapid response teams. Retrieved from http://www.ihi.org/engage/initiatives/completed/5MillionLivesCampaign/Pages/default

Institute for Healthcare Improvement. (2017). *IHI seven spreadly sins*. Retrieved from http://www.ihi.org/resources/Pages/Tools/IHISevenSpreadlySins.aspx

Institute of Medicine. (2000). *To err is human: Building a safer health system*. Washington, DC: National Academies Press.

Institute of Medicine. (2001a). *Crossing the quality chasm: A new health system for the 21st century*. Washington, DC: National Academies Press.

Institute of Medicine. (2001b). *Envisioning the national health care quality report*. Washington, DC: National Academies Press.

Juran, J. M., & Godfrey, A. B. (1999). *Juran's quality handbook* (5th ed.). New York, NY: McGraw-Hill.

Leape, L., Berwick, D., Clancy, C., Conway, J., Gluck, P., Guest, J., . . . Isaac, T. (2009). Transforming healthcare: A safety imperative. *Quality and Safe Health Care, 18*(6), 424–428. doi:10.1136/qshc.2009.036954

Long, K. A. (2003). The Institute of Medicine Report: Health professions education: A bridge to quality. *Policy, Politics, & Nursing Practice, 4*(4), 259–262. doi:10.1177/1527154403258304

Massoud, M. R., Nielsen, G. A., Nolan, K., Nolan, T., Schall, M. W., & Sevin, C. A. (2006). *A framework for spread: from local improvements to system-wide change*. Cambridge, MA: Institute for Healthcare Improvement.

Melnyk, B. M., Gallagher-Ford, L., Long, L. E., & Fineout-Overholt, E. (2014). The establishment of evidence-based practice competencies for practicing registered nurses and advanced practice nurses in real-world clinical settings: Proficiencies to improve healthcare quality, reliability, patient outcomes, and costs. *Worldviews Evidence Based Nursing, 11*(1), 5–15. doi:10.1111/wvn.12021

Melnyk, B. M., Gallagher-Ford, L., Thomas, B. K., Troseth, M., Wyngarden, K., & Szalacha, L. A. (2016). Study of chief nurse executives indicates low prioritization of evidence-based practice and shortcomings in hospital performance metrics across the United States. *Worldviews Evidence Based Nursing, 13*(1), 6–14. doi:10.1111/wvn.12133

Melnyk, B. M., Gallagher-Ford, L., Zellefrow, C., Tucker, S., Thomas, B., Sinnott, L. T., & Tan, A. (2018). The first US study on nurses' evidence-based practice competencies indicates major deficits that threaten healthcare quality, safety, and patient outcomes. *Worldviews Evidence Based Nursing, 15*(1), 16–25. doi:10.1111/wvn.12269

National Academies of Sciences, Engineering, and Medicine. (2018). *Crossing the global quality chasm: Improving health care worldwide*. Washington, DC: National Academies Press.

Rogers, E. M. (2004). A prospective and retrospective look at the diffusion model. *Journal of Health Communication, 9*(Suppl 1), 13–19. doi:10.1080/10810730490271449

Salas, E., Sims, D. E., & Burke, C. S. (2005). Is there a "big five" in teamwork? *Small Group Research, 36*(5), 555–599. doi:10.1177/1046496405277134

Scoville, R., & Little, K. (2014). *Comparing lean and quality improvement: IHI white paper*. Cambridge, MA: IHI.

Scoville, R., Little, K., Rakover, J., Luther, K., & Mate, K. (2016). *Sustaining improvement: IHI white paper*. Cambridge, MA: IHI.

Stumbo, S. P., Ford, J. H., & Green, C. A. (2017). Factors influencing quality improvements made in addiction treatment facilities: A qualitative study. *Addiction Science and Clinical Practice, 12*(1), 26. doi:10.1186/s13722-017-0093-x

ANSWERS TO CASE STUDY QUESTIONS

CHAPTER 2: EFFECTIVE LEADERSHIP

1. R.B. can work to develop relationships with mentors, seek feedback from her team, continue her work to finish her DNP, build networks among the hospital leaders, and work to develop broader competency in leadership. As she progresses in her personal power, her next step may include an increased emphasis on self-reflection, continuing to collaborate with wise mentors, and continuing to be part of the leadership network in the hospital.

2. R.B. can schedule a staff meeting with the neurology unit to provide face-to-face announcement of her new role as manager. She can provide a confident, poised, positive statement about assuming the manager's role. She can articulate that her role has shifted from peer to manager, so her relationship will change, and her intention is to empower the team to maintain and improve high-quality patient care. She will promote a just culture in which individuals are not blamed and everyone works to improve system issues. She will use an open-door policy so anyone can come to her and discuss issues, suggestions, and successes. She wants her team members to be prepared with solutions when they identify a problem. She will let staff know when decisions are open to input and when decisions are closed to negotiation.

3. R.B. can use structural empowerment by providing staff: (a) access to information; (b) constructive feedback and guidance; (c) adequate resources, including staffing, supplies, technology; and (d) culture of personal growth and development. For instance, R.B. will share mean absolute error (MAE) metrics with the team at each staff meeting and post the metrics on a visually appealing poster in the break room. She will share success by publicly recognizing actions leading to improvements. R.B.

can use relational empowerment by being very intentional in building relationships with her team. She can meet one on one on a regular basis with all individuals to learn their goals and aspirations, strengths, communication preferences, frustrations. She can guide team members to write development plans and review progress every 6 months.

4. An important outcome used to assess the success of R.B.'s leadership will be the number of MAEs on the unit. Assessing baseline MAE data before R.B.'s transition into the managerial role is important. Nursing satisfaction with interventions that R.B. chooses to address MAEs is also an important indicator of R.B.'s leadership success. R.B. may further assess the effectiveness of her leadership by using a safety culture assessment tool to measure safety culture on her unit. Staff satisfaction with the microsystem culture, as well as nurse turnover, may also provide some insight into the effectiveness of R.B's work as the unit's manager.

CHAPTER 3: LEADERSHIP AND SYSTEMS THINKING

1. You organize a QI team: a nurse manager, medical director, activity nurse, restorative nurse, physical therapist, and a certified nursing assistant (CNA).

   Because the CNAs provide most of the ADL care, it is important you interview them. You interview a few CNAs and learn that it is more convenient for staff to wheel residents from one place to the other than assist them with walking.

2. Over the course of a week and 21 meals, you observe how residents get to their meals, to obtain baseline data for breakfast, lunch, and dinner. You find that only an average of 3 (15%) patients is walked down to the dining area per meal.

3. Goals for your improvement project may include increasing the percentage of LTC residents who walk to each meal to exceed the 15% baseline.

4. The Fishbone diagram might be populated with data from the following items:

   People

   • The floor is sometimes understaffed

   • CNAs turnover is high

   • A third manager was hired within last 2 months and is still getting oriented

   • Family members request wheelchairs for residents to take residents to meals

Policies

- CNAs think that it is restorative staff function to provide walking activity to residents
- Two restorative nurses are in charge of the Walk to Dine program in the entire facility (230 beds)
- Family members request wheelchairs for residents to take residents to meals

Workflow

- There is no clear workflow process of walking a resident from an activity to a meal
- There is no clear process for identification of residents who want to walk to meals
- Many residents have dementia and they tell you they were assisted with walking even though you are told by staff they did not walk
- Two restorative nurses are in charge of the Walk to Dine program in the entire facility (230 beds)
- Family members request wheelchairs for residents to take residents to meals

Equipment

- There are not enough walkers for residents who can ambulate with a walker
- Family members request wheelchairs for residents to take residents to meals

Measurement

- There is no log to track who walks to meals
- No one knows which residents are able to ambulate to meals
- There is no monitoring in how the residents that ambulate to meals tolerate the ambulation

5. SMART = Specific, Measurable, Achievable, Relevant, Time bound

A smart goal for this project may be:

Within 6 months, 20% of Unit A residents who are able to ambulate to meals will participate in the Walk to Dine program five times a week.

6. Data collected may include:

- Percentage of Unit A residents who ambulate to meals five times a week
- For Unit A residents who are oriented, resident satisfaction with the Dine to Walk program
- CNA satisfaction with the Dine to Walk program

- Restorative Nurse satisfaction with the Dine to Walk program
- Resident family satisfaction with the Dine to Walk program

CHAPTER 4: QUALITY IMPROVEMENT: THE ESSENTIALS

1. J.B. will want to see what quality data is collected on catheter-associated urinary-tract infections (CAUTI) at the hospital level and at the unit level. She will want to assess how her medical/surgical unit compares to other similar units in her hospital.

2. The Centers for Disease Control and Prevention (CDC) collects hospital-acquired infection data every year. J.B. can see find out what the standardized infection ratio (SIR) is for her hospital, and compare those results to national statistics. The CDC hospital acquired infections report is availab e online (gis.cdc.gov/grasp/PSA/HAIreport.html).

3. The American Nurses Association has partnered with Agency for Healthcare Research and Quality (AHRQ) and the Centers for Medicare & Medicaid Services (CMS) to develop toolkits that are ready for practice, and that synthesize the best evidence available in preventing hospital-acquired conditions (HACs). A CAUTI Prevention Toolkit is available, with a CAUTI resource site, and abundant evidence on the background and best practices in preventing CAUTI (www.nursingworld.org/practice-policy/work-environment/health-safety/infection-prevention/ana-cauti-prevention-tool).

   Johns Hopkins also has a robust website that offers evidence-based practice for CAUTI prevention, and a compendium of strategies to prevent CAUTI. These resources can be found at: www.hopkinsmedicine.org/heic/infection_surveillance/cauti.html

4. J.B.'s CAUTI team might include:
   - Bedside RNs from her unit
   - Infectious disease nurse from the hospital
   - Providers who often admit to J.B.'s med/surg unit and order urinary catheters
   - Process improvement expert who can guide the team in establishing current state and possible foci for improvement
   - Electronic health record (EHR) expert who can identify data that are accessible in the EHR and easily mined.

5. What kind of data tools might J.B. use to analyze the cause of CAUTI on her unit and display CAUTI data over six months?
   - A flow chart will help J.B. identify the current state of placing, maintaining, and discontinuing urinary catheters on her unit. A flow

chart will also help identify whether the occurrence of CAUTI is connected to incorrect placement, inadequate maintenance, or delay in discontinuing catheterization.

- A check sheet will be helpful once J.B. establishes a standardized approach to urinary catheter care. The check sheet will not only identify the standardized processes, but can be used to track adherence.

- A cause-and-effect diagram will help J.B. and her team map all of the contributing factors to CAUTI on her unit.

- Once a standardized process has been determined for urinary catheter placement, care and discontinuance, a run chart of CAUTI rates will be helpful in reflecting the improvement or lack of improvement over time.

CHAPTER 5: LEADING PROCESS IMPROVEMENT

1. Y.H. can represent the family nurse practitioners (FNPs) in the clinic. Her team will also need to include the clinic manager, and the medical assistant or other staff who assist in clinic visits and with patients.

2. A process map of the current state would allow Y.H.'s team to assess where the delays are occurring (before the waiting room, in the waiting room, in the exam room), and what ineffective processes are contributing to the delays.

   A time–motion study of patients from their time of arrival at the clinic until their departure would provide valuable information for sources of delay or inefficiencies.

Use of the "5 Whys" would get to root causes of delay.

3. Processes that occur before the FNP visit that might be contributing to long wait times include:
- Cumbersome, ineffective previsit paperwork
- No clear communication to the clinic staff that a patient has arrived
- Appointment times that do not allow the FNP to provide adequate care or that do not reflect the full set of individuals who need time with the patient
- Poor coordination or handoffs between clinic staff and the FNP
- Inadequate clinic space
- Problems with rooming patients due to an insufficient number of scales or vital sign monitors
- Inadequate notification process for FNP that patient is in the exam room ready to be seen

4. Data could include wait times in the waiting room, wait times in exam room, patient satisfaction, FNP satisfaction, team members' satisfaction, number of patients seen/day, time spent with patients versus the time scheduled, average time FNPs and team need to stay past close of clinic to finish patient appointments.

CHAPTER 6: IMPROVEMENT, EVIDENCE-BASED PRACTICE, AND RESEARCH

1 and 2. **DNP Essentials I, II, III** are met by James in his review of the clinical problem and use of evidence to guide practice excellence. James demonstrated understanding of organizational health systems leadership, ways to obtain internal and external hospital data concerning falls, and he partnered with key stakeholders in the organization (i.e., chief quality officer, nurses, patients, etc.) to understand the clinical problem. He systematically analyzed the clinical problem to include understanding the patient's perspective, which is key to evidence-based practice (EBP) and critically reevaluated the evidence to improve practice through de-implementation and EBP implementation strategies. **DNP Essential VI** was demonstrated by James's request to develop an interprofessional team to implement a mobility protocol and to stop the practice of encouraging limited mobility in older patients.

      DNP Essential IV was not overtly discussed beyond James ensuring the electronic health reord matched the policy expectations. Competencies **V and VII** were not evident given the local, micro level of the clinical practice problem focus. And **DNP Essential VII** may be assumed in the success of James's efforts to successfully implement EBP.

3. **DNP Essential I and III** were demonstrated by James in his personal realization that the role of the DNP is to translate evidence into practice rather than conduct research. He reached out to his research professor for guidance and to collaborate on a research study should evidence to change practice remain lacking. His continued path to implement EBP would not require institutional review board (IRB) oversight, thus he would need to circle back to the leadership team to explain his decision to forgo an IRB review. Discussing the project with the providers, however, would be essential to ensure all healthcare team members understood the evidence to guide the practice change. He further used his skills to critically review and analyze the body of evidence concerning falls in older adults and discovered practice at his organization was not evidence based. This prompted him to propose de-implementation of a practice tradition that was causing patient harm and to implement an EBP practice initiative, aligning with **DNP Essentials I, II, III, and VIII**.

4. The case study lacks depth of discussion to fully evaluate practice out-comes to demonstrate **DNP Essential II and III.** However, given the sys-tematic method in which James explored finding, analyzing, and using data to address a patient outcome concern, one can assume he will use objective and subjective data to measure the practice change successes. For example, he most likely will continue to track fall rates, specifically, fall rates by age, and compare the hospital fall rates to National Database of Nursing Quality Indicators (NDNQI) benchmarks. Because he is de-implementing the practice of keeping older patients immobilized and implementing a mobility protocol, he will need to develop practice pol-icy, electronic health record interface, and audit mechanism to determine effective EBP adoption into daily practice. Last, garnering nursing prac-tice understanding of the practice change and patient perceptions though conversations will be important to garner buy in and to understand pos-sible barriers and overall satisfaction.

CHAPTER 7: LEADING WITH QUALITY METRICS

1. The two databases available at Mercy Hospital are the electronic clinical quality measures (eCQM) Feedback Report provided to Mercy Hospital, as well as the Quality Check website.

2. The eCQM pertinent to this project is the ED-1 Median Time from ED Arrival to ED Departure for Admitted ED Patients.

3. The DNP student can use minimum performance standards set by The Joint Ciommission as well as average wait times from other eCQM reporting facilities to determine a reasonable goal for Mercy Hospital emergency departmment wait times.

CHAPTER 8: LEADERSHIP AND TEAM SCIENCE

1. The team brainstormed ideas to address the issue. Three ideas were agreed upon by the team. The first suggestion was for better orienta-tion of new team members, including shadowing other team members to better understand their roles. Adding new members to a team can frequently cause disruption in usual processes. Realizing the deficits of the current orientation process shows that the team realized the impor-tance of defining clear expectations and team ground rules with new members of the team. The second suggestion was to build ongoing team training into regular meetings as well as to ask the education depart-ment to provide simulation training around interprofessional commu-nication in intensive care (see section Training to Improve Teamwork

for more details). Last, but not least, over a few weeks, the group used improvement tools to map the current process for establishing the plan of care and did several iterative PDSA (plan-do-study-act) cycles to improve the process.

2. In this situation using the check-back technique could ensure effective communication between the two providers. Check-back uses closed-loop communication to verify and confirm the information exchanged. So in this case the attending physician initiates the communication, then the advanced practice provider (APP) confirms what was communicated, and then the attending physician verifies that the communication received was correct. More dialogue can occur than just giving and receiving orders in this interaction, but using the check-back technique at the conclusion of the conversation ensures that all of the information discussed is mutually understood and agreed upon.

3. During this case study, it appears psychological safety is present in the group as the APPs had the capability to express concerns without being judged or punished. Due to this psychological freedom, discussion of the problem could be initiated. The team was able to have open dialogue to better understand each other's different perspectives of the issue and work together to address it. Without the APPs having this sense of safety and freedom to express their concerns, the issue would have never been addressed and the negative effects on the patients, team, and hospital would have continued to occur if the APPs did not feel safe enough to take the risk to address this issue.

4. Team leadership is an essential part of a highly functioning team. Leadership provides direction by clearly defining the goals and objectives for the team, communicating the expected outcomes of the team's work, and by holding others accountable for their efforts. Every team member should know his or her role on the team and actively participate in team activities. Deliberate team-building activities help team members get to know each other and begin to develop mutual respect and trust.

It is also necessary that team leadership uses role modeling and shows commitment to quality. This can inspire others within the team and help achieve buy in from all members of the team.

CHAPTER 9: LEADING PROGRAM EVALUATION

1. The choice of program evaluation will depend on many things, including the amount of time that is given to work on the project. The DNP-prepared nurse must first think about whether this is (a) a scholarly

school project that has defined time limits or (b) a project that he or she will lead in the work setting. Budget concerns and role responsibilities must be evaluated before a decision about program evaluation method can be made. What data can be obtained to evaluate the length of stay? Once permission is obtained to conduct the evaluation, any of the evaluation types can be utilized to get to the outcome defined. It is important to begin early to seek, review, and evaluate the evidence and develop the program theory.

2. There are many departments within a hospital system that can be involved in this program evaluation, including maternal outpatient methadone treatment clinics. A choice of what part of the system can be impacted by the evaluation must be made with input from the interdisciplinary team with a focus on budget, time, and span-of-control. For example, there may be multiple obstetric clinics that see pregnant women; will this evaluation focus on just one clinic or multiple clinics? Does the DNP leader have authority to change practice or implement evidence-based guidelines in all of these areas? Often, a program evaluation can begin with one obstetric clinic and then expand after changes are implemented and evaluated in that one clinic. This might be done as a formative evaluation.

3. The actual problem should be defined by those involved in the program evaluation, including the mothers who either will give birth or have given birth to a baby exposed to substances while in utero. Will the evaluation attempt to decrease length of stay for the exposed newborn? Will the project attempt to get more mothers treated in a methadone clinic while pregnant, thereby limiting infant symptoms of withdrawal? A driver diagram would be a beneficial tool. A driver diagram is a visual display of the team's theory of what "drives," or contributes, to the project aim. Key drivers may include nonpharmacological interventions, simplified assessment of infants, decreased use of morphine, and enhanced communication among units.

4. Begin with the outcome of the project, and work backward, identifying all of the processes that are in effect from when the mother enters the healthcare system (e.g., timing of screening for substance use, sharing of treatment options for substance use, timing of information on neonatal abstinence symptoms, plans to room-in). Map each part of a process, crossing units, inpatient and outpatient, as well as lines of authority. A process map would be a beneficial tool to use. Identify leaders of each process. The DNP scholar will coordinate the entire evaluation.

5. Once a change is decided on, the DNP project leader must decide on a change theory to implement the change. For example, the neonatal intensive care unit nurse can be asked to stop using NAS scoring to score

withdrawal behavior and instead implement a functional assessment. How will this change happen? Lewin's Change Model will frame the change and help identify the need for change, educational strategies, and measurement of success.

CHAPTER 10: IMPROVEMENT AND BIG DATA

1. A project this complex, using big-data techniques, can pose multiple challenges to the local team and project collaborators. First, it may be difficult to know and understand all of the idiosyncrasies of the data and linkages prior to data extraction. Electronic health record (EHR) and other data systems are designed for a specific purpose: to support patient care and the overall operation of the clinical enterprise. Using these data for other purposes can be challenging and time-consuming. Data for this evaluation must come from multiple sources, including the pharmacy database, bar code medication administration (BCMA), and human resources systems data.

2. With very large data, it may be difficult to find errors. Validation of the final extracted dataset will require sustained effort to ensure that the final file supports the planned analysis. Without rigorous, meticulous processes for cleaning and transforming data, the analysis could be corrupted or biased, leading to erroneous interpretations and conclusions.

3. The number of resources needed to extract and analyze large datasets should be considered. Even simple construction of tables and figures can be very time-consuming without the necessary computational resources. Big-data projects and analyses—especially when multiple, diverse datasets can be linked—have enormous potential value. These projects can provide new insights, methods, and results that to date have not been possible. The DNP-prepared nurse provides a bridge between and among researchers, clinicians, information technology personnel, and healthcare leaders. The DNP-prepared nurse plays a pivotal role in facilitating analysis of big data and interpreting results within a clinical and leadership context. As a result, the DNP-prepared nurse can promote actionable strategies, interventions, and practices that can enhance and improve healthcare.

CHAPTER 11: VALUE-BASED PAYMENT MODELS IN HEALTHCARE

1. The certified nurse midwives (CNMs) at ABC Clinic appreciate the flexibility the bundled payment model provides them in providing patient-centered care. Without rigid care parameters, providers at ABC Clinic have been able to adjust their care, based on patient preferences and

needs. This flexibility in care has contributed to the clinic's strong reputation in the community for providing effective patient-centered care.

2. Challenging aspects of the bundled payment model include the limited
value of bundled payments for maternity care because of the perception that the reimbursement amount is not adequate. Limits of the bundled payment model include the CNMs wanting their integrated care
reflected in the performance measures used within their payer contracts.
CNMs believe that they help their patients and families thrive, not just
avoid harm, and many aspects of their integrated care are not included
in the performance measures.

3. If ABC clinic wants to expand its practice to include Women's Health
Nurse Practitioners (WHNP) to offer primary care to women of all ages,
the practice would need to explore expanded episode definitions, episode
timing, patient population, patient engagement, and quality metrics.

4. ABC Clinic would need to expand its quality metrics to include quality metrics specific to primary care. Primary care value is being guided
by patient-centered medical home (PCMH) elements. Thus, instead of
episodic care, ABC clinic would need to shift its care model to where
patients received more continuous care, instead of episodic care focused
on reproductive care needs.

CHAPTER 12: THE DNP PROJECT—THE ESSENTIALS

1. **A.D. partially meets DNP Essential I.** A.D. initially identified a gap in
practice using scientific evidence: New evidence-based practice (EBP)
protocols and bundles were not being used on patients with central
venous catheters (CVCs). A lack of using EBP protocols and bundles
for patients with CVCs could be a contributing factor to the increase in
hospital readmissions for central line-associated bloodstream infections
(CLABSI). Although A.D. used scientific concepts as the underpinnings
of her project, she failed to correctly incorporate the scientific concepts
into the outcome measure. Subsequently, her project centered on hand
hygiene versus a gap in practice related to CLABSI protocols and bundles. A.D.'s project should have centered on the implementation and
evaluation of new EBP CLABSI protocols and bundles, and thus her outcome measure should have been decreasing CLABSI in patients with a
CVC on the oncology unit.

    A.D. partially meets DNP Essential II. A.D. did not address account-
ability in the project. Her approach was more autocratic than inclusive
with little effort expended to understand care delivery approaches in the
oncology unit, or gain insight from opinion leaders or content experts.
Some organizational and system leadership was evident in A.D.'s

incorporation of the hand-hygiene campaign throughout the unit; however, she lacks the input of organizational leadership in her approach to improve hand hygiene. There is also little initiative to expand the project on a system-wide scale. A lack of sustainability was evident in A.D.'s final email to the nursing staff indicating the project was complete rather than initiating a plan to continue to monitor hand -hygiene practices.

A.D. did not meet DNP Essential III. The problem identified in A.D.'s practice was an increase in CLABSI. A.D.'s literature search revealed a gap in EBP and research; however, her initial focus related to CLABSI was side tracked by the literature pertaining to hand hygiene and bacteremia. A.D.'s outcome measure was related to hand hygiene instead of the appropriate outcome measure of decreasing CLABSI. If the correct outcome measure was originally targeted, A.D. would have ample opportunities to create process measures that align with national benchmarks, including EBP protocols and bundles to prevent CLABSI.

Data collection in this project reflected research, not quality improvement. Research methodology was reflected in patients being randomly assigned to control and noncontrol groups, and the use of nondescriptive statistics in data interpretation. There was also a lack of dissemination of the project findings other than to the group of hospitalists she practices with on the oncology unit.

A.D. did not meet DNP Essential IV. There was no mention of the use of technology to assess, implement, or evaluate the project.

A.D. did not meet DNP Essential V. An existing policy did not address the use of new EBP protocols or bundles. This would have been an excellent opportunity for A.D. to update the existing policy or create a new policy to support patient advocacy to prevent CLABSI.

A.D. did not meet DNP Essential VI. A.D. did not create an interdisciplinary team, but rather enlisted nursing colleagues to implement the process measures of placing reminders in the break room and on patient doors. She did not enlist the support of stakeholders on her team, nor did she enlist champions and content experts. Dissemination of the findings of the project was limited to her immediate practice group of hospitalists.

A.D. partially meets DNP Essential VII. Although A.D.'s project focused on hand hygiene instead of decreasing CLABSI, either idea involves improving patient health through health promotion measures. The project, however, does not acknowledge the environmental and cultural concepts contributing to the gap in practice.

A.D. partially meets DNP Essential VIII. A.D. identified gaps in practice, but does not mentor or guide an interdisciplinary team. There is no evidence that A.D. has identified organizational priorities or initiatives that complement the project outcome measures. This is an important piece of gaining stakeholder buy-in, as well as making connections among organizational priorities, practice, patient needs, and policy issues.

Other factors to consider:

- A.D.'s project does not meet the definition of *quality improvement* due to a randomized methodology, and the intervention being delivered only to some patients.

- Rapid-cycle changes needed to drive the improvement were not identified. A.D. collected data at one point in time, versus monitoring changes over time to realize what change prompted improvement. A pre-/post design was not part of the methodology as data was collected once after the process measures were implemented.

2. Practices to promote stakeholder buy-in include coupling project outcomes to organizational or unit initiatives, missions, and goals and reporting project outcome measures to stakeholders to demonstrate project effectiveness (Brown, 2010). A good "fit" between the organizational structure and the EBP must also be considered. If the system and work flow is not synergistic with the EBP, it is less likely to be adopted (Titler, 2007). Stakeholder buy-in begins by building relationships with stakeholders through attending meetings in person, shadowing clinicians, and being courteous (Brown, 2010; Becker, Renger, & McPherson, 2015). The art of self-reflection in communicating project outcomes and process measures to stakeholders is also a key part of stakeholder buy-in and is accomplished by evaluating "what we do, how we look, what we say, and how we say it" (Brown, 2010, p. 38).

3. A.D. identified a gap in practice: EBP protocols and bundles shown to decrease CLABSI were not used. Instead of making this her outcome measure, she chose hand hygiene as the outcome measure. A more appropriate outcome measure would have been decreasing CLABSI in oncology patients with a central venous catheter. Hand hygiene would be a good process measure for A.D.'s project as this intervention could have been implemented in addition to the CLABSI protocols and bundles used to support the outcome measure of decreasing CLASBI. Balancing measures for this project could include increased time for nurses to perform hand hygiene before and after CVC dressing change.

4. Strategies to promote sustainability include having change champions on the oncology unit to continue supporting the change after the project is complete, gaining organizational leadership buy-in, aligning organizational goals with project goals, gaining staff buy-in by highlighting improved patient outcomes and improved workflow, and incorporating reminders in electronic medical records regarding interventions to decrease CLABSI.

5. Team members to include in A.D.'s project would be an infectious disease provider, unit and organizational leadership, as well as staff from the hospital infection control department.

6. A.D. formulates an outcome measure for her DNP project: Decrease CLABSI in oncology patients with CVC by May 14, 2018. Her process measures include increase hand hygiene of nurses by 20% when changing CVC dressings, educate the nurses on the oncology unit about the importance of good hand hygiene, educate the nurses about sterile technique when changing a CVC dressing, and use reminders on bulletin boards posted in the nurse's break rooms and on patient doors to perform hand hygiene before and after the CVC dressing change.

   A.D. formulates a team of nurses, infectious disease providers, and organizational and unit-based leaders to help implement the project. She strengthens buy-in from her team stakeholders by aligning her goals for the project with organizational goals and initiatives to decrease hospital-acquired infections, and attending monthly meetings with the infection control department at the hospital. A.D. collects data on CLABSI rates prior to implementation of her process measures and 9 months after implementation of her process measures. She uses run charts to track the implementation of her process measures to see what change contributed to the improvement. After several PDSA (plan-do-study-act) cycles over multiple months, using descriptive statistics, A.D. was able to see a 20% reduction in the CLABSI rate in the oncology unit.

   Following data collection, A.D. sends an email to her interdisciplinary team thanking them for their time and energy. She presents her findings at Grand rounds at the hospital, as well as through a poster presentation at the EBP conference at the hospital. To prompt sustainability, A.D. continues to meet with the infection disease department and unit leadership to monitor CLABSI rates on other units in the hospital. She also implements a reminder system in the electronic medical record used throughout the hospital to prompt the nursing staff and providers to follow the EBP protocol and bundle to prevent CLABSI. A.D. updates the unit policy on CVC care to include the new DBP bundles.

REFERENCES

Becker, K. L., Renger, R., McPherson, M. (2015). Indicators of buy-in to gauge evaluation success. *Evaluation Journal of Australasia, 15*(2), 12–21. doi:10.1177/1035719X1501500203

Brown, J. (2010). Compliance effectiveness: How do we get there? *Journal of Health Care Compliance, 12*(4), 37–63.

Titler, M. (2007). Translating research into practice. *American Journal of Nursing, 107*(6), 26–33. doi:10.1097/01.NAJ.0000277823.51806.10

CHAPTER 13: USING AN EVIDENCE-BASED APPROACH TO DEVELOP A DNP PROJECT

1. J.C. invites all disciplines that potentially "touch" the patients of interest to join the work group, thereby gaining trust and fostering a team-based approach to improve care for the individual patients (lower risk of adverse reaction to an antibiotic that is not necessary and fewer return visits to the emergency department [ED]) and for populations (decrease population-based antibiotic resistance and overall healthcare costs) to achieve the IHI Triple Aim of improved care for the population, engaging patients in their health, and lowering costs (Swensen, Pugh, McMullan, & Kabcenall, 2013).

2. The utility of gathering data in set, reasonable time intervals and plotting the findings each month in this case is that it allows for a more nuanced understanding of variation in the processes within the organization that impact the outcomes. For example, if at 3 months into the project, the EHR order set is impacted by an upgrade to the entire EHR system and it is discovered after a few weeks that one of the orders in the set is not active, the team can explain the impact on the outcome measures. Identifying where along the run-chart timeline this occurred to show how it impacted the monthly data gives context to the process in the "real life" clinical environment.

3. DNP Essential III: Clinical Scholarship and Analytic Methods for Evidence-Based Practice. The DNP scholar in practice uses scientific methods to address complex clinical questions. The rigor of the project design starting with a well-thought-out PICO (population/problem, intervention, comparison, outcome) question and literature search, followed by EBP statistical processes, will have a direct impact on the outcome, magnitude of change, and whether the change is sustainable or practice quickly returns to its prior state when the project is completed. If the team does not see the value of changing practice based on evidence, the goal is less clear and providers may fall back to prior practice patterns.

4. The dissemination of the local project outcomes within the organization and in peer-reviewed journals that publish quality improvement outcomes projects will advance nursing practice by promoting DNP-prepared APRNs as leaders of interdisciplinary teams to lead change. Often strategies that are used in one setting can be adapted to other similar clinical settings and shared ideas among nursing professionals supports the enhancement and recognition of nursing leadership in healthcare, encouraging others to follow suit to build a future nursing workforce that is ready to address the ongoing demands of our rapidly changing systems.

REFERENCE

Swensen, S., Pugh, M., McMullan, C., & Kabcenall, A. (2013). *High impact leadership: Improve the health of populations, and reduce costs*. Cambridge, MA: Institute for Healthcare Improvement.

CHAPTER 14: FINDING EVIDENCE TO IMPROVE PROCESSES

1. The exact PICOT (population/problem, intervention, comparison, outcome, time) question will depend on whether all children (from infants to 18 year olds) are included or only a subset of ages. Other considerations are inclusion of type of headache and also types of electronic devices.

   In children and adolescents, how much screen time is shown to cause headache?

   In children aged 10 to 18, is electronic screen use positively associated with headaches or migraines?

2. This topic is within the scope of content for the following databases: MEDLINE/PubMed, CINAHL (Cumulative Index of Nursing and Allied Health Literature), Scopus or Embasem PsycINFO. Each of these databases is the premier database in its area and should be searched to avoid missing key citations.

   Additional databases could be considered.

3. P (Patient): Children

   Child OR children OR preteen OR preteens OR adolescent OR adolescents OR teenagers

   I (Risk Factor): Electronic screen use
   Computer use OR smartphone OR internet OR video games OR television
   C (Absence of Risk Factor)
   Left blank as it is difficult to search for null.
   O (Outcomes): Headaches
   Headache OR headaches OR migraine OR migraines
   Consider also narrowing headache to etiology, epidemiology, or risk.

   Possible combination of terms:
   A simple search could use the following strategy, utilizing multiple terms and relying on the default fields searched in the databases:
   (Child OR children OR preteen OR preteens OR adolescent OR adolescents OR teenagers) AND (Computer use OR smartphone OR internet OR video games OR television) AND (Headache OR headaches OR migraine OR migraines)

A more targeted search could use subject terms to narrow the citations retrieved. The following is a search run in PubMed using the MeSH terms and subheading for headache and etiology:

(Child OR children OR preteen OR preteens OR adolescent OR adolescents OR teenagers) AND (Computer use OR smartphone OR internet OR videogames OR television) AND ("Headache/epidemiology"[Mesh] OR "Headache/etiology"[Mesh] OR "Migraine Disorders/epidemiology" [Mesh] OR "Migraine Disorders/etiology"[Mesh])

4. This case is looking at risk or etiology, and is most likely to be covered by cohort study, case control, or case series designs.

CHAPTER 15: COST ANALYSIS IN DNP PROJECTS

1. Because health literacy involves how patients encounter the clinic from the start of the visit through return to home to implement the treatment plan, perhaps a billing specialist could be added. If additional disciplines are located within the clinic, representatives from those specialties could be included.

2. There are several basic process-modeling techniques, including brainstorming, cause-and-effect diagrams, a flow diagram, a deployment flowchart, and a work-flow diagram (Ogrinc et al., 2018). In this case, D.B. chose a flow diagram. Once the improvement plan is developed, other modeling tools, like the cause-and-effect diagram, might be more appropriate.

3. It is important to incorporate the amount of time required for data collection for the health literacy needs assessment as well as any technological or statistical services required. The Agency for Healthcare Research and Quality (AHRQ, 2015) indicates that the assessment tool is available in a free Survey Monkey format, so that might facilitate gathering data with little resource use. It is also important to include the time and resources required to track progress. As a reminder, this is the cost estimate for the launch of the project. Once a plan is developed and new tools are launched, an incremental adjustment for staff time should be added.

REFERENCES

Agency for Healthcare Research and Quality. (2015). *Health literacy universal precautions toolkit* (2nd ed.). Rockville, MD: Author. Retrieved from http://www.ahrq.gov/professionals/quality-patient-safety/quality-resources/tools/literacy-toolkit/healthlittoolkit2.html

Ogrinc, G. S., Headrick, L. A., Barton, A. J., Dolansky, M. A., Madigosky, W. S., & Miltner, R. S. (2018). *Fundamentals of health care improvement: A guide to improving your patient's care* (3rd ed.). Oak Terrace, IL: Joint Commission Resources.

CHAPTER 16: THE DNP PROJECT DELIVERABLES: SUSTAINABILITY AND SPREAD

1. The implementation will be tracked through formalization of the dysphagia recommendations in organization-wide staff education policies and procedures, reflecting hierarchical control. Tracking of the dysphagia toolkit downloads from the hospital system intranet will be analyzed. P.G. will lead meetings to share the progress.

2. A supportive management structure is already in place. Plans to put together the team should be a priority. Include patients or patient's family members. Understanding what disciplines need to be involved and having the their representatives at the meetings is key to success. Process mapping would be the next step. Structures to fool proof the change must be decided on and implemented, keeping in mind the context of individual unit's needs. Organized meetings with agendas are important to keep everyone on track.

3. P.G. must decide what the key elements are for each individual or discipline to get them engaged. For example, why would the nurses on the units where these patients stay want to implement such a new framework? Is there something that P.G. can share with them that would help them see the benefit? Of course the evidence, but what about how the project would make the nurses work more efficiently? How will this project bring joy to their work? Possibly by seeing a patient with dysphagia learn to eat safely?

INDEX

AAACN. *See* American Academy of Ambulatory Care Nursing
AAP. *See* American Academy of Pediatrics
academic detaining, 232
academic practice partnership, 37–38
acceptance sampling, 62
Accountable Care Organization (ACO) model, 202
  age-appropriate screening, 210
  commercial and public payer, 211
  Medicare, 209–210
  Physician Group Practice demonstration project, 209
  preventive screening, 210–211
  providers, 209
  quality metrics, 210
  shared savings, 211
ACEP. *See* American College of Emergency Physicians
ACGME. *See* American College of Graduate Medical Education
ACO model. *See* Accountable Care Organization model
ACOVE quality indicators. *See* Assessing Care of Vulnerable Elderly quality indicators
activity-based costing, 298–299
Acute Care Episode (ACE) Demonstration Project, 207
acute care quality metrics
  chart-abstracted measures, 112
  data reporting, 112
  electronic clinical quality measures, 111–112
  ORYX Performance Measurement program, 110–111
  resources, 112
  significance, 111
adaptive system model, 46–47
advanced public health nurse (APHN), 124, 126–127
Agency for Health Care Policy and Research, 66
Agency for Healthcare Research and Quality (AHRQ)
  indicators, 116
  patient safety indicators, 123

Pediatric Quality Measures Program, 115
AGREE II. *See* Appraisal of Guidelines for Research and Evaluation II
ambulatory care nurse-sensitive indicators, 128
ambulatory care, quality metrics, 127–129
American Academy of Ambulatory Care Nursing (AAACN), 127–129
American Academy of Pediatrics (AAP), 114
American College of Emergency Physicians (ACEP), 120
American College of Graduate Medical Education (ACGME), 56
APEX-PH. *See* Assessment Protocol for Excellence in Public Health
Appraisal of Guidelines for Research and Evaluation II (AGREE II), 101
Assessing Care of Vulnerable Elderly (ACOVE) quality indicators, 120
Assessment Protocol for Excellence in Public Health (APEX-PH), 127
authentic leadership, 23

baccalaureate programs, 99
balanced scorecard, 301
bar coding of medication administration (BCMA), 172
BCMA. *See* bar coding of medication administration
Beers Criteria, 124
big data
  BCMA system, 172
  case study, 185–186
  categorical data, 181
  core EHR components, 172
  data cleansing, 180–181
  data dictionary, 178–180
  data-analysis plan, 182–183
  data-entry error, 181
  dissemination plan, 183
  DNP practice, 174–176
  DNP-prepared nurse's role, 172–174
  ID_Patient and ID_Nurse Extracted Data, 178
  information technology programmers, 179
  issues, 183–184

big data (*cont.*)
    Nursing Value Data Model, 177
    patient- or provider-level data, 179
    relational database, 176
    transformations and new variables, 181–182
Black Belt, Six Sigma organization, 83
BPCI. *See* Bundled Payments for Care
    Improvement Initiative
budget basics, 296–297
budget-impact analysis (BIA), 297
bundled payment models
    BPCI episodes, 208
    commercial health plans, 207–208
    maternity care, 208
    Medicare PPS program, 206
    PROMETHIUS bundled payment model
      project, 208
    public and private payers, 207
Bundled Payments for Care Improvement
    Initiative (BPCI), 208

CADIMA tool, 290
call-out technique, 138
CALNOC. *See* Collaborative Alliance for Nursing
    Outcomes
cause-and-effect diagram, quality improvement,
    70
CBA. *see* cost–benefit analysis
Center for Medicare and Medicaid Innovation
    (CMMI), 201
Centers for Medicare & Medicaid Services (CMS),
    110
CEP. *See* clinical episode payments
Certificate of Need (CON) concept, 194
certificate of professional nursing (CPN), 8
certified nurse midwives (CNMs), 212
chart-abstracted measures, 112
check sheet, quality improvement, 70
check-back technique, 138
chief nursing executives (CNEs), 314
Child Health Insurance Program, 113
Children's Health Insurance Program
    Reauthorization Act (CHIPRA), 113, 114
CINAHL. *See* Cumulative Index of Nursing and
    Allied Health Literature
clinical doctorate degree, 3
    and clinical professions, 4
    non-PhD doctorate, 3–4
    nursing doctorate (ND), 4–13
clinical episode payments (CEP), 206–209
Clinical Microsystem Assessment Tool, 50
clinical practice guidelines (CPG), 101
CMMI. *See* Center for Medicare and Medicaid
    Innovation
CNMs. *See* certified nurse midwives
Cochrane Review, 260

cognitions, teamwork, 138–139
cohort studies, 284–285
Collaborative Alliance for Nursing Outcomes
    (CALNOC), 129
collaborative practice change models, 247–248
commercial health plans, 207–208
Commission on Collegiate Nursing Education
    (CCNE), 9
common cause variation, 63
Common Risky Behaviors Checklist, 115
communication, 32–33, 137–138
community-based education program, 148
complex healthcare system, 46–48
CON concept. *See* Certificate of Need concept
Consolidated Standards of Reporting Trials
    (CONSORT) guidelines, 71
constructive feedback and guidance, 31
continuous quality improvement (CQI), 67–68
control chart, quality improvement, 70
cost analysis, DNP projects
    budget basics, 296–297
    exemplary case study, 299–303
    models, 297
    time-driven activity-based costing, 297–299
cost–benefit analysis (CBA), 297
cost–consequence analysis, 297
cost-effectiveness analysis (CEA), 297
cost-minimization analysis, 297
cost-of-illness analysis, 297
cost–utility analysis (CUA), 297
CQI. *See* continuous quality improvement
creative leaders, 26
critical appraisal, 286
CUA. *see* cost–utility analysis
culture change, 35
Cumulative Index of Nursing and Allied Health
    Literature (CINAHL), 260, 280, 286–288
customer delighters, 88–89

data cleansing, 180–181
data collection and reporting
    balancing measures, 266
    outcome measure, 264
    process measures, 264–266
    standardized accepted methods, 266–267
data dictionary, 178–180
data mining, 171
data reporting, quality metrics, 112
data transparency, 31
define, measure, analyze, improve, and control
    (DMAIC), 83
de-implementing practices, 103
Deming Model of Quality Management, 64
Deming plan-do-study-act cycle, 63
Deming, W. E., 63, 64, 67
descriptive statistics, 62

diagnosis-related groups (DRGs), 198, 199
Diffusion of Innovation (DOI) theory, 314
direct costs, 296
dissemination plan, 183
DMAIC. *See* define, measure, analyze, improve, and control
Doctor of Nursing Practice (DNP) degree
  AACN recommendations, 15
  DNP/PhD nurse collaboration, 18–19
  growth of, 16–17
  nursing education, 18
Doctor of Nursing Practice (DNP) portfolio, 226
Doctor of Nursing Practice (DNP) Project Team, 227
Doctor of Nursing Practice (DNP) projects
  AACN DNP Essentials, 222
  case study, 248–249
  collaborative practice change models, 247–248
  core elements, 251, 252
  cost analysis (*see* cost analysis, DNP projects)
  definition, 221
  DNP Implementation Task Force recommendations, 225–228
  Enhances, Culmination, Partnerships, Implements, Evaluates method, 242–244
  evidence search (*see* evidence search techniques)
  evidence-based best practice, 221–222
  evidence-based practice (*see* evidence-based practice)
  Institute for Healthcare Improvement (IHI) model, 237, 239–242
  institutional guidelines, 254
  Iowa model, 245–247
  lack of consistency, 222, 224
  potential outcomes, 223–224
  purpose, 253
  reference manager, 262
  scientific reports and clinical research, 252
  self-reflection, 254
  stakeholder buy-in, 228–234
  sustainability and spread (*see* sustainability and spread, evidenced-based projects)
  U.S. healthcare system, 252
  Zaccagnini and White DNP project process model, 234–239
Donabedian, A., 65, 67
Donabedian model, 65, 151
DRGs. *See* diagnosis-related groups

EBP. *See* evidence-based practice
EC as PIE method. *See* Enhances, Culmination, Partnerships, Implements, Evaluates method
eCQMs. *See* electronic clinical quality measures
effect theory, 160
effective leadership

integrative leadership framework, 24–27
  leadership model, 27–39
  leadership theory, 23–24
egocentric leaders, 26
EHR. *See* electronic health record
electronic clinical quality measures (eCQMs), 111–112
electronic health record (EHR), 114, 171
elemental innovation, 34
emergent geriatric general care indicators, 120–121
empathy map, 36, 37
empowerment
  communication, 32–33
  relational, 32
  structural, 30–32
Enhances, Culmination, Partnerships, Implements, Evaluates (EC as PIE) method, 242–244
Enhancing the QUAlity and Transparency Of health Research (EQUATOR) network, 289
entrepreneur, characteristics, 39
Envisioning the National Health Care Quality Report, 310–311
episode-based payments, 206–209
esthetic leadership, 23
evidence search techniques
  background questions, 278
  case study, 292
  databases, 286–288
  documentation, 289–291
  field searching, 283
  filters, 283–284
  grey literature, 288
  intervention table, 291
  keyword searching, 279–280
  levels of evidence, 284–286
  operators, 281–282
  PICOT question, 278–279
  subject searching, 280–281
  truncation and wild cards, 282–283
evidence-based practice (EBP)
  adoption, 96–98
  case example, 271–272
  case study, 105–106
  clinical practice guidelines, 96
  data collection and reporting, 264–266
  definition, 97
  guidelines, 263
  institutional review boards resources, 104
  level of evidence grading, 255, 261–262
  models, 99–102
  patient preference, 262–263
  PICOT question (*see* PICOT question)
  practice and systems, 269
  project dissemination, 270

evidence-based practice (EBP) (*cont.*)
    project limitations, 269–270
    project meetings, 263
    QI initiatives, 102–104
    research, 98–99, 103
    research literature, 260–262
    seminal publication, 95–96
    stakeholder buy-in, 231, 232
    statistical and clinical significance, 268–269
    theoretical model, 255, 259
executing phase, process improvement, 91–92
expenses, 296

face-to-face communication, 33
Federal Tort Claims Act, 212
federally qualified health center (FQHC), 212, 299
fee-for-service (FFS) model, 194
FFS model. *See* fee-for-service model
field searching, 283
filters, 283–284
fishbone diagram, quality improvement, 70
fixed costs, 296–297
flowchart, quality improvement, 70
formal capacity-building programs, 317
formative evaluations, 154
full-time equivalent (FTE), 296

gait-and-motion program, 148
general geriatric care quality, 117–119
geriatric quality metrics
    emergency care, 120–121
    five Ds, 115–116
    general geriatric care quality, 117–119
    home care, 119
    practice and care recommendations, 116–117
    quality indicators, 116
    quality outcomes, 116
    safety, 122–124
geriatric safety collaborative management
    indicators, 123–124
graduate entry DNP Program, 9
group communication, 33
group conflict, 137
group/team projects, 226–227

HCD. *See* human-centered design
HCP LAN. *See* Health Care Payment Learning &
    Action Network
Health and Human Services (HHS), 201
Health Care Payment Learning & Action
    Network (HCP LAN), 207
Health Insurance Portability and Accountability
    Act (HIPAA) Privacy Rule, 176
health literacy project budget, 306
health maintenance organizations (HMOs) Act,
    198

Health Planning and Resource Development Act
    of 1974, 194
Healthcare Effectiveness Data and Information
    Set (HEDIS), 113–114
healthcare financing and insurance
    healthcare delivery and payment reform,
        200–201
    healthcare legislation in 21st century, 202–203
    industrial era and modern medicine, 191–192
    public and private insurance expansion, 192–200
    value-based payment models, 201, 203–214
healthcare systems
    AACN DNP essentials, 45–46
    care delivery, 44
    high-quality care, 43
    large-scale projects, 44
    leadership roles, 44
    medical errors, 43
    quality and safety, 44, 45
HEDIS. *See* Healthcare Effectiveness Data and
    Information Set
hierarchical systems, 42
highly reliable processes, 79
Hill–Burton Act, 192, 194, 198
HIPAA Privacy Rule. *See* Health Insurance
    Portability and Accountability Act Privacy
    Rule
histogram, quality improvement, 70
HMOs Act. *See* health maintenance organizations
    Act
home care, geriatric quality metrics, 119
home care quality indicators (HCQIs), 119
Hospital Quality Incentive Demonstration
    (HQID) program, 204–205
Hospital Survey and Construction Act, 192
Hospital Value-Based Purchasing (HVBP)
    program, 205
4-hour educational strategy, 52
HQID program. *See* Hospital Quality Incentive
    Demonstration program
human-centered design (HCD)
    components, 36
    culture change, 35
    design thinking, 35
    empathy map, 36, 37

ICHOM. *See* International Consortium for Health
    Outcomes Measurement
IHI. *See* Institute for Healthcare Improvement
income, 296
incremental innovation, 34
independent practice association (IPA), 199
information technology programmers, 179
initiate phase, process improvement
    "5 Whys" technique, 84–85
    SWOT analysis, 85, 86

innovation
  elemental, 34
  human-centered designs, 35–36
  incremental change, 34
  monumental change, 34–35
inpatient quality indicators (IQIs), 116
input—process—output (IPO) model, 135
Institute for Healthcare Improvement (IHI), 48,
    69, 81, 101, 237, 239–242, 263, 311, 312
Institute of Medicine (IOM), 95–96
institutional review board (IRB), 179
integral leaders, 26
integrative leadership framework
  developmental stages, 25–26
  holistic nursing, 25
  knowledge formation, 24
  metaparadigm concepts, 25
  paradigm shift, 24
  task and relationship concepts, 25
  Wilber's four quadrant model, 24–25
International Consortium for Health Outcomes
    Measurement (ICHOM), 117–118
International Resident Assessment Instrument
    (interRAI), 119
interpersonal communication, 33
interprofessional teams, 135
interprofessional teamwork, 47
intrapersonal communication, 33
introduction, methods, results, and discussion
    (IMRaD) organization, 74
invisible architecture, 38
Iowa evidence-based practice model, 245–247

Joanna Briggs Institute (JBI) Levels of Evidence,
    285
Juran, J. A., 66, 67

Kano model, 87–88
Kaplan and Norton's balanced scorecard, 302–
    303, 305
Kerr–Mills program, 193
key performance indicators (KPIs), 149–150
keyword searching, 279–280
knowledge discovery, 171
knowledge, skills, and abilities (KSAs), 71, 139
KPIs. See key performance indicators
Kurt Lewin's Change Model, 164

leadership
  complex healthcare system, 46–48
  definition, 45–46
  support, teamwork, 136–137
  systems thinking (see systems thinking)
  theory, 23–24
leadership model
  empowerment, 30–33

innovation, 33–36
  organizational transformation, 36–39
  personal power, 27–30
Lean method, 82
Lean Six Sigma, 159
Learning Organization Model, 48
Little's Law, 159
Logic modeling, 158
logic models, 158–159

macrosystem, 49
managed care models, 199
MAPP. See Mobilizing for Action through
    Planning and Partnerships
mass communication, 33
master's programs, 99
MATCH. See Mobilizing Action for Community
    Health
maternity care episode recommendations,
    212–213
Medical Literature Analysis and Retrieval System
    Online (MEDLINE) database, 280, 288
Medicare, 66, 209–210
Medicare Access and CHIP Reauthorization Act
    (MACRA), 202
Medicare and Medicaid Act, 193–197
Medicare Utilization and Quality Control Peer
    Review Organization, 66
Medicare's Physician Group Practice (PGP)
    demonstration project, 209
merit-based incentive payments (MIPS), 202
mesosystem, 49
microsystem, 35, 49, 50, 79
Minimum Data Set—Home Care (MDS-HC), 119
mistake proofing, 82
Mobilizing Action for Community Health
    (MATCH), 126, 127
Mobilizing for Action through Planning and
    Partnerships (MAPP), 127
Model for Improvement, 81–82
monitoring phase, process improvement, 92
monumental innovation, 34–35
multiteam system, 136

National Academy of Medicine (NAM), 95
National Committee for Quality Assurance
    (NCQA), 113, 205
National Database of Nursing Quality Indicators
    (NDNQI), 151, 314
National Institute for Health and Care Excellence
    (NICE), 291
National Network of Libraries of Medicine
    (NNLM), 277
National Patient Safety Foundation's Lucian
    Leape Institute (LLI), 311
National Quality Forum (NQF), 151

NDNQI. *See* National Database of Nursing Quality Indicators
need-finding, HCD, 36
neonatal abstinence syndrome (NAS), 165–166
NICE. *See* National Institute for Health and Care Excellence
Normative theory, 157
NQF. *See* National Quality Forum
number needed to treat (NNT) measures, 268
nurse-led quality behavioral health services, 300
nurse-value equation, 32
nursing, ANA's definition, 44
Nursing Doctorate (ND) degree
    Case Western Reserve University (CWRU), 5–7
    classification, 4
    Colorado's ND curriculum, 9–13
    Graduate Entry DNP Program, 9
    postlicensure component, 9
    Post-MSN DNP Program, 9
    prelicensure component, 8
    3-year and 4-year DNP programs, 8
Nursing Value Data Model, 177
Nursing Worklife Model, 30

odd ratios, 268
opportunity assessment, 162
organizational communication, 33
organizational culture, teamwork, 136
organizational transformation
    academic practice partnership, 37–38
    changing culture, 38
    entrepreneurial and intrapreneurial nursing initiatives, 39
ORYX Performance Measurement program, 110–111
outcome, Donabedian model, 65

Pareto diagram, quality improvement, 70
Partnership for Patients (P4P), 44
Patient Protection and Affordable Care Act (ACA), 112–113, 201
patient safety indicators (PSIs), 116
Patient-Centered Medical Home (PCMH), 205–206
pay-for-performance (P4P) programs, 204–205
PCMH. *See* Patient-Centered Medical Home
PDSA cycle. *See* plan-do-study-act cycle
pediatric quality metrics
    AHRQ Pediatric Quality Measures Program, 115
    American Academy of Pediatric measures, 114
    federal agencies, 113
    Healthcare Effectiveness Data and Information Set measures, 113–114
    mental healthcare, 114–115
    quality indicators, 113
    U.S. healthcare system, 112–113

performance management
    Donabedian's linear evaluation model, 151
    key performance indicators, 149–150
    metrics, 150–151
    National Database of Nursing Quality Indicators, 151
    National Quality Forum, 151
performance measures, 110
personal power
    Hagberg's six stages, 28–29
    self-awareness, 30
PHAB. *See* Public Health Accreditation Board
PhD degree, 17–19
PHI. *See* protected health information
Physician Group Practice (PGP) demonstration project, 209
PICOT question
    comparison, 257
    digital age, 258
    evidence table, 261
    format, 100–101
    intervention, 256–257
    key words identifying, 260
    outcomes, 257
    population, 256
    structured format, 258
    templates, 258–259
    time frame, 258
"Plan for Progress" of Nursing Education, 5–6
plan-do-study-act (PDSA) cycle, 68, 81–82, 91
planning phase, process improvement
    customer delighters, 88
    customer's perspective, 86
    inputs, process steps, and outputs, 86–87
    Kano model, 87–88
    objective data, 90
    process map, 89–90
    tampering, 89
    time-motion study, 90
policy, regulatory, and organizational constructs in educational and environmental development (PROCEED), 161, 162
polypharmacy, 124
poorly designed processes, 79
population health, 125
population-focused care, 125
Post-MSN DNP Program, 9
power, definition, 30
powerlessness, 28, 29
P4P. *See* Partnership for Patients
PPOs. *See* preferred provider organizations
PPS. *See* prospective payment system
practice doctorate, 3
practice doctorate degree, 13–16
practice-focused doctorate, 99

PRECEDE. *See* predisposing, reinforcing, and enabling constructs in educational diagnosis and evaluation
predisposing, reinforcing, and enabling constructs in educational diagnosis and evaluation (PRECEDE), 161, 162
preferred provider organizations (PPOs), 199
Preferred Reporting Items for Systematic Reviews and MetaAnalyses (PRISMA), 289–290
prevention quality indicators (PQIs), 116
PRISMA. *See* Preferred Reporting Items for Systematic Reviews and MetaAnalyses
PROCEED. *See* policy, regulatory, and organizational constructs in educational and environmental development
process conflict, 137
process, Donabedian model, 65
process evaluation, 155–156
process improvement
    continual improvement, 78–79
    definition, 78
    fundamental ideas, 79
    high quality and low cost, 80–81
    Lean method, 82
    length of stay and readmissions, 80
    mission, 77
    Model for Improvement, 81–82
    multiple interrelated processes, 78
    process design, 79
    process flaws, 80
    projects, 84–93
    and quality improvement, 78
    Six Sigma method, 82–84
process map, 89–90
process theory, 159
program evaluation
    case study, 165–166
    Change Model, 164
    community-based education program, 148
    decision-making, 151–152
    effect theory, 160
    ethical standards, 152
    evidence-based program, 152
    formative evaluations, 154
    gait-and-motion program, 148
    impact evaluation, 156–157
    inputs and process, 148
    logic models, 158–159
    nonprofit organization, 148
    outputs and outcomes, 148
    performance management, 149–151
    PRECEDE–PROCEED model, 161
    problems, 162–163
    process evaluations, 155–156
    process mapping, 160
    process theory, 159
    program theory, 157–158
    research, 153
    stakeholders, 152
    summative evaluation, 154
    Tar Wars Program, 149
    viable project settings, 161–162
program theory, 157–158
project charter, 93
projects, process improvement
    executing phase, 91–92
    initiate phase, 84–86
    monitoring phase, 92
    planning phase, 86–90
PROMETHEUS payment project, 207
prospective payment system (PPS), 198, 199
protected health information (PHI), 176
PSIs. *See* patient safety indicators
psychological safety, teamwork, 136
Public Health Accreditation Board (PHAB), 126
Public Health Foundation, 127
Public Health Improvement Resource Center, 127
Public Health Quality Improvement Exchange, 127
public health quality metrics
    clinical doctorate programs, 126–127
    definition, 125
    quality improvement, 126
    in United States, 124
PubMed, 260

QI. *See* quality improvement
QIC. *See* quality improvement collaboratives
QSEN initiative. *See* Quality and Safety Education for Nurses initiative
Quality and Safety Education for Nurses (QSEN) initiative, 44, 45, 71–74
quality control, 66
quality gurus, 64
quality healthcare, 310–311
quality improvement (QI), 66. *See also* teamwork
    continuous quality improvement, 67–68
    evidence-based practice, 102–104
    history, 61–67
    knowledge, skills, and attitudes, 71
    Model for Improvement, 69–70
    standards, 71–72, 74–75
quality improvement collaboratives (QIC), 242
quality metrics
    acute care quality metrics, 110–112
    ambulatory care, 127–129
    case study, 129
    clinical outcomes, 109–110
    geriatric quality metrics, 115–124
    pediatric quality metrics, 112–115
    performance measures, 110
    public health quality metrics, 124–127

quality planning, 66
quality trilogy, 66
quality work, 65

RBRVS. *See* Resource-Based Relative Value Scale
reactive leaders, 26
relational database, 176
relational empowerment, 32
relationship conflict, 137
relative risk, 268
Relative Value Scale Update Committee (RUC), 192
relative value units (RVUs), 192, 193
research-focused doctorate, 99
resonant leadership, 24
Resource-Based Relative Value Scale (RBRVS), 200
Rogers's translation research model, 231
Rounding to Influence practice, 31
RUC. *See* Relative Value Scale Update Committee
run chart, quality improvement, 70

SAEM Geriatric Task Force. *See* Society for Academic Emergency Medicine Geriatric Task Force
safety culture, 35
SBAR. *See* situation–background–assessment–recommendation
scholarly project, 225–226
Screening Tool of Older Persons' potentially inappropriate Prescriptions (STOPP), 124
Screening Tool to Alert doctors to the Right Treatment (START), 124
self-awareness, 30
self-organizing systems, 47
self-reflection, 254
shared mental model, 138
shared savings, 211
Shewhart, W. A., 62, 63, 67
situation–background–assessment–recommendation (SBAR), 138
Six Sigma method, 82–84
SMART goal. *See* specific, measurable, achievable, realistic, and time-specific goal
Social Security Act, 191, 193
socially responsible leadership, 24
Society for Academic Emergency Medicine (SAEM) Geriatric Task Force, 116–117, 120
SPC. *See* statistical process control
special cause variation, 63
specific, measurable, achievable, realistic, and time-specific (SMART) goal, 69
SQC. *See* statistical quality control
SQUIRE guidelines. *See* Standards for Quality Improvement Reporting Excellence guidelines

Stabilization Act of 1942, 192
stakeholder buy-in
    Iowa Model, 231
    monitoring tool, 233–234
    organizational structure and readiness, 232–233
    potential user strategies, 232
    Rogers's translation research model, 231–232
    stakeholder, 228–231
Standards for Quality Improvement Reporting Excellence (SQUIRE) guidelines, 71–72, 74–75
START. *See* Screening Tool to Alert doctors to the Right Treatment
statistical process control (SPC), 62
statistical quality control (SQC), 62
statistical sampling techniques, 62
STOPP. *See* Screening Tool of Older Persons' potentially inappropriate Prescriptions
Strategies and Tools to Enhance Performance and Patient Safety (TeamSTEPPS) program, 139
STrengthening the Reporting of OBservational studies in Epidemiology (STROBE) guidelines, 71
strengths/weaknesses, opportunities/threats (SWOT) analysis, 85, 86
STROBE guidelines. *See* STrengthening the Reporting of OBservational studies in Epidemiology guidelines
structural empowerment
    adequate resource needs, 31
    constructive feedback and guidance, 31
    data transparency, 31
    Nursing Worklife Model, 30
    personal growth and development culture, 32
    staff access to information, 31
    structural factors, 30
subject headings searches, 280–281
summative evaluation, 154
supportive management structure, 314–315
sustainability and spread, evidenced-based projects
    campaign interventions, 317–319
    case study, 320
    deeply engaged staff, 316–317
    "foolproof" change, 315
    formal capacity-building programs, 317
    plan for sustainability, 309–310
    quality healthcare, 310–311
    service organization, 311–313
    shared sense of the system, 316
    supportive management structure, 314–315
    transparent feedback systems, 315
SWOT analysis. *See* strengths/weaknesses, opportunities/threats analysis
system, 80
systematic review, 285

Systems Level Awareness Model, 51, 52
systems thinking
  ACGME competencies, 56
  attributes, 51
  elements, 52–55
  framework, 48
  instrument, 51–52
  Learning Organization Model, 48
  long term care, 57–58
  macrosystem, 49
  mesosystem, 49
  microsystem, 49
  resources, 49–50
  Systems Level Awareness Model, 51, 52
Systems Thinking Scale, 51

tampering, 89
Tar Wars Program, 149
task conflict, 137
TDABC. *See* time-driven activity-based costing
team building, 139–140
team debriefing, 140
TeamSTEPPS program. *See* Strategies and Tools
    to Enhance Performance and Patient Safety
    program
teamwork
  actions and improvements, 140–142
  case study, 142–143
  cognitions, 138–139
  communication, 137–138
  conceptual model, 135
  conflict, 137
  definition, 134
  inputs, 135–137
  outputs, 135
  principles, 134
  processes, 135
  training, 139–140

transactive memory system, 139
The Joint Commission (TJC), 110, 111
Theory of Change (ToC), 158, 164
Theory of Profound Knowledge, 63
time-driven activity-based costing (TDABC),
    297–299, 304
TJC. *See* The Joint Commission
TMS. *See* transactive memory system
ToC. *See* Theory of Change
Total Quality Management (TQM), 64, 312
TQM. *See* Total Quality Management
transactive memory system (TMS), 139
transformational leadership, 24
transparent feedback systems, 315
Triple Aim, 1, 200, 295
truncation and wild cards, 282–283
two-way communication, 92

U.S. healthcare system, 190

Value-Based Modifier System (VBMS), 202
value-based payment (VBP), 190
  ACO models, 209–211
  bundled payment models, 206–209
  case study, 212–214
  characteristics and core elements, 201
  FFS model, 203
  Patient-Centered Medical Home, 205–206
  pay-for-performance programs, 204–205
  performance-based strategies, 203
variable costs, 297
VBMS. *See* Value-Based Modifier System
VBP. *See* value-based payment
visual accounting system, 233

well-designed processes, 79
Wilber's Integrative Model for Knowledge
    Development, 24–25

CPSIA information can be obtained
at www.ICGtesting.com
Printed in the USA
BVHW071233181020
591228BV00009B/29